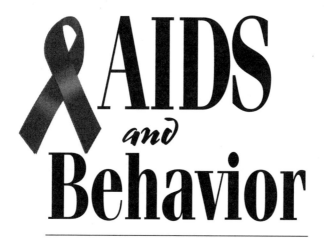

AIDS *and* Behavior

An Integrated Approach

Judith D. Auerbach, Christina Wypijewska,
and H. Keith H. Brodie, Editors

Committee on Substance Abuse and Mental Health
Issues in AIDS Research

Division of Biobehavioral Sciences and Mental Disorders

INSTITUTE OF MEDICINE

NATIONAL ACADEMY PRESS
Washington, D.C. 1994

National Academy Press • 2101 Constitution Avenue, N.W. • Washington, D.C. 20418

NOTICE: The project that is the subject of this report was approved by the Governing Board of the National Research Council, whose members are drawn from the councils of the National Academy of Sciences, the National Academy of Engineering, and the Institute of Medicine. The members of the committee responsible for the report were chosen for their special competencies and with regard for appropriate balance.

This report has been reviewed by a group other than the authors according to procedures approved by a Report Review Committee consisting of members of the National Academy of Sciences, the National Academy of Engineering, and the Institute of Medicine.

The Institute of Medicine was chartered in 1970 by the National Academy of Sciences to enlist distinguished members of the appropriate professions in the examination of policy matters pertaining to the health of the public. In this, the Institute acts under both the Academy's 1863 congressional charter responsibility to be an adviser to the federal government and its own initiative in identifying issues of medical care, research, and education. Dr. Kenneth I. Shine is president of the Institute of Medicine.

Support of this project was provided by the National Institute on Alcohol Abuse and Alcoholism, the National Institute on Drug Abuse, and the National Institute of Mental Health.

Library of Congress Cataloging-in-Publication Data

AIDS and behavior : an integrated approach / Judith D. Auerbach,
    Christina Wypijewska, and H. Keith H. Brodie, editors ; Committee on
    Substance Abuse and Mental Health Issues in AIDS Research, Division
    of Biobehavioral Sciences and Mental Disorders, Institute of
    Medicine.
        p. cm.
    Includes bibliographical references and index.
    ISBN 0-309-05093-6
    1. AIDS (Disease)—Prevention—Research—Government policy—United
States. 2. Health behavior. I. Auerbach, Judith D.
II. Wypijewska, Christina. III. Brodie, H. Keith H. (Harlow Keith
Hammond), 1939– . IV. Institute of Medicine. Division of
Biobehavioral Sciences and Mental Disorders. Committee on Substance
Abuse and Mental Health Issues in AIDS Research.
    [DNLM: 1. National Institute on Alcohol Abuse and Alcoholism
(U.S.). 2. National Institute on Drug Abuse. 3. National Institute
of Mental Health (U.S.). 4. Acquired Immunodeficiency Syndrome.
5. Health Services Research—organization & administration—United
States. 6. HIV Infections—psychology. 7. Substance Abuse. 8. Sex
Behavior. WD 308 A28774 1994]
RA644.A25A342   1994
616.97'92—dc20
DNLM/DLC   94-3786
for Library of Congress   CIP

The serpent has been a symbol of long life, healing, and knowledge among almost all cultures and religions since the beginning of recorded history. The image adopted as a logotype by the Institute of Medicine is based on relief carving from ancient Greece, now held by the Staalichemuseen in Berlin.

Edward H. Kaplan, Professor of Management Sciences, Yale School of Organization and Management, and Professor of Medicine, Yale School of Medicine, New Haven, Connecticut

Richard W. Price, Professor and Head, Department of Neurology, University of Minnesota, Minneapolis, Minnesota

Alfred Saah, Associate Professor of Epidemiology, School of Hygiene and Public Health, and Associate Professor of Medicine, School of Medicine, Johns Hopkins University, Baltimore, Maryland

Peter Selwyn, Associate Director, AIDS Program, and Associate Professor of Internal Medicine, Epidemiology, and Public Health, Yale University School of Medicine, New Haven, Connecticut

LIAISON TO THE COMMITTEE

Susan Folkman, Co-Director, Center for AIDS Prevention Studies, and Professor of Medicine, University of California, San Francisco, San Francisco, California

STUDY STAFF

Judith D. Auerbach, *Study Director*
Christina Wypijewska, *Project Officer*
Karen Autrey, *Project Assistant*
Holly Dawkins, *Research Assistant*
Robert Cook-Deegan, *Director, Division of Biobehavioral Sciences and Mental Disorders*
Constance M. Pechura, *Associate Director, Division of Biobehavioral Sciences and Mental Disorders*

OTHER IOM STAFF

Michael A. Stoto, *Director, Division of Health Promotion and Disease Prevention*
Leslie Hardy, *Study Director, AIDS Activities*
Gail Spears, *Administrative Assistant, Division of Biobehavioral Sciences and Mental Disorders*

Preface

In its FY 1992 appropriations bill for the Departments of Labor, Health and Human Services, and Education (P.L. 102-170), Congress called for an assessment of the AIDS research programs of the Alcohol, Drug Abuse, and Mental Health Administration (ADAMHA). This action resulted in part from a long-standing concern among members of Congress, the behavioral and social science community, and AIDS advocates that insufficient attention was being paid by federal research agencies to the potential contributions of behavioral and social science research to AIDS prevention efforts.

Congress specifically directed ADAMHA to contract with the Institute of Medicine (IOM) to undertake a study that was to "include, but not be limited to an assessment of the mission, programs, management, and funding levels" of the ADAMHA AIDS research and services programs. The mandate specifically required that the evaluation of ADAMHA's AIDS programs be similar to the previous IOM assessment (1991a) of the AIDS programs of the National Institutes of Health (NIH) and that it (1) assess the balance between biomedical and behavioral research in the AIDS research programs, (2) pay particular attention to behavioral-science-based AIDS prevention efforts at ADAMHA, and (3) assess the links between AIDS research and services programs in ADAMHA (Senate Report 102-104:154).

In order to conduct the study, IOM convened the Committee on Substance Abuse and Mental Health Issues in AIDS Research, which was composed of fourteen members with expertise in clinical medicine, epidemiology, neurology, neuroscience, nursing, operations research, psychiatry, psychology, public advocacy, public health, and sociology. Many committee members also had extensive experience in the areas of AIDS, mental health and illness, and substance abuse.

Once the study was under way, however, two events occurred that had a direct effect on the ability of the committee to conduct the project as mandated. First, after a year of debate and consideration, Congress passed the ADAMHA Reorganization Act of 1992, which, effective October 1, 1992 (the day after the IOM contract began), restructured ADAMHA by separating out its research and services functions. The three research institutes—National Institute on Alcohol Abuse and Alcoholism (NIAAA), National Institute on Drug Abuse (NIDA), and National Institute of Mental Health (NIMH)—were transferred to NIH. The two services offices—Office of Substance Abuse Prevention (OSAP) and Office of Treatment Improvement (OTI)—were renamed Centers (CSAP and CSAT) and, along with a newly created Center for Mental Health Services (CMHS), were reconstituted as the Substance Abuse and Mental Health Services Administration (SAMHSA).

As a result of the reorganization of ADAMHA, the IOM study was refocused to assess the AIDS research portfolios of NIAAA, NIDA, and NIMH with respect to balance between biomedical and behavioral research, attention to behavioral preventive interventions, and the relationship between research at the institutes and AIDS-related mental health and substance abuse services programs at SAMHSA and elsewhere in the Public Health Service (PHS).

The second event of consequence to this study was the passage of the NIH Revitalization Amendments (P.L. 103-43) on July 10, 1993. That bill substantially increased the authority of the NIH Office of AIDS Research (OAR) to determine budgeting and, to some degree, program priorities for AIDS research at all NIH institutes effective FY 1994 (October 1, 1993). Because the former ADAMHA institutes had become part of NIH, the "mission, program management, and funding levels" of their AIDS portfolio were affected by the new OAR authority during the course of this study.

Together, the changes at ADAMHA and NIH produced a set of difficulties not only for the institutes themselves—which were forced to operate for several years in a climate of uncertainty—but also for the study committee, which had to deal with a "moving target" throughout the course of its efforts. Although these legislative changes were not intended to be the focus of the study, the committee decided that their consequences for the AIDS programs of NIAAA, NIDA, and NIMH could not be ignored. Therefore, the implications of this set of circumstances for both the institutes' programs and the committee's work are noted, where relevant, throughout this report.

After revising the contract to reflect these structural changes, the charge to the committee became to assess: (1) the scope and content of each institute's AIDS research program activities; (2) the relationship between their research and the services-oriented programs at SAMHSA, Centers for Disease Control and Prevention (CDC), and Health Resources and Services Administration (HRSA); (3) the balance among various research categories (e.g., biomedical, neuroscientific, neuropsychiatric, and behavioral research) and research mechanisms; (4) the role of behavioral-science-based preventive interventions in the institutes' research programs; (5) the role of the public and field opinion in influencing the direction of AIDS research; (6) the adequacy of the administrative structure to support the institutes' AIDS programs; and (7) the adequacy of interagency coordination of AIDS activities.

In order to address the various elements of the study charge, the committee and the study staff engaged in a range of data collection activities. These included: creating an electronic database of abstracts of all AIDS grants funded by the three institutes between FY 1983 and FY 1992; reviewing strategic planning, conference summary, and other relevant documents related to their AIDS programs; conducting interviews with federal agency staff, external researchers, AIDS advocates, and other interested persons; visiting four institute-funded AIDS research centers; holding a public meeting; and conducting widespread literature searches. These diverse methods yielded a wealth of information and insights into the accomplishments and the shortcomings of the institutes' AIDS programs *vis-à-vis* the epidemic.

The resulting report is divided into two parts. Part I, "Research Findings and Opportunities," presents an overview of findings from neurobiological, psychological, and social science research related to the substance use, sexual behavior, and mental health aspects of HIV. Much, but not all, of this research has been supported by NIAAA, NIDA, and NIMH. These findings provide a useful backdrop against which to assess the AIDS programs of the institutes, and they help to point out future directions for AIDS research. Moreover, the committee felt it was important to identify the scientific contributions of the former ADAMHA institutes as they integrate into the larger context of NIH and its AIDS research agenda. Part II, "Managing the AIDS Research Programs at NIAAA, NIDA, and NIMH," provides information about the context in which the institutes' AIDS programs have been operating and presents the committee's assessment of their actual AIDS programs.

Throughout the report, the committee makes a number of recommendations related to advancing the scientific agenda and improving the management of AIDS research at NIAAA, NIDA, and NIMH. The committee wishes to note here that these recommendations are not prioritized or ranked; rather, they follow the order of the text in each chapter. Furthermore, because the three institutes were reviewed simultaneously, the recommendations reflect both their unique and their overlapping missions.

Although this report contains a number of important findings and recommendations, the committee wishes to stress that many of the scientific fields relevant to this study, such as neuro-AIDS, behavioral epidemiology, and qualitative sociology, are still in the early stages of their development and application. The AIDS epidemic requires better integration of these basic biological, psychological, and social science perspectives in order to achieve the complex understanding that will lead to more appropriate and effective AIDS prevention and intervention efforts.

H. Keith H. Brodie, *Chair*
Judith D. Auerbach, *Study Director*

Acknowledgments

The committee's efforts were enabled by the extraordinary work of an excellent project staff under the insightful leadership of Judy Auerbach. We are indebted to Christina Wypijewska for her excellent skills in collecting, analyzing, and presenting a range of information and for her oral and written contributions to the structure and substance of the report. Holly Dawkins brought notable research skills to our efforts, including intensive literature searches and the retrieval of numerous documents from the institutes under review and elsewhere. Karen Autrey provided the committee with extraordinary attention to the logistics of our meetings and to the production of the report, including the documentation of all of our references. Constance Pechura, Robert Cook-Deegan, Mike Stoto, and Leslie Hardy, all members of the IOM staff, contributed constructively to our committee's deliberations and provided necessary guidance in informing the committee of our responsibilities in developing a report worthy of publication.

The committee also benefitted from excellent background research provided by Robert Walkington and Beth Kosiak. Additional thanks are owed to Linda Humphrey for carefully editing and improving the structure of many sections of the report, to Mike Edington for coordinating editing and publication, to Claudia Carl for coordinating the review process, to Nina Spruill for guiding the budget, and to Gail Spears for providing a range of administrative assistance.

We are also indebted to the many federal agency and congressional staff, external researchers, AIDS advocates, and representatives of other interested groups who provided input into the committee's deliberations. These individuals are acknowledged by name in Appendix C. One of these people, however, deserves special mention. William A. Bailey, a legislative affairs officer for the American Psychological Association, contributed greatly to this study, by lobbying Congress to mandate the IOM examination of the AIDS programs at the former ADAMHA, by presenting memorable testimony at the committee's public meeting, and by facilitating communication among the committee, the AIDS research and advocacy communities, and the federal government. Bill was a tireless advocate for AIDS prevention, a generous commitment from someone already afflicted with the disease. AIDS claimed Bill's life on April 23, 1994. The committee notes his passing with sadness and remembers his work with thanks.

Finally, the committee wishes to express its deep appreciation for the leadership, insight, and extraordinary diligence of our project director, Judy Auerbach, who instilled in us all a commitment to produce a report of which we could be proud. In addition to writing significant sections herself, she brought out our best efforts and was consistently able to produce the information we required to make this report responsive to our charge and, we hope, helpful to the field.

Contents

PART II
MANAGING THE AIDS RESEARCH PROGRAMS
AT NIAAA, NIDA, AND NIMH

List of Boxes, Figures, and Tables

TABLES

AIDS and Behavior

Executive Summary

Since it appeared in the early 1980s, the acquired immune deficiency syndrome (AIDS), and the human immunodeficiency virus (HIV) that causes it, have wrought alarming physical and social devastation around the world. The number of people afflicted by the illness has increased markedly, and the range of communities affected has expanded. In the United States, while AIDS was first considered a disease of gay men, the reach of the epidemic now has expanded to injection drug users and their sexual partners, heterosexual partners of non-drug-using HIV-infected persons, infants born to mothers infected with HIV, and hemophiliacs and others exposed to blood products or blood transfusion.

The number of AIDS cases reported in the United States has grown rapidly, surpassing 100,000 in 1988, 200,000 in 1990, and 300,000 in 1992. The rate of increase is alarming—the first 100,000 reported cases occurred within an eight-year period, while the second 100,000 cases occurred in only a two-year period (CDC, 1992a). By the end of 1992, AIDS had become the leading cause of death for men between the ages of 25 and 44 and the fourth leading cause of death for women in that age group. By the end of 1992, over 200,000 people in the United States had died of complications related to AIDS (CDC, 1994).

Despite extensive efforts to develop effective treatments as well as a vaccine for HIV/AIDS, a fully effective treatment, cure, vaccine, or other medical intervention appears to be years away. In conjunction with such developments, efforts to prevent the transmission of HIV through the cessation of behaviors that contribute to it must be expanded. This requires a commitment to understanding and intervening in human behavior.

This report surveys the AIDS research programs of the National Institute on Alcohol Abuse and Alcoholism (NIAAA), National Institute on Drug Abuse (NIDA), and National Institute of Mental Health (NIMH). Much of the AIDS research supported by these institutes is dedicated to developing and implementing (and to a lesser extent, evaluating) HIV preventive interventions in different populations. These interventions should be driven by basic behavioral and social science research on the determinants of behavior and behavior change; and to a great extent they are. Yet much of this basic research is still in its early stages, its development inhibited by a political climate during the first decade of the epidemic that made it difficult, and on some occasions impossible, to conduct research on the very behaviors in question: drug use and sex. For example, although numerous scientific and policy reports called for a federally sponsored, national survey of sexual behavior to help determine the nature and level of risk for HIV transmission in the general population, federal and congressional restrictions did not allow it.

The absence of information about the actual sexual behaviors in which people are engaging has hampered AIDS prevention efforts during this period. Now, although the current climate is more supportive of such research, basic behavioral and social science research is having to catch up. Moreover, much-needed efforts to integrate this research with basic biomedical research to obtain a more complete understanding of the complex factors that contribute to the transmission, disease progression, and prevention of HIV/AIDS among different people are still just beginning.

Part I of this report presents an overview of findings from relevant research to date. The committee felt it was important to elucidate the status of knowledge about the substance abuse and mental health aspects of HIV/AIDS first, as a backdrop to its assessment of the specific research programs of NIAAA, NIDA, and NIMH, which appears in Part II. This was thought to be a constructive approach, as it provides a baseline for assessing contributions, gaps, and future directions for AIDS research at the institutes.

Chapter 1 provides a general introduction to the report and its organization. Chapter 2 reviews the extent of knowledge about the range and contexts of sexual and substance-using behaviors by which HIV is transmitted. Although attempts to conduct large-scale projects on the specific behaviors involved have been hampered, significant contributions to the knowledge base have come from individual studies using the methods of qualitative, social science research and behavioral epidemiology. Chapter 3 reviews what is known about the neurobiological, psychological, and social determinants of HIV risk behavior and examines the application of that basic knowledge to interventions directed at changing behavior in positive ways.

While preventing the initial transmission of HIV is the top priority from a public health perspective, it is equally important to develop effective treatment interventions for those people who are already infected. This requires knowledge about disease progression and how it might differ among individuals and populations. With respect to mental health and substance abuse, a key issue is the relationship between HIV, the brain, and behavior. This is explored in Chapter 4.

After highlighting some of the significant developments and outstanding gaps in AIDS-related behavior, mental health, and substance abuse research, the report moves in Part II to a discussion of the specific AIDS programs of NIAAA, NIDA, and NIMH. Chapter 5 describes the general context within which these programs have been operating. The most salient elements of that context are: (1) the recent reorganization of the Alcohol, Drug Abuse, and Mental Health Administration (ADAMHA); (2) the new budget and program authority of the Office of AIDS Research (OAR) at the National Institutes of Health (NIH); (3) the budget process; and (4) the grant review process. Chapter 6 contains the committee's assessment of the content and management of the institutes' AIDS programs themselves, focusing on balance among scientific approaches, the use of various funding mechanisms to support research, and the overall funding picture. Finally, Chapter 7 explores the relationship between the AIDS research programs of NIAAA, NIDA, and NIMH and the services programs formerly at ADAMHA and now at SAMHSA (and elsewhere in the Public Health Service).

PART I
RESEARCH FINDINGS AND OPPORTUNITIES

UNDERSTANDING HIV TRANSMISSION

Although the general categories of risk behavior are well known, the specific acts responsible for HIV transmission—use of injection drugs and sexual practices, for example—have not been adequately researched or discussed because of their sensitive nature. Yet, in order to develop effective prevention and treatment strategies, it is crucial to understand the specific behaviors involved. As described in Chapter 2, knowledge gained to date from the biological, epidemiological, psychological, and social sciences— much of it supported by NIAAA, NIDA, and NIMH—has helped elucidate the specific behaviors responsible for transmitting HIV. However, much remains to be learned. In particular, the prevalence and spread of those behaviors within certain communities is unknown.

SEX, DRUG USE, AND HIV TRANSMISSION

As with any sexually transmitted disease, the transmission of HIV is highly dependent on the number of partners one has and the specific types of sexual practices in which one engages. Anal intercourse carries the highest risk for HIV acquisition, followed by penile-vaginal and oral-genital intercourse. These sexual behaviors can place anyone at high risk for HIV, regardless of his or her sexual orientation or gender. However, having a large number of sexual partners, and having a concurrent or prior infection (such as those associated with syphilis, gonorrhea, anal and genital warts, and herpes), may increase one's susceptibility to infection (CDC, 1987).

With respect to drug use, the sharing of hypodermic needles, syringes, and other injection paraphernalia is the most likely route of HIV transmission. The vector is the exchange of the blood of the previous user that is lodged in the paraphernalia. Certain methods of injection drug use are believed to be more risky than others, but any method that involves contact with potentially infected blood is dangerous (Grund, Kaplan, and Adriaans, 1989; Grund et al., 1990; Inciardi, 1990a; Inciardi and Page, 1991; Jose et al., 1993).

Much high-risk sexual and drug-using behavior in urban locales takes place in specific settings, such as "shooting galleries" and "crack houses." Although these settings have not yet been systematically studied, emerging ethnographic research has revealed some of the particular practices that contribute to the potential for HIV transmission among patrons (Marmor et al., 1987; Murphy and Waldorf, 1991; Schoenbaum et al., 1989). This research suggests that these dangerous settings would be particularly promising sites in which to prevent HIV transmission. A better understanding of the character and dynamics of such settings is required to develop fully effective preventive interventions.

In order to understand the potential course of the epidemic, behavioral epidemiologists have focused on determining the likelihood that infected individuals in one group will have contact with uninfected individuals in another; identifying the contexts that influence risk taking; investigating whether people in high- and low-risk groups are adopting recommended preventive behaviors; and examining how the spread of HIV infection will be altered by changing patterns in concurrent epidemics of drug use and infectious diseases.

In Chapter 2, after reviewing the status of knowledge on HIV transmission through sexual and drug-using behaviors, the committee makes several recommendations:

2.1 The committee recommends that a national survey be undertaken to determine the prevalence and correlates of HIV risk-taking behavior. NIAAA, NIDA, and NIMH should collaborate to sponsor such a survey.

2.2 The committee recommends that NIAAA, NIDA, and NIMH support studies of the social, psychological, and biological determinants of HIV risk-taking behavior using a variety of methods complementing the national survey. These studies would allow an understanding of the detailed mechanisms of such behavior, the social dynamics within which they occur, the differing conceptualization and terminology in specific communities, and the role of concurrent health events.

2.3 The committee recommends that NIAAA, NIDA, and NIMH develop studies of the high-risk settings, such as shooting galleries and crack houses, that may contribute to epidemic spread and implement prevention efforts in those settings.

2.4 The committee recommends that NIAAA, NIDA, and NIMH support research that integrates basic biological, epi-

demiological, psychological, and social research to better understand transmission of HIV through sex and drug use.

2.5 The committee recommends that NIAAA, NIDA, and NIMH support research on AIDS risk and behavior change among seriously mentally ill men and women and people with other cognitive impairments, including those not in psychiatric treatment. Such research should be conducted in a range of geographic locations.

2.6 The committee recommends that the Public Health Service coordinate interagency efforts to monitor and respond to concurrent epidemics (such as drug use, violence, and infectious diseases) that will alter the course of the HIV epidemic.

UNDERSTANDING THE DETERMINANTS OF HIV RISK BEHAVIOR

Human behavior is determined by multiple factors in the individual and the environment, ranging from the micro-level molecular biological to the macro-level social and environmental. These factors often interact in mutually reciprocal relationships such that one factor both influences and is influenced by another.

Much has been learned from research on the psychosocial determinants of AIDS-related sexual and drug-using behaviors. However, research on the brain biology of sexuality and drug addiction has rarely been integrated into these studies, even though it may be critical for understanding and preventing high-risk behavior.

Neurobiological Determinants of Risk Behavior

While impressive strides have been made in the area of sexuality, the brain, and behavior, much remains to be learned. Characterization of sexual dimorphism at the genomic, molecular, cellular, behavioral, and social levels is still in its early stages. In the absence of this basic information, the very existence of a biology of high-risk sexual behaviors—a central missing element in basic biomedical and neurobiological AIDS research—cannot be approached.

Some outstanding issues include: identifying the neurochemical molecular substrates, if any, associated with sexual risk taking; determining how insights from the studies of the neurobiology of sexuality would relate to high-risk sexual behavior and to sexually transmitted diseases, including AIDS; and determining how society might best integrate the study of the biology of sexuality and sexual risk taking into the broader context of sexuality, sexual behavior, and sexually transmitted diseases.

Understanding the biological basis of drug addiction is an important link to understanding drug abuse behaviors, and unlike the biology of sexuality has been the object of a great deal of research. Recent studies on the cellular and molecular basis of dependence and tolerance suggest that the processes are separate and distinct, and are mediated by different brain systems. The actual anatomical circuits in the brain that participate in the addictive process have been identified in some detail, although the story is not yet complete. The neuroanatomic and molecular bases of the withdrawal syndrome are less clearly understood.

PSYCHOSOCIAL DETERMINANTS OF RISK BEHAVIOR

Theoretical models, primarily from psychology, have been used either to predict risk behavior or to predict behavior change and, less frequently, maintenance of positive behavior change. Such models focus on the individual's perception of susceptibility, perception of benefits, constraints, and intentions to behave in particular ways (Fishbein et al., 1991). The concept of self-efficacy— the individual's belief that he or she can effectively carry out a desired behavior in a particular setting—is central to most models.

Despite their conceptual contributions, current theoretical models are limited in their ability to predict risk behavior for two main reasons. First, with respect to sexual behavior, the models are based on the assumption that sexual encounters are regulated by self-formulated plans of action, and that individuals are acting in an intentional and volitional manner when engaging in sexual activity. However, sexual behavior is often impulsive and, at least in part, physiologically motivated.

Second, the dominant theoretical models of behavior do not easily accommodate contextual personal and sociocultural variables such as gender, race/ethnicity, culture, and class. For example, gender roles and cultural values and norms influence the behavior of women and men and the nature of the relationships in which sexual activity occurs. Unsafe sexual practices often are not the result of a deficit of knowledge, motivation, or skill, but instead have meaning within a given personal and sociocultural context. A great deal of work remains to be done to better integrate theories of gender and culture with models of behavior change.

Additionally, models designed to explain or predict risk behavior tend to focus only on one level of analysis—the individual—without regard for other levels, such as the culture and community to which an individual belongs. This focus on the individual has obscured the influence of social factors.

SOCIAL SCIENCE PERSPECTIVES ON BEHAVIOR AND BEHAVIOR CHANGE

Social science perspectives, which only recently have been applied broadly to AIDS research, have the potential for productively refocusing the investigation of AIDS to reveal the complex, yet powerful linkages between individuals and their social structure, and to suggest how specific social changes can inspire individual changes (Adam, 1992; Friedman, Des Jarlais, and Ward, 1994).

Several levels of social arrangements can affect behaviors related to the transmission of HIV—ranging from couples to social networks to the community to society as a whole. At the broadest level, social conditions, such as the lack of universal access to health care, racial and ethnic discrimination, unemployment, and a lack of public monies to promote AIDS prevention, contribute to a social context in which HIV transmission is prone to occur.

The smallest unit of social interaction that may influence one's participation in risk-taking behavior is the dyad—the two-person relationship. However, social influence does not begin and end with a partner. The scope and character of one's broader social network—the array of individuals upon whom one relies for support, who serve as reference groups, and who establish group standards of conduct (social norms) and sanction behavior—are central to understanding the behavior that puts one at risk for HIV infection (Klovdahl, 1985; Klovdahl et al., 1994; Neaigus et al., 1994). It is at this level that the operation of social norms can best be observed and understood, and where intervention to change norms may be most feasible.

Social networks and the norms that govern the behavior of their members exist within communities, including those defined by culture. Sensitivity to the values and historical experiences of cultural communities is essential for designing and implementing appropriate AIDS interventions. At the same time, cultural values may be at cross-purposes with public health interests, as is the case with the opposition among many racial/ethnic community leaders to needle exchange programs in areas with significant drug-using populations (Bayer, 1994). How the various interests of different communities and of members within them are best mediated in the context of HIV/AIDS is an important area of further study.

Theoretical models and constructs from the psychological and social sciences, notwithstanding their limitations, have been applied to the design of preventive interventions and behavior change strategies in an attempt to prevent further transmission of HIV. AIDS prevention intervention research typically focuses on identifying and modifying behaviors—usually those related to drug use and sex—known to be associated with HIV infection and targets both uninfected and infected persons in a range of populations and settings. Although most studies target individuals, some recently have begun to focus on the community as the target for intervention, recognizing the importance of socially created norms as determinants of behavior.

AIDS intervention studies employ a range of methodologies. Although experimental studies that randomize subjects into control and experimental groups have been considered to be the "gold standard," most studies do not adhere to this rigid design because of the difficulties associated with maintaining experimental conditions in the settings involved. Moreover, in some cases the randomized controlled trial is simply not appropriate for the question under study (Oakley, 1989). Rather, simple pre-post comparison studies are the most common means of assessing the effects of prevention programs, and specific changes (such as increased condom use) and mediating variables (such as demonstrated self-efficacy) have been the standard outcome measures for determining whether or not a particular intervention has been successful.

Even though many intervention studies have demonstrated behavior change, they may be limited in a few ways: (1) most rely solely on self-reported data; (2) for the most part they have not yet demonstrated long-term behavior change (beyond 6 months); (3) it is not yet known whether they work with populations outside of their target groups; (4) many interventions may not be cost-effective to implement on a larger scale; and (5) with few exceptions, they do not measure HIV transmission and do not necessarily indicate that HIV infection has been averted.

The mixed results of interventions informed by basic psychological and social research suggests that much remains to be learned—including how the psychological and social dimensions of behavior interact with the biological to encourage or prevent risky behavior and to initiate and maintain positive behavior change. Cross-disciplinary research in this regard will play an important role in improving the design, application, and evaluation of HIV prevention interventions.

After reviewing relevant neurobiological, psychological, and social research supported by NIAAA, NIDA, and NIMH in Chapter 3, the committee makes the following set of recommendations:

3.1 The committee recommends that NIAAA, NIDA, and NIMH expand basic research on the biology of sexuality as it potentially relates to high-risk sexual behaviors. This might include research on the central nervous system (CNS) sexual systems that mediate sexual behaviors, the CNS neural systems underlying sexual behavior, and the molecular genetics of sexual behaviors.

3.2 The committee recommends that NIAAA, NIDA, and NIMH expand research on the biology of substance abuse to provide additional knowledge for approaching high-risk behaviors. This might include research to define structure-activity relationships in the function of dopamine systems; the role of noradrenergic systems and molecular mechanisms in the components of addiction (including euphoria, tolerance, sensitization, and withdrawal); the role of opiate peptide receptor subtypes in components of the addiction-abuse syndrome; as well as research to identify mechanisms of cocaine addiction.

3.3 The committee recommends that, where appropriate, NIAAA, NIDA, and NIMH coordinate their efforts with other relevant federal agencies (e.g., other NIH institutes, the National Science Foundation) that are also attempting to integrate biological, behavioral, and social research to define high-risk behaviors.

3.4 The committee recommends that NIAAA, NIDA, and NIMH support AIDS research that integrates theories of gender (identity, development, and dynamics) and behavior change models.

3.5 The committee recommends that NIAAA, NIDA, and NIMH expand the research effort examining social and structural factors (such as class, race/ethnicity, gender relations, and community) that increase risk for AIDS, affect progression of disease, and provide points of intervention. This

might require research that takes as the unit of analysis the social context and relationship (e.g., dyads, families, communities) in which HIV occurs—as opposed to the individual at risk of or who has HIV.

3.6 The committee recommends that NIAAA, NIDA, and NIMH, in conjunction with other NIH institutes, develop new and existing woman-controlled HIV/STD prevention methods (e.g., female condoms and microbicides) and examine the social and behavioral issues related to their use.

3.7 The committee recommends that NIAAA, NIDA, and NIMH support basic and applied research on the maintenance of behavior change, for example, risky sexual behavior and alcohol and other drug-using behavior, including the prevention of relapse. (The committee notes that this has been recommended in previous NRC reports—*AIDS: The Second Decade*, 1990; *AIDS, Sexual Behavior, and Intravenous Drug Use*, 1989—but has not been attended to adequately.)

3.8 The committee recommends that NIAAA, NIDA, and NIMH expand funding for HIV intervention research initiatives, particularly those that: (1) have rigorous evaluation components; (2) investigate motivations, intentions, and barriers in addition to behavior change; (3) include outcome measures in addition to behavior change, such as HIV seroprevalence, STD rates, and pregnancy rates; and (4) target a full range of racial/ethnic, gender, and cultural groups for the purpose of assessing between-group differences.

3.9 The committee recommends that NIAAA, NIDA, and NIMH support research that estimates the number of HIV infections averted by current prevention efforts and that includes cost estimates for these efforts.

DISEASE PROGRESSION AND INTERVENTION

Although every effort must be made to prevent new transmission of HIV, it is equally important to diagnose, treat, and care adequately for people who already are infected. Research on the pathogenesis and disease progression of HIV/AIDS relevant to mental health and substance abuse has developed quickly over the past decade. This research, which ranges from basic molecular and cellular biology to clinical pathology to social psychology, has provided some important clues about the relationship between

HIV, the brain, and behavior, and most importantly, about their interactive nature. Chief interactions discussed in Chapter 4 include: (1) HIV infection of the brain and the effects it has on the central nervous system; (2) effects of interactions among HIV infection, substance use, and mental illness, and the unique medical care and treatment issues associated with such interactions; and (3) the relationship between psychosocial factors and HIV infection for individuals with the disease, as well as for their loved ones and caregivers.

THE RELATIONSHIP BETWEEN HIV AND THE CENTRAL NERVOUS SYSTEM

HIV-associated conditions affecting both the central nervous system (CNS) and the peripheral nervous system (PNS) are common and result in considerable morbidity and mortality. Some conditions are secondary complications of HIV infection, resulting from opportunistic infections or systemic organ dysfunction that follows from immune deficiency induced by HIV infection. Among these are cerebral toxoplasmosis, primary CNS lymphoma, cryptococcal meningitis, and progressive multifocal leukoencephalopathy.

Other conditions likely result directly from HIV infection itself. The pathogenesis of these primary complications is not yet clearly understood, but they are thought to be sequelae of interactions among HIV, the immune system, and various components of the nervous system. These conditions include, at the early stage of HIV infection, mild meningitis with headache. As the infection progresses, patients may experience "aseptic" meningitis, peripheral neuropathy, and, most significantly, a set of afflictions collectively known as AIDS dementia complex (ADC).

In its mild form, ADC syndrome slows intellectual processing, blunts concentration and impairs rapid and fine motor control. When more severe, it can dull the personality and cause truly devastating dementia that reduces the patient to a shell of his or her former self, impairs walking, and, eventually, leaves the victim bedridden, incontinent, and mute (Navia et al., 1986; Navia, Jordan, and Price, 1986; Price and Sidtis, 1992). ADC can be a source of protracted and severe disability, modifying and markedly diminishing the quality of remaining life, reducing enjoyment of work and daily life, depriving the patient of social and intellectual pleasures, and requiring emotionally and financially costly care.

The core features of the ADC have now been well characterized, and a descriptive staging system, useful to provide a common vocabulary for both clinical practice and clinical investigation, has been developed (see Price, 1994; Sidtis, 1994). However, the character of HIV infection of the CNS is not yet fully understood. Changes in the virus, with respect to both predominant cell tropism and virulence may be important. A number of studies have shown early invasion of the CNS and early local host immune responses in the cerebrospinal fluid (CSF). A critical question remaining to be answered is whether the virus then persists in the CNS in latent form or as an indolent infection that is asymptomatic. If it can remain latent, it is important to know what cells might harbor the proviral DNA: microglia, astrocytes, or other CNS cells. Pathological observations to date suggest that the virus *indirectly* injures the brain rather than *directly* killing or infecting nerve cells. This distinguishes HIV from other viral infections of the brain, such as those caused by poliovirus or herpes simplex virus.

Understanding the pathogenic mechanisms has great potential importance for treating ADC patients not only using methods that interfere with the virus, but also strategies directed at interrupting some of its toxic processes. Indeed, these considerations underlie some of the approaches now being taken to treat ADC, including treatment protocols using nimodipine, a calcium channel blocker that can prevent gp120-induced neuronal death *in vitro*, and pentoxyphilline, an antagonist of Tumor Necrosis Factor.

Research on ADC and CNS HIV infection has biological importance not only for understanding the nature and course of HIV infection, but also more generally for suggesting mechanisms involved in other infectious, immunological, and neurodegenerative diseases. The early penetration of the blood-brain barrier by HIV, the local immune response detected in the spinal fluid, and the subsequent active replication of HIV in the brain late in infection hold clues regarding the CNS ecology of HIV.

INTERACTIONS AMONG HIV, SUBSTANCE USE, AND MENTAL ILLNESS

The second type of interaction among brain, behavior, and HIV relates to the unique issues associated with multiple diagnoses, that is diagnosis of any combination of HIV, drug or alcohol abuse, and mental illness.

Drinking alcohol to excess has been shown to cause damage to the immune system (Kruger and Jerrells, 1992). It therefore seems reasonable to assume that alcohol consumption in significant amounts might also make an individual more vulnerable to HIV infection and facilitate the transition from HIV infection to AIDS. Alcohol may increase the susceptibility of phagocytes to initial infection, impairing their ability to eliminate the virus in the early stages of infection, and thus increasing their potential to function as reservoirs for HIV (Kruger and Jerrells, 1992).

Alcohol also reduces the number of T-cells in the spleen, lymph nodes, thymus, and blood (Jerrells, Smith, and Eckardt, 1990; Saad and Jerrells, 1991). This loss of cells in the immune system may accelerate the onset of clinical manifestations among HIV-infected people, but research on this issue is inconclusive. Although it is clear that excessive alcohol consumption can impair cell-mediated immunity, this has not translated into accelerated clinical progression of HIV to AIDS in reports to date (Isaki and Gordis, 1993; Kaslow et al., 1989). The precise relationship between alcohol use and HIV/AIDS remains to be elucidated.

Treatment of drug users who are at risk for or already infected with HIV is complicated by many factors: the fact that the clinical course of HIV infection may have special characteristics among drug injectors, the existence of complex medical and psychosocial comorbidities, and the often tenuous relationship between drug users and the health care system. Although a significant body of research has been conducted on clinical aspects of HIV disease and its management among drug users, a number of key research areas require further examination. These include: charting changes in the spectrum of HIV disease over time, such as, the emergence or disappearance of AIDS-related illnesses in this group as a result of medical interventions or other differences; further epidemiologic and clinical study of tuberculosis among HIV-infected drug users; and clarifying further the clinical expression and outcome of hepatitis C infection in co-infected groups (Donahue et al., 1991; Haverkos and Lange, 1990; Novick et al., 1988; van den Hoek et al., 1990).

Pharmacokinetic and other pharmacologic studies involving drugs of abuse and medications used for the treatment of HIV-related disease, as well as prescribed opioids such as methadone used to treat opiate addiction, will help determine whether interactions have potential clinical significance. With the increasing number of medications continually being added to the standard therapeutic regimens of HIV-infected patients, it will be even more important in the future to assess these agents pharmacologically in relation to psychoactive drugs, both prescribed and over-the-counter drugs. Because most of the therapies used for HIV infection and related conditions (e.g., tuberculosis) require long-term medical regimens, often involving multiple medications, the levels of adherence to medical care among drug users in a variety of treatment settings must be examined. Finally, because drug injectors as a group are likely to have a high lifetime prevalence of depression, anxiety, personality disorder, and other psychiatric diagnoses (Batki, 1990a; Rounsaville et al., 1991), the comorbidity of drug abuse and psychiatric disorders must be studied further. On this point, a research and clinical agenda that brings together mental health services, drug abuse treatment, and medical care for HIV should be pursued. This will frequently require crossing categorical boundaries that separate research and services programs.

The convergence of psychiatric disorders, substance abuse, and HIV among those already infected who are also severely mentally ill raises difficult questions about appropriate treatment, similar to those related to injection drug users. For example, possible toxic reactions between antipsychotic and anti-HIV medications, and perhaps even antinarcotic medications, require further investigation. Moreover, little if anything is yet known about HIV disease progression among the seriously mentally ill. Given what has already been learned about the interactions of the virus and the CNS, it is possible that there are unique manifestations among people already suffering brain disorders. Yet, this area remains remarkably understudied.

THE RELATIONSHIP BETWEEN PSYCHOSOCIAL FACTORS AND HIV INFECTION

The final type of brain, behavior, and HIV interaction addressed in Chapter 4 is the relationship between HIV infection and certain psychiatric disorders, behavioral states, or reactions. For example, concern about HIV infection can lead to anxiety or depression. The stress of coping with the illness is not confined to the person infected, but also encompasses those who care for him or her. While not directly related to HIV infection *per se*, there are both diagnostic and therapeutic implications in the management of HIV infection.

The bidirectional relationship between psychosocial factors and HIV infection may influence disease progression and the ability to effectively treat related symptoms. These phenomena primarily have been informed by two types of research: psychoneuroimmunology and psychosocial research on coping and caregiving.

In the context of HIV/AIDS, psychoneuroimmunology is the study of how mental states might modify immune defenses and even viral replication within the immune system. Depression and other mental states may have an impact on the immune system through the hypothalamic-pituitary-adrenal axis, the autonomic nervous system, and other pathways. Stress and other nervous system perturbations may alter immune function in both animal models and humans. The complex interactions among HIV infection, immune function, and mental states have been a major theme of AIDS-related research, particularly at NIMH. Although much has been learned about the effects of HIV on psychosocial factors, less is known about the effects of psychosocial factors on HIV.

A number of studies have looked at the psychiatric implications of HIV/AIDS, but they have not been able to determine whether psychiatric disorder is an effect of HIV or existed prior to HIV. For example, among gay men, psychiatric morbidity rates are relatively high regardless of HIV serostatus. This may be due to the fact that these men have to deal with a host of psychological issues related to being gay and their consequent status in society (Atkinson et al., 1988; Tross et al., 1987; Williams et al., 1991). This finding suggests the need to understand how the context of HIV affects psychiatric symptoms among gay men, that is, what disclosure and recognition of both being gay and having HIV may mean.

After learning that they are HIV positive, most people employ strategies of coping and social support that vary at different stages of the disease. Studies of asymptomatic HIV-positive people suggest that "avoidant coping"—screening out the negative implications and focusing instead on the positive—does not protect them from emotional distress (Joseph et al., 1990; Nicholson and Long, 1990; Rabkin et al., 1990; Storosum, Van Den Boom, and Beauzekom, 1990). Cognitive coping strategies, however, such as positive reinterpretation, sense of control over events, and positive changes in daily life, seem to promote psychological well-being throughout the course of the disease (Hart et al., 1990; Rabkin et al., 1991; Storosum, Van Den Boom, and Beauzekom, 1990).

To date, nearly all of the research on coping—including that on bereavement after the death of someone with AIDS—has focused on gay men. Much remains to be learned about how people from various gender, racial/ethnic, and cultural groups cope with their own and others' HIV status, including not only general psychological strategies, but also motivation or resistance to adherence to medical treatment and its implications for disease progression.

People who provide care to those with HIV/AIDS also experience its psychological impact. Most informal AIDS caregivers (relatives, lovers, and friends) are forced to learn a range of technical and emotional skills on the job, and many experience dysphoria—an emotional state of depression, anxiety, and restlessness (Folkman, Chesney, and Christopher-Richards, 1994).

Although stress experienced by formal HIV caregivers is reported in professional and lay articles, research has not included systematic documentation of the incidence and prevalence of physical, psychological, occupational, or interpersonal symptoms or disorders in health care professionals who devote a substantial amount of their clinical activities to patients with HIV illness (Silverman, 1993). Anecdotal reports of various symptoms, such as AIDS-related nightmares and psychological numbing, together with other symptoms related to stress and depression, suggest that some caregivers might be experiencing a form of posttraumatic stress disorder. However, according to Silverman (1993), only one published psychiatry article has addressed this possibility (Horstman and McKusick, 1986).

The psychological and physical implications of AIDS caregiving for health professionals undoubtedly is affected by their attitude toward AIDS. Surveys among nurses, physicians, dentists, social workers, psychiatrists, and health profession students are notable for revealing a consistent aversion among caregivers to the HIV/AIDS disease, to patients and their lifestyles, and to caregiving work itself, much of it based on fear of contagion (Silverman, 1993). A related issue is the psychological and social consequences (including occupational stress) of dealing with HIV/AIDS among outreach workers and service providers (Broadhead and Fox, 1993).

After reviewing the literature on disease progression and intervention in Chapter 4, the committee makes a number of recommendations:

4.1 The committee recommends that NIMH continue research on the pathogenesis of HIV infection of the brain, including the factors controlling virus replication such as local immune defenses and changes in the viral genome determining neuropathogenicity.

4.2 The committee recommends that NIMH continue research on the pathobiology of nervous system injury underlying the AIDS dementia complex, including the morphological, biochemical, and molecular basis of neuronal dysfunction related to viral and cellular gene expression.

4.3 The committee recommends that NIMH support collab-

orative studies of the prevention and treatment of the AIDS dementia complex and other central nervous system complications of HIV infection.

4.4 The committee recommends that NIAAA, NIDA, and NIMH continue supporting research on the development of animal models for examining the basic neurochemical and behavioral changes associated with HIV/AIDS.

4.5 The committee recommends that NIAAA, NIDA, and NIMH expand research on the natural history of HIV infection among various populations, including injection drug users, other substance abusers, and the seriously mentally ill.

4.6 The committee recommends that NIAAA, NIDA, and NIMH support research on the relationship between the medical consequences of substance abuse and related behaviors and the clinical expression of HIV among the drug-using population.

4.7 The committee recommends that NIAAA, NIDA, and NIMH support research at the intersection of AIDS treatment and clinical care for substance abusers, addressing, for example, how to treat HIV/AIDS in mental health and substance abuse treatment programs.

4.8 The committee recommends that NIAAA, NIDA, and NIMH collaborate on research to investigate interactions among psychotropic (including illicit) drugs, antinarcotic and antipsychotic medications, and drugs used to treat HIV and opportunistic infections—for example, the effect of methadone on zidovudine (AZT)—including research on toxicities that might develop through such drug interactions.

4.9 The committee recommends that NIAAA, NIDA, and NIMH support more research on the neuropharmacology of anti-HIV medication.

4.10 The committee recommends that all relevant NIH institutes eliminate systemic barriers to the inclusion of injection drug users and other substance abusers in AIDS and AIDS-related clinical trials.

4.11 The committee recommends that NIAAA, NIDA, and NIMH support research on the utilization of health resources by people with AIDS, including substance abuse and mental health treatment programs. This research might include studies of the extent and manner in which the medical system acts (intentionally or not) to exclude drug users from care.

4.12 The committee recommends that NIAAA, NIDA, and NIMH support research on the relationship between adherence to HIV/AIDS medical treatment and disease progression among individuals from diverse gender, racial/ethnic, and cultural groups.

4.13 The committee recommends that NIAAA, NIDA, and NIMH support research that integrates substance abuse and mental health treatment; in particular, demonstration projects for integrated multidisciplinary treatment systems that include mental health.

4.14 The committee recommends that NIMH support research on positive as well as negative consequences of HIV, for example, how people with AIDS and their caregivers maintain positive coping strategies in the face of the disease.

4.15 The committee recommends that NIAAA, NIDA, and NIMH support research on how families (broadly defined to include persons who consider themselves to be family through mutual commitment) from diverse racial/ethnic, socioeconomic, and sexual orientation backgrounds cope with the reality of having family members who are infected with HIV or have AIDS. Special attention should be given to patterns and consequences of caregiving in such families.

PART II
MANAGING THE AIDS RESEARCH PROGRAMS AT NIAAA, NIDA, AND NIMH

THE CONTEXT OF AIDS PROGRAMS AT NIAAA, NIDA, AND NIMH

In order to analyze the AIDS research programs of NIAAA, NIDA, and NIMH, one must understand the larger context in which they have been operating. The most significant elements for this study are: (1) the passage of the ADAMHA Reorganization Act of 1992 (PL 102-321), which separated ADAMHA's research and services entities into two different agencies (NIH and SAMHSA respectively); and (2) the NIH Revitalization Act of 1993 (PL 103-43), which assigned the NIH Office of AIDS Research (OAR)—housed in the office of the NIH director—new budgetary authority over

the AIDS programs of all NIH institutes.   Other factors, such as
the overall federal budget process and procedures for program planning
and grant review, affect the nature of the AIDS programs of NIAAA,
NIDA, and NIMH. Chapter 5 discusses these contextual factors.

EFFECTS OF THE ADAMHA REORGANIZATION AND
NIH REAUTHORIZATION

Overall, the reorganization appears to have had only a limited
effect on the research programs of the three institutes to date.
Their organizational structure and staffing have been left largely
intact, and their review processes remain the same as they were
at ADAMHA for the period FY 1993 through FY 1996, as mandated by the reorganization legislation.

ADAMHA never had an official, authorized, functioning AIDS
office. Because the Department of Health and Human Services
(HHS) was considering reorganization, ADAMHA created an acting AIDS office rather than a permanent one. This office was
headed by a part-time acting coordinator, who also directed the
NIMH AIDS office. Each institute at ADAMHA devised its own
way to manage its AIDS program: NIAAA had only one or two
staff acting as AIDS coordinators on a part-time basis; NIDA had
an official AIDS coordinator located within one of its regular divisions; and NIMH had a formal Office on AIDS Programs with a
full-time director. These organizational structures were maintained after reorganization. Only three of the 24 programs that
were transferred from ADAMHA to SAMHSA as a result of the
reorganization are directly related to AIDS: AIDS health care
worker training (moved from NIMH to CMHS); AIDS health care
worker training/AIDS hotline (moved from NIDA to CSAT); and
AIDS service delivery demonstrations (also moved from NIDA to
CSAT).

Simultaneous to the ADAMHA reorganization, NIH underwent
changes in its leadership, and under the NIH reauthorization bill
passed in 1993 developed a much more centrally managed AIDS
research effort as new and greater authority over the AIDS budget
was given to OAR. The bill requires a comprehensive plan for the
expenditures of appropriations, and authorizes an emergency discretionary fund for the director of OAR. According to the legislation, the plan must: (1) provide for the conduct and support of all
AIDS activities at NIH; (2) prioritize the various AIDS activities,
which are required to have objectives, measures, and a time frame;
(3) ensure that the budget is allocated accordingly; (4) be updated

annually; (5) ensure that approval of specific projects and ongoing operation remain with the individual institute, center, and division directors; and (6) include a full range of research (including basic, applied, intramural, extramural, investigator-initiated, NIH-directed, and behavioral and social science research). This comprehensive plan is meant to be the basis for developing the annual budget requests for AIDS research.

Beginning in FY 1995, when AIDS funds are appropriated to NIH by Congress they will go directly to the director of OAR. The director will allocate to the individual institutes, centers, and divisions all of the funds received in accordance with the previously approved comprehensive plan for expenditures and appropriations.

THE BUDGET PROCESS

The specific funding of ADAMHA and NIH AIDS activities over time has taken place within the larger context of the overall federal budget process and has been directly affected by it. Appreciating the length and complexity of the budget process is critical for understanding the problems faced by rapidly changing and expanding research areas such as AIDS and by organizations that are in the process of restructuring, as were ADAMHA and NIH during the course of this study.

At any one point in time, an institute (whether at ADAMHA or NIH) must consider its research program in relation to *three* separate budgets. For example, at the end of calendar year 1993, an institute would have been in the midst of utilizing its current funds (which were allocated through September 30, 1994), presenting and defending its next year's (FY 95) budget to reviewers ranging from HHS and the Office of Management and Budget (OMB) to various congressional committees and interest groups, and planning the subsequent year's (FY 96) budget request.

NIAAA, NIDA, and NIMH joined in the FY 1994 NIH budget process after the major internal HHS decisions already had been made about the NIH AIDS budget, although they still were affected by those decisions. In FY 1994, as in all preceding years, once the institute received its budget allocation, the determination of the specific projects to fund was mostly a function of the grant review process.

THE GRANT REVIEW PROCESS

The ADAMHA Reorganization Act provided that the ADAMHA peer review systems, advisory councils, and scientific advisory committees would remain in effect through FY 1996 (ending September 30, 1996).

In most ways, the review procedures of the former ADAMHA research institutes are similar to the procedures at NIH. ADAMHA, like NIH, used a dual review system that separated technical and scientific assessment of projects from subsequent policy decisions concerning programmatic, scientific areas in which projects would be supported. This dual technical and programmatic review has been retained at the institutes. The scientific review process is kept separate from funding in part to ensure that program officials are not involved in making determinations on the scientific merit of research applications.

The first level of grant review is conducted by technical experts, largely from outside the federal government, and is designed to evaluate competing applications based on scientific and technical merit. The second level of review is conducted by advisory councils to assess the quality of the first-level review and to offer recommendations based on the relevance of the research to the institute's mission. The recommendations of both levels of review are advisory to the federal government and the final funding decisions reside with the institute director. Funding decisions are based not only on scientific merit and policy consideration, but may also consider administration policy, funding availability, and other factors.

Although the ADAMHA Reorganization Act mandated that the review processes (both at the first and second levels) be maintained through 1996, it is not yet clear how AIDS research applications at the three institutes will be reviewed when this period ends.

Given the composition of the NIH-wide AIDS study sections, some have expressed concern that applications related to the biobehavioral and social-behavioral research foci of NIAAA, NIDA, and NIMH—that is, the cross-disciplinary focus—will not fare well should the three institutes be subject to the overall NIH review process. While it is too soon to determine if this concern is well founded, the committee is aware that such concern is widespread among the institute program staff and the external research community.

It is the perception of many people, including some members of the committee and researchers interviewed for the study who have sat on study sections, that the current NIH review and scoring procedures are inherently prejudicial to innovative and collaborative proposals. Review panel members are likely to regress the scores that they give to proposals involving disciplines other than their own. They often are not in a position to know what constitutes an "extremely good" proposal in another discipline. As a result, a single-discipline proposal will be less competitive to the extent that it is judged by specialists from other disciplines. A cross-disciplinary proposal is almost guaranteed to contain elements that will be unfamiliar to each reviewer.

These problems can be addressed either by working within the existing review procedures or by changing them. Within the system, one possibility is to weight ratings by the disciplinary competence of the raters or rescale scores so that they are standardized within different categories. More fundamental changes might include convening special review panels, affording votes to ad hoc reviewers, and dedicating funds to unconventional proposals (so that they compete only amongst themselves). Implementing these proposals would require considering the appropriateness of existing review staff for creating the appropriate panels and procedures. It also would have to be in accord with the scientific principles of evaluation. As this report was being written, the current NIH director established a series of inter-NIH panels to examine the ways in which the peer review process could be streamlined and more innovative projects rewarded.

From its overview of funding and administration of AIDS research, presented in Chapter 5, the committee makes two recommendations:

5.1 The committee recommends that NIAAA, NIDA, and NIMH develop new programs and grant review procedures to encourage and facilitate innovative, collaborative, and cross-disciplinary proposals.

5.2 The committee recommends that the NIH task force charged with streamlining peer review consider alternative scoring schemes that would favor cross-disciplinary and innovative research proposals.

RESEARCH FUNDING, PROGRAMS, AND PRIORITIES AT NIAAA, NIDA, AND NIMH

The specific AIDS programs and priorities of NIAAA, NIDA, and NIMH are analyzed in Chapter 6. The committee was asked to assess the adequacy of the response of these three institutes to the AIDS epidemic by evaluating the scope and content of their AIDS research program activities and the balance between bio-medical and behavioral research. The committee conducted a grant-by-grant analysis of all AIDS research projects funded by NIAAA, NIDA, and NIMH from FY 1983—the first year of AIDS funding—through FY 1992—the most recent year for which complete data were available. In addition, the committee reviewed a range of documents and plans produced by the institutes that describe their AIDS programs and priorities and interviewed a number of researchers, federal agency staff, and public advocates.

When the committee began to address the balance between bio-medical and behavioral AIDS research at NIAAA, NIDA, and NIMH early in the study, it quickly realized that the categories were too limiting, because the definitions of "biomedical" and "behavioral" were not clear and because counterpoising these two categories masked the true level of cross-disciplinary research supported by the institutes. As the committee began to review the research portfolios grant by grant, it became apparent that labeling a project as either biomedical or behavioral was misleading, because significant portions of many projects included both.

As a consequence, the committee developed its own simple matrix, using four domains of science: biomedical/biobehavioral, epidemiological, psychosocial, and social-structural. These domains were cross-cut by two types of research: basic and applied. "Biomedical/biobehavioral" research focuses on improving knowledge about basic biological mechanisms and processes, disease pathogenesis, and clinical issues related to progression and treatment of HIV/AIDS. "Epidemiological" research focuses on transmission of HIV and the natural history of infection and disease progression. This category also includes biostatistical research to develop and refine mathematical modeling techniques for improved forecasting of HIV seroprevalence. "Psychosocial" research includes efforts to understand psychological determinants of behavior and behavior change and to develop and evaluate preventive interventions, the effect of psychosocial variables on disease progression, and the impact of HIV/AIDS on behavior and psychological functioning. "Social-structural" research examines the social context in which HIV/AIDS is transmitted and experienced, by focusing on relationships, families, communities, institutions, and cultures rather than on individuals. Social-structural research includes research on health services, evaluation, and operations. "Basic" research studies the basic mechanisms underlying biological, neurological, behavioral, and social processes and outcomes, and includes theoretical work. "Applied" research encompasses projects that test interventions.

The committee constructed an electronic database from abstracts of funded, extramural grants at NIAAA, NIDA, and NIMH from FY 1983 to FY 1992. Each AIDS grant was either single-coded with one of the four science categories or, where appropriate, multi-coded in two or more of the science categories. These latter were considered by the committee to be cross-disciplinary research. In addition, each grant was coded as either basic or applied. Grants also were coded according to their funding mechanism.

A significant proportion of AIDS research at NIAAA, NIDA, and NIMH is cross-disciplinary, according to the committee's coding scheme. The committee's analysis also discovered that most extramural AIDS research grants funded by NIAAA, NIDA, and NIMH involve basic research.

Although NIAAA, NIDA, and NIMH have utilized all mechanisms for supporting extramural AIDS research, they have done so in different proportions. For example, the majority of NIAAA's extramural research grants and dollars have been committed to investigator-initiated grants (R01s); NIMH AIDS extramural funding has been largely committed to R01s and research centers (P50s); and NIDA's extramural program has employed the widest variety of mechanisms, particularly by committing resources to research demonstration projects (R18s).

When compared to non-AIDS research, a greater proportion of AIDS research at NIAAA, NIDA, and NIMH has been directed in some way by the institutes. The level of directed research in the AIDS programs—as evidenced by program announcements (PAs), requests for applications (RFAs), and the funding of core and center grants—suggests active leadership among the institute staff in encouraging investigations of specific AIDS-related topics. This kind of leadership may be more necessary in a new research field, such as AIDS, when it becomes important to recruit investigators who have been establishing careers in other, related areas of science.

NIAAA

Because of the small size of its AIDS program, NIAAA has never established an Office of AIDS and has never had any full-time AIDS staff. Currently, NIAAA has two "part-time" coordinators—one for social and behavioral research and one for bio-

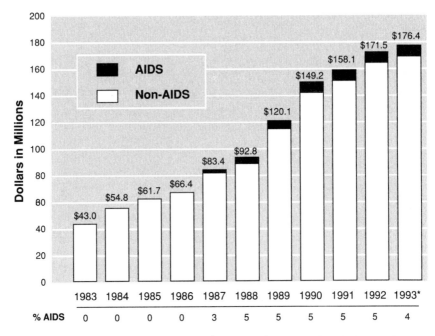

FIGURE S.1 NIAAA Expenditures (AIDS/Non-AIDS), 1983-1993. *Estimate. Source: NIAAA Budget Office.

medical research. AIDS funding at NIAAA increased from $2.4 million in FY 1987 (when the institute began its AIDS program) to $8 million in FY 1993, while total NIAAA funding (AIDS and non-AIDS) grew from $43 million to $176 million in the same period (Figure S.1).

Since NIAAA initiated its AIDS program, it has devoted much of its extramural and intramural research efforts to biomedical issues. NIAAA's broad research goal in this area is to elucidate how alcohol alters the immune system in ways that may compromise host defense against HIV. By 1990, NIAAA's research portfolio shifted so that half of the research grants had a biomedical component, half had a psychosocial component, and approximately one-fourth had an epidemiological component. None of the NIAAA research grants included a social-structural component until 1992.

NIDA

Although NIDA has had an AIDS coordinator since the mid-1980s, the institute only formally established an Office of AIDS

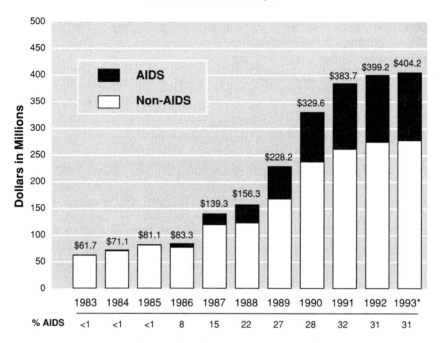

FIGURE S.2 NIDA Expenditures (AIDS/Non-AIDS), 1983-1993. *Estimate. Source: NIDA Budget Office.

in FY 1993, as required by the ADAMHA Reorganization Act. NIDA's AIDS program is designed to be decentralized and it appears that the office has a fairly limited coordinating role. NIDA's Office of AIDS has no budgetary or oversight authority for the wide range of AIDS activities. The current director of the Office of AIDS is also the acting director of the Division of Clinical Research. Although AIDS made up less than 1 percent of the total NIDA budget in FY 1983 (when NIDA's AIDS program began), it now constitutes approximately one-third ($127 million) of NIDA's budget, making it the third largest AIDS budget among the NIH institutes (Figure S.2). NIDA's AIDS portfolio has included a significant proportion of research demonstration projects (R18s) and cooperative agreements (U01s), in addition to traditional investigator-initiated grants (R01s). The bulk of NIDA's AIDS budget, however, remains allocated to research project grants (RPGs).

During the first decade of AIDS research funding at NIDA, a significant proportion of AIDS grants were biomedical and psychosocial, according to the committee's coding. Beginning in 1987, behavioral interventions aimed at reducing high-risk drug-using and sexual behaviors became a significant focus of the AIDS program. Some also included a social-structural component.

NIDA-supported biomedical research focuses on: the interrelationships among HIV infection and effects of drugs of abuse on the immune, neuroendocrine, and central nervous systems; vertical transmission of HIV (pediatric AIDS projects); nonreusable syringe development; medications development to create new pharmacological agents for treating substance abuse and addictive disorders; and treatment to reduce drug use and related risky behaviors.

Epidemiological research supported by NIDA monitors HIV infection and risk behaviors among injection drug users through surveillance efforts that are an integral part of various program initiatives, including natural history studies, community-based outreach studies, and research on the sex-for-crack phenomenon.

NIDA supports basic psychosocial research on the determinants of AIDS risk behaviors (including sexual and drug-using behaviors) and applied research on AIDS preventive interventions, in particular, community-based AIDS programs to get people into drug treatment to reduce their AIDS risk behaviors. Social-structural research supported by NIDA investigates community and relationship factors that influence high risk behaviors among drug users and their affiliates. Although NIDA has not yet been able to support such research, the institute's five-year strategic plan also emphasizes the need for research to examine HIV risk behaviors over time and under different social circumstances using multidimensional, longitudinal studies.

One of NIDA's main priorities for AIDS extramural and intramural research includes strategies for increasing the effectiveness of drug abuse treatment. Although treatment research has always existed as a priority for NIDA, the AIDS epidemic has heightened its importance. Drug addiction often involves physical and psychiatric health problems in addition to environmental and social conditions that may contribute to addiction; therefore, effective treatment requires a comprehensive approach. Indeed, because treatment research utilizes both pharmacologic and behavioral approaches, it is an area that was not easily categorized into one of the four scientific domains identified by the committee matrix. In fact, what makes these NIDA-funded research projects so unique is their emphasis on employing various combinations of pharmacologic, behavioral, and social approaches to improve the effectiveness of addiction treatment.

NIMH

Unlike NIDA and NIAAA, the AIDS research program at NIMH has for some time been managed by a central AIDS office, which develops the AIDS plan (with input from outside consultants and the various divisions and offices in NIMH), develops the annual AIDS budget, and directs the AIDS extramural program. The total NIMH budget increased from $191.5 to $560.5 million between FY 1983 and FY 1992. The AIDS budget increased from $200,000 to $76.2 million in the same period, making it the fourth largest AIDS budget among the NIH institutes. AIDS accounted for less than 1 percent of the total NIMH budget from FY 1983 through FY 1985 and rose to 14 percent by FY 1990 (Figure S.3).

NIMH funding generally has been committed to traditional investigator-initiated grants (R01s) and research center grants (P50s). NIMH has supported more AIDS training grants than the other two institutes. With respect to representation across fields, the most significant single domain of extramural research at NIMH,

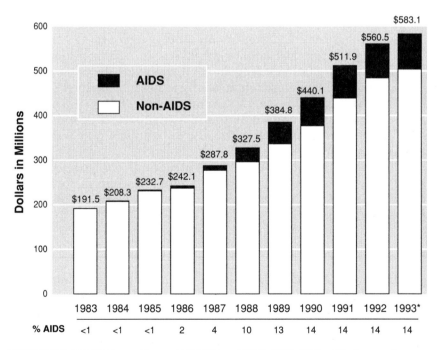

FIGURE S.3 NIMH Expenditures (AIDS/Non-AIDS), 1983-1993. *Estimate. Source: NIMH Budget Office.

according to the committee coding scheme, is psychosocial, followed closely by biomedical. In fact, the NIMH AIDS portfolio is relatively well-balanced between the two areas. Psychosocial research grants at NIMH include basic research on psychological mechanisms that underlie behavioral outcomes (including such topics as stress and coping processes and decision-making processes), behavioral and psychological responses to HIV testing and HIV status, and stress and coping among caregivers. Applied psychosocial research grants include behavioral interventions for HIV prevention. NIMH also supports behavioral epidemiology research to identify specific populations at risk for HIV/AIDS and to understand the specific high-risk behaviors of various populations. Biomedical/biobehavioral grants at NIMH examine the effects of HIV/AIDS on CNS function, the neuropsychological, neuropsychiatric, and neurological sequelae of HIV infection on the CNS, and the biological interface of stress and immune function (psychoneuroimmunology).

Many NIMH research grants have both biomedical and psychosocial research components. Applied biomedical/psychosocial grants include: behavioral interventions for HIV prevention that incorporate outcome measures such as HIV seropositivity rates and/or sexually transmitted disease (STD) rates in addition to behavioral outcome measures; and treatments and interventions for AIDS-related depression and emotional distress. Basic biomedical/psychosocial grants include: natural history and descriptive studies examining the neuropsychological and neurobehavioral sequelae of HIV infection and research examining the relationship between psychosocial factors and the immune system generally and/or with HIV disease progression specifically (in humans and nonhuman primates).

NIMH's few grants with a social-structural component are all basic research and focus on understanding the role of social relationships and social networks in shaping an individual's HIV risk-related behavior.

COLLABORATIVE PROJECTS

NIAAA, NIDA, and NIMH have collaborated on a number of AIDS research activities. Perhaps most significant are the jointly sponsored multidisciplinary extramural AIDS research centers, first initiated in 1986. Most funding for the centers has come from NIMH, but NIDA contributed some support to three centers from 1986 through 1991. In many instances, individual researchers affiliated with the AIDS research centers also are supported with additional R01s from NIAAA, NIDA, or NIMH. Currently, NIMH is funding five AIDS research centers, each with a different focus, ranging from the basic cellular mechanisms underlying ADC to basic and applied research on HIV risk behaviors.

THE NIH CONTEXT

Total NIH funding increased more than 100 percent between 1983 and 1993 (from $4.3 billion to $10.3 billion). While growth in AIDS research in the same period appears to be explosive by absolute measures, it reflects the requirement to respond rapidly to a new disease with major public health implications. Seven NIH institutes (including NIDA and NIMH) together received the vast majority of AIDS funding during this period: 90 percent of the total AIDS budget for FY 1992 and over 90 percent of the cumulative total since 1983 (Figure S.4).

While NIAAA, NIDA, and NIMH represent a significant portion of the NIH AIDS budget, their funds are distributed quite differently from most of the other institutes. In FY 1992, NIAAA, NIDA, and NIMH together comprised approximately 20 percent of the total NIH AIDS budget (NIAAA was a relatively minor portion of this). According to estimates for FY 1993, the three institutes continued to account for 11 percent of the total NIH budget and 20 percent of the AIDS budget. Yet they funded more than 97 percent of NIH's AIDS-related behavioral research, 64 percent of surveillance, 54 percent of neuroscience and neuropsychiatric research at NIH, and over 30 percent of health services research and research training (as defined by categories used by the Public Health Service). On the other hand, NIAAA, NIDA, and NIMH account for less than one percent of the funding for therapeutic agents and 12 percent of the funding for biomedical research, two categories that together represent nearly 60 percent of the total NIH AIDS budget. It is clear that NIAAA, NIDA, and NIMH play a critical role in the overall NIH AIDS research agenda and in its biobehavioral and behavioral agenda in particular.

After reviewing the content and management of the AIDS research portfolios of the NIAAA, NIDA, and NIMH in Chapter 6, the committee makes several recommendations:

6.1 The committee recommends that NIAAA, NIDA, and NIMH each establish a position for a full-time AIDS coordinator. The coordinator should be provided appropriate re-

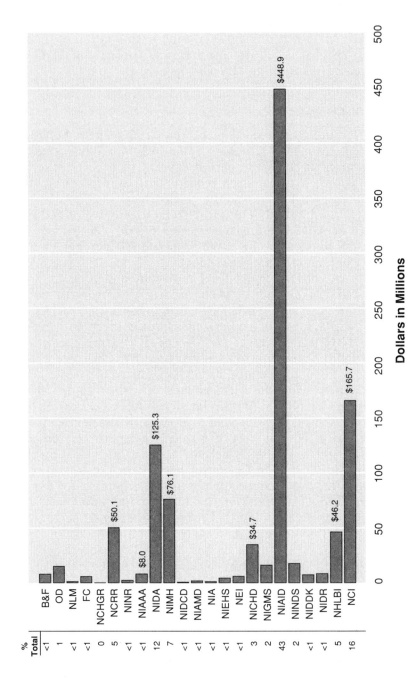

% Total	
<1	B&F
1	OD
<1	NLM
<1	FC
0	NCHGR
5	NCRR
<1	NINR
<1	NIAAA
12	NIDA
7	NIMH
<1	NIDCD
<1	NIAMD
<1	NIA
<1	NIEHS
<1	NEI
3	NICHD
2	NIGMS
43	NIAID
2	NINDS
<1	NIDDK
<1	NIDR
5	NHLBI
16	NCI

Dollars in Millions

FIGURE S.4 NIH AIDS Research Funding by Component, 1992. Source: OAR and Division of Financial Management, NIH.

32

sources to develop and coordinate the institute's AIDS programs in cooperation with division and branch staff. The coordinator also should be linked to the NIH Office of AIDS Research.

6.2 The committee encourages OAR to serve as a catalyst for cross-institute and cross-PHS agency research collaborations through its funding authority and leadership role.

6.3 The committee recommends that the OAR leadership include competence in biomedical, neuroscience, behavioral, and social science perspectives.

6.4 The committee recommends that NIAAA, NIDA, and NIMH ensure the maintenance of the behavioral and social science research programs of the three institutes within the NIH context. The committee supports the recommendation of the National Commission on AIDS (1993b) to expand research in the following behavioral and social science research perspectives: behavioral epidemiology; cognitive science; cultural and ethnographic studies; intervention research; mental health research; behavioral aspects of technological interventions; and organizational studies. The committee adds to that list cost-effectiveness research and evaluation research.

6.5 The committee notes that, of all the types of AIDS research at NIAAA, NIDA, and NIMH, social science research is the most underfunded. The committee therefore recommends that the three institutes develop new initiatives to support research on the role of social, cultural, and structural factors in HIV/AIDS transmission, prevention, and intervention.

6.6 The committee recommends that, given the prominent role of drug injection in HIV transmission and given the considerable evidence that has been assembled over the past several years regarding the efficacy of needle exchange, the U.S. government remove current restrictions barring federal funding for needle exchange programs, promote services-oriented research to help implement such programs where warranted, and evaluate these programs with an eye toward maximizing their preventive impact.

6.7 The committee recommends that drug abuse treatment research at NIDA be continued to support the design and evaluation of innovative and cross-disciplinary drug abuse treatment strategies, including collaborative efforts with SAM-HSA. These strategies should include those targeted to high-risk populations, such as drug-involved offenders, prisoners, women and crack-cocaine users. The committee urges NIDA to pay particular attention to developing treatment strategies for crack-cocaine.

6.8 The committee recommends that NIAAA, NIDA, and NIMH restore support for research demonstration projects, using a mechanism similar to the R18 that facilitates cooperation between the NIH research institute and the relevant PHS services agency or agencies.

6.9 The committee recommends that an effort be made to coordinate between institutes that have overlapping AIDS research programs (for example, HIV and CNS function at NIMH and NINDS) by collaborating in the program development, review, and funding processes.

6.10 Given the disproportionate impact of the epidemic on men, African Americans, and Hispanics/Latinos, it is important to understand the sociocultural-specific factors—including gender, race/ethnicity, and class—that play a role in the behavioral aspects of AIDS. Therefore, the committee recommends that NIAAA, NIDA, and NIMH, with input from appropriate experts, develop a mechanism for collecting and reporting data on the gender, race/ethnicity, and socioeconomic status (class) of study populations in projects supported by the institutes. Such data collection and reporting should be guided by clear articulation of the role of these variables in the epidemic.

LINKAGES BETWEEN RESEARCH AND SERVICES

With respect to AIDS prevention and intervention, research findings must be disseminated to the field as quickly and as effectively as possible. At the same time, service providers often are in a unique position to discover new, researchable questions. How the two worlds of researchers and service providers interact is of great concern to all those involved in AIDS activities and is addressed in Chapter 7. To facilitate the exchange of ideas, federal agencies charged with missions for research and services must overcome differences and develop strategies for effective coordination and communication.

AIDS Programs at SAMHSA

The integration of substance abuse and mental health services into the general health care system is the primary goal of the SAMHSA AIDS office, which was created in 1992 by the ADAMHA Reorganization Act. Currently, SAMHSA has an associate administrator for AIDS who is located in the office of the SAMHSA administrator. The associate administrator works with the three center offices on AIDS. These, too, were established by the ADAMHA reorganization bill, and are responsible for ensuring that HIV/AIDS issues are addressed and integrated into the overall programs of the center.

SAMHSA's total budget (comparable to the ADAMHA services programs' budget before FY 1993) increased from $794.7 million in FY 1988 to a $2.1 billion appropriation in FY 1993. During the same time period, specifically identified AIDS funding decreased from $42.5 million to $28 million (falling from 5 percent of the total budget to 1 percent). To some degree, the small proportion of the SAMHSA budget devoted to AIDS is a legacy of the ADAMHA years, during which the vast majority of AIDS funding at the agency was allocated to research activities (Figure S.5). These research activities are now located at NIH.

As of FY 1994, only four programs are recognized in SAMHSA's formal budget as AIDS-related. Two of these programs—which constitute the bulk of the agency's specific HIV/AIDS funds—are located in CSAT (formerly OTI). These are the Demonstrations and Training Program and the Treatment Improvement Demonstration Program, also known as the Comprehensive Community Treatment Program (CCTP). The CMHS AIDS program includes Training and AIDS Training, which began at NIMH in FY 1990, and a new AIDS Mental Health Services Demonstration Program, which was initiated in FY 1994. CSAP (formerly OSAP) had no AIDS program until FY 1994, when it proposed providing supplements to the Prevention Demonstrations for High Risk Youth Program to fund outreach and risk reduction activities related to HIV/AIDS, including skills building, pre-post HIV test counseling, outreach to resistant populations, and services to those who have lost people to AIDS.

Collaborations Between Research and Services

A major concern about the ADAMHA Reorganization Act of 1992 (see Chapter 5) was how it would effect the relationship

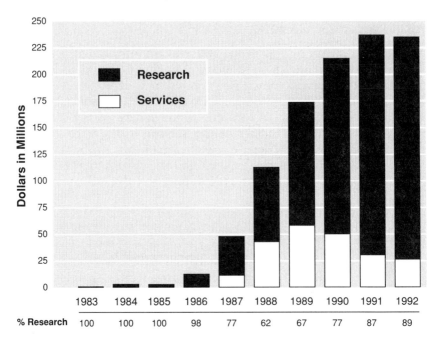

| % Research | 100 | 100 | 100 | 98 | 77 | 62 | 67 | 77 | 87 | 89 |

FIGURE S.5 ADAMHA AIDS Budget Authority, 1983-1992. Note: "Research" includes former ADAMHA research activities currently with NIH (NIAAA, NIDA, NIMH, Office of Director, Buildings and Facilities); "Services" include former ADAMHA services activities currently with SAMHSA. Source: SAMHSA Budget Office.

between research and services, with regard to the rapid, bidirectional transmission of information, that is, the transfer of research findings "from bench to bedside" and observations and concerns from practitioners to the research community. Those concerned about the splitting of the research and services programs of ADAMHA expressed fears that such separation could disrupt the linkages that existed within a single agency and make the process of "technology transfer" more difficult. Those favoring the reorganization argued that separating the programs might well enhance relationships and thus improve linkages.

The problem of a lack of collaboration between research and services communities exists beyond the federal agencies, and is based in great part on different professional cultures. The two salient features of the research culture are the drive for "knowledge for knowledge's sake" and the existence of a reward system based on amount and type of publications. The pursuit of knowledge involves the employment of a scientific method that emphasizes conducting controlled experiments, limiting randomness of outcomes, and producing findings that can be replicated by other scientists.

In contrast, the services world is driven by a desire to provide direct services to as many people as possible. Although the methods of service delivery are planned and evaluated, their internal integrity is often less important than the number of clients served. And while extensive reporting is often required by funding sources, this too is seen as less important to the mission of service providers than actually rendering the services—indeed, it is often seen as a distraction. Furthermore, unlike researchers, service providers are trained to be subjective, to identify with and to advocate for their clients. These fundamental differences in culture and orientation between researchers and service providers result in significant barriers to collaboration.

This situation is experienced at the federal level among agencies charged respectively with supporting research and services programs and is evidenced by the relatively limited collaborations between the AIDS research programs at NIAAA, NIDA, and NIMH and the AIDS services programs of SAMHSA, Centers for Disease Control and Prevention (CDC), and the Health Resources and Services Administration (HRSA), and the broader service-providing community. Even information exchange is limited. For example, each year the three research institutes sponsor many research exchange meetings, including research planning meetings, technical review meetings, workshops, and symposia. However, most of these meetings are designed to bring researchers together and very few reach beyond the research community to include service providers.

All but one (the CMHS demonstrations) of the examples of collaborations between research and services noted in Chapter 7 predate the reorganization of ADAMHA. Moreover, according to institute and agency staff, these collaborations came about as a result of informal communications between individual staff. No formal mechanism existed—or yet exists—to encourage interagency cooperation. Although within ADAMHA there had been tension between the research and services entities, some fear that the organizational separation of those entities will make collaboration even more difficult. In addition to cultural differences, legal and regulatory barriers also hinder collaboration between the institutes now at NIH and the services entities at SAMHSA (as well as HRSA and CDC).

COORDINATION OF AIDS ACTIVITIES WITHIN THE PUBLIC HEALTH SERVICE AND THE DEPARTMENT OF HEALTH AND HUMAN SERVICES

The possibility of collaborative activities between NIAAA, NIDA, and NIMH and SAMHSA, CDC, and HRSA is framed within the larger context of PHS and HHS AIDS activities. Coordination of PHS programs has resided for the past number of years with the National AIDS Program Office (NAPO), and cross-agency coordination has been the function of the Federal Coordinating Committee on AIDS, chaired by PHS. In 1993, however, the Clinton administration elevated the status of federal AIDS coordination to a White House position with the appointment of a National AIDS Policy Coordinator responsible for all federal AIDS policy and program. The activities of the newly titled Office of National AIDS Policy (ONAP) and the structures of organization and coordination within PHS and across federal agencies were still being determined at the time this report was written.

Having reviewed in Chapter 7 the scope of collaborations and exchanges between the AIDS research programs of NIAAA, NIDA, and NIMH and the services programs of SAMHSA and other PHS entities, the committee makes the following recommendations:

7.1 The committee recommends that NIAAA, NIDA, and NIMH ensure adequate follow-up time and money in their AIDS intervention research grants to accelerate information dissemination activities, including technical assistance.

7.2 The committee recommends that formal mechanisms be developed within the NIH institutes and other PHS agencies to foster linkages between AIDS research and services.

7.3 The committee recommends that NIAAA, NIDA, and NIMH sponsor regular research exchange meetings with services agencies and service providers, including local, regional, and national meetings.

7.4 The committee recommends that the Assistant Secretary for Health of HHS and the Director of the Office of National AIDS Policy continue to develop a specific strategic plan for interagency cooperation and coordination among PHS AIDS activities, including an implementation plan.

1

Introduction

Since it appeared in the early 1980s, the acquired immune deficiency syndrome (AIDS) and the human immunodeficiency virus (HIV) that causes it have wrought physical and social devastation around the world. The number of people afflicted by the illness has increased markedly, and the range of communities affected has expanded. In the United States, while AIDS was first considered a "gay" disease because of the predominance of cases among men who had sex with men, the reach of the epidemic now has expanded to intravenous drug users and their sexual partners, heterosexual partners of non-drug-using HIV-infected persons, infants born to mothers infected with HIV, and hemophiliacs and others exposed to blood products or blood transfusion.

The number of AIDS cases reported in the United States has grown rapidly, surpassing 100,000 in 1988, 200,000 in 1990, and 300,000 in 1992. The rate of increase is alarming: the first 100,000 reported cases occurred in an eight-year period, while the second 100,000 cases occurred in only a two-year period. The demographic makeup of the epidemic has seen rapid changes as well. Although men continue to constitute over 85 percent of the adults diagnosed with AIDS, the proportion of women is increasing: from 9 percent among the first 100,000 cases to 15 percent among the third. The proportion of cases among African Americans and Hispanic/Latino Americans has also increased, from 42 percent in

1988 to 48 percent in 1990 (CDC, 1992a). By the end of 1992, AIDS had become the leading cause of death for men aged 25-44 years and the fourth leading cause of death for women in the same age group. By the end of 1993, over 200,000 people in the United States had died of complications related to AIDS (CDC, 1994).

Reported AIDS cases tell only a piece of the story: the prevalence and incidence of HIV infection—the precursor to AIDS—is even more telling. However, truly accurate data are unavailable because not everyone is tested for HIV and not all results from those who are tested are reported. Available data show that the epidemic initially spread rapidly among fairly large, tightly knit, geographically concentrated networks of gay men and injection drug users, but now is expanding outward. Aside from hemophiliacs, the highest seroprevalence rates documented have been among drug users in the New York metropolitan area. As early as 1984, studies reported a rate of infection as high as 50 percent among this group (Marmor et al., 1987). However, alarming HIV seroprevalence rates also have recently been observed among other groups, including female Job Corps students, young gay men, alcoholics in treatment, and psychiatric patients.

Despite extensive efforts to develop effective treatments as well as a vaccine for HIV/AIDS, a fully effective treatment, cure, vaccine or other medical intervention appears to be years away. In conjunction with such developments, efforts to prevent the transmission of HIV through the cessation of behaviors that contribute to it must be expanded. This requires a commitment to understanding and intervening in human behavior.

Much of the AIDS research supported by the institutes under review here (NIAAA, NIDA, and NIMH), is dedicated to developing and implementing (and to a lesser extent, evaluating) HIV prevention interventions within various populations. These interventions should be driven by basic behavioral and social science research on the determinants of behavior and behavior change, and to a great extent they are. Yet much of this basic research is still in its early stages, its development inhibited by a political climate during the first decade of the epidemic that made it difficult, at times impossible, to conduct research on the very behaviors in question: drug use and sex. For example, although numerous scientific and policy reports called for a federally sponsored national survey of sexual behavior to help determine the nature and level of risk for HIV transmission in the general population, federal and congressional restrictions have not allowed it.

The absence of information about the specific sexual behaviors in which people are engaging has hampered AIDS prevention efforts. Now, although the current climate is more supportive of such research, basic behavioral and social science research is having to catch up. Moreover, much-needed efforts to integrate this research with basic biomedical research to obtain a more complete understanding of the complex factors that contribute to the transmission, disease progression, and prevention of HIV/AIDS among different people are still just beginning.

An overview of the extent of knowledge about the range and contexts of sexual and substance-using behaviors by which HIV is transmitted is presented in Chapter 2. Although attempts to conduct large-scale projects on the specific behaviors involved has been hampered, significant contributions to the knowledge base have come from individual studies using the methods of qualitative, social science research and behavioral epidemiology.

As the state of knowledge about the psychological and social determinants of HIV-related behavior improves, it will become increasingly important to investigate how these determinants interact with neurobiological factors to influence the specific behaviors of individuals in social contexts. Even though basic neurobiological, psychological, and social data about the determinants of risk behavior remain to be gathered, behavioral and social science-based AIDS prevention interventions have been developed and employed by NIAAA-, NIDA-, and NIMH-supported researchers, and they are yielding some important findings. Chief among these is the fact that behavior can be changed, even among people perceived as being especially hard to reach, such as injection drug users and homeless and runaway youths. At least, research has found that behavior can be changed for the short term; more research is necessary to determine if behavior change can be maintained over time. Additionally, assessing the relationship between behavior change and actual avoidance of HIV infection is an important component of AIDS prevention research that has been relatively underexplored to date. These issues are the focus of Chapter 3.

While preventing the initial transmission of HIV is the top priority from a public health perspective, it is equally important to develop effective treatment interventions for people who are already infected. This requires knowledge about disease progression and how it might differ among individuals and populations. Although major advances have been made in understanding the basic biological mechanisms of the virus in the body, the issue of how the virus relates to the brain and to behavior is just beginning to be explored. Recent and current research suggests a bidirectional relationship: that is, the virus may affect the brain (e.g., infected cells produce neuropathology, such as dementia) and the brain may in turn effect the virus (e.g., psychosocial coping strategies boost immune system functioning). Unlocking some of the remaining mysteries about the complicated relationship between HIV, the brain, and behavior requires cross-disciplinary research, research at the intersection of biology and behavior. Ultimately, this should lead to the development of appropriate interventions, pharmacologic, psychosocial, and social-structural. These issues are addressed in Chapter 4.

After highlighting some of the significant developments and outstanding gaps in AIDS-related behavior, mental health, and substance abuse research, the report moves in Part II to a discussion of the context in which this research has been supported. Chapter 5 describes the general context within which the NIAAA, NIDA, and NIMH AIDS programs have been operating. The most salient elements of that context are: (1) the recent reorganization of the Alcohol, Drug Abuse, and Mental Health Administration (ADAMHA); (2) the new budget and program authority of the Office of AIDS Research (OAR) at NIH; (3) the budget process; and (4) the grant review process. A discussion of these elements makes evident the level of complexity and uncertainty at the institutes while they were part of ADAMHA and as they were being transferred to NIH.

The committee was asked to assess the balance between biomedical and behavioral AIDS research in the portfolios of NIAAA, NIDA, and NIMH (notwithstanding this fluctuating context). The committee began by examining the programs and priorities for AIDS research as articulated in various planning and reporting documents produced by the institutes. In addition, the committee engaged in a grant-by-grant analysis of the three institutes' AIDS programs. Together, these efforts yielded some interesting findings. In particular, the committee determined that the very act of counterpoising these two categories of "biomedical" and "behavioral" research—while common in health science policy discussions—not only is inadequate for describing the nature of research supported by the institutes, but also undermines the possibilities of advancing the very sort of cross-disciplinary research needed to address the AIDS epidemic. In order to address the spirit of the question, but to more adequately describe the institute programs, the committee developed its own simple scheme for categorizing research approaches, which is presented in Chapter 6.

In the course of its analysis, the committee discovered that cross-disciplinary research that traverses the biomedical-behavioral boundaries to examine the relationships among the brain, behavior, and HIV is underway at NIAAA, NIDA, and NIMH. However, although increased attention is being paid to links between the biological and the psychological aspects of HIV/AIDS on the individual level, very little research has been conducted on the social factors and context in which individuals contract, transmit, and experience the disease. Chapter 6 elucidates this analysis of the balance among research perspectives in the three institutes' portfolios. The management of the AIDS programs of the institutes is also discussed, with respect to specific budgets for AIDS and non-AIDS research and the organizational structure of each institute's AIDS program.

Finally, in Chapter 7, the relationship between the AIDS research programs of NIAAA, NIDA, and NIMH and the services programs formerly at ADAMHA and now at SAMHSA (as well as relevant programs elsewhere in PHS) is discussed. With respect to AIDS prevention and intervention, it is very important to disseminate research findings to the field as quickly and as effectively as possible. At the same time, service providers often are in a unique position to discover new, researchable questions. How these two worlds of researchers and service providers interact—including how the federal agencies responsible for research and service programs coordinate their activities—is of great concern to all those involved.

This report presents both an overview of salient research on mental health, substance abuse, and other behavioral factors associated with AIDS, and an analysis of the context in which that research has taken place. It aims to provide a critical assessment—and an appreciation—of the efforts of the federal research enterprise to respond to and anticipate new directions in an epidemic that has burst quickly upon the scene and has already wreaked havoc on individuals, families, and communities around the world.

PART I

Research Findings and Opportunities

2

Understanding HIV Transmission

This chapter presents an overview of knowledge about the transmission of HIV, focusing on the sexual and substance-using behaviors that have been most implicated in the spread of the disease. Although the general categories of risk behavior are well known, the specific acts responsible for HIV transmission—use of injection drugs and sexual practices, for example—have not been adequately researched or discussed publicly because of their sensitive nature. Yet, in order to develop effective prevention and treatment strategies, it is crucial to understand the specific behaviors involved. A review of knowledge gained to date from biological, epidemiological, psychological, and social research on HIV transmission—much of it supported by NIAAA, NIDA, and NIMH—has helped to elucidate relevant behaviors. However, much remains to be learned. In particular, the prevalence and spread of those behaviors within certain communities is unknown.

SEXUAL TRANSMISSION

In 1992, the World Health Organization estimated that as many as 10 million people around the globe were infected with HIV, and that 40 million would be infected by the end of the century (Eckholm, 1992). Although this estimate is indefinite (for reasons described below), it reflects the general consensus that in the ab-

47

sence of effective intervention, the epidemic will spread vastly and rapidly, primarily through sexual transmission.

As with any sexually transmitted disease (STD), transmission of HIV is highly dependent on the number of sex partners one has and the specific types of sexual practices in which one engages. Sexual intercourse has been and continues to be a very important mechanism of HIV transmission. In particular, anal intercourse carries the highest risk for HIV acquisition, for both receptive and insertive partners. Penile-vaginal intercourse places individuals at next highest risk for HIV transmission, and is followed by oral-genital intercourse. These sexual behaviors can place anyone at risk for HIV, regardless of his or her sexual orientation or gender.

In major studies of prevalent HIV infection among gay men, receptive anal intercourse has been the primary mode of transmission when researchers controlled for other risk factors, including number of sex partners (Winkelstein et al., 1987). Similarly, receptive anal intercourse has been shown to be the primary mode of transmission of HIV among gay men in cohort studies in which seroconversion has been analyzed during follow-up (Kingsley et al., 1987; Winkelstein et al., 1989).

Among people who engage in anal intercourse, a series of cofactors for HIV infection affect transmission. Cofactors include any physical conditions, behavioral practices, or microbiological agents that facilitate the transmission of HIV. Two major categories of cofactors have been investigated: those that might affect acquisition of HIV before or during sexual contact (such as foreplay and other ancillary sexual practices) and those, of a more general nature, that might enhance susceptibility. Cofactors include two major types of ancillary sexual practices: those that are likely to disrupt sensitive tissues in the rectum, thereby facilitating infection, and those that interfere with judgment, thereby rendering sex partners less likely to take precautions against acquiring infection. Under the first group of sexual practices that place individuals at risk are anal intercourse itself, rectal douching, and "fisting." The tissues inside the rectum are highly delicate, and minor tearing of these sensitive membranes is possible during any form of anal intercourse. Even when lubricants are used, vigorous intercourse can cause rectal trauma. Moreover, it is not uncommon for people to insert fingers and dildos into the rectum during sexual activity, which contributes to the potential for trauma. Data from various longitudinal studies have documented that enemas and douching before sexual contact increase the risk of HIV infection during receptive anal intercourse (Kingsley et al., 1987;

Polk et al., 1987). The findings of a large-scale study of risk factors for STD infection in gay men attending five public health clinics for STD treatment were consistent with observations of an association between douching and hepatitis B virus (HBV) infection (Schreeder et al., 1980). Specifically, men who practiced rectal douching in association with receptive anal-genital intercourse were found to be at greater risk for HBV infection. One can logically speculate that if this practice provides both a source of HBV-infectious blood and a point of introduction for HBV infection, the same would be the case for HIV infection. Finally, likelihood for rectal injury exists with "fisting," anal penetration by the fingers or hand into the rectum and possibly into the sigmoid colon (Browning, 1993). As with rectal douching, receptive fisting has been found to be significantly related to HBV infection (Schreeder et al., 1980).

Under the second group of ancillary sexual practices, those that interfere with judgment, are the use of psychoactive drugs such as nitrite inhalants. The nitrites—principally amyl and butyl nitrite—are liquid compounds that were first introduced into medicine more than a century ago for the treatment of angina. They have had other therapeutic uses, as muscle relaxants and vasodilators. The primary effect of these drugs is the relaxation of all smooth muscles in the body, including those in the blood vessels, thus allowing a greater flow of oxygenated blood to the brain (Nickerson, 1975). Amyl and butyl nitrite are quick-acting drugs, taking effect in 15 to 30 seconds, with a duration of two to three minutes. On inhalation, there is a distinct "rush." The recreational popularity of the nitrites results from their reputation as aphrodisiacs (Louria, 1970; Seymour and Smith, 1987). Nitrites—and their association with the sexual activities of homosexual men—have received a great deal of attention, especially with respect to their potential role as a cofactor in Kaposi's sarcoma (Archibald et al., 1992; Haverkos, 1990; Ross and Drew, 1991). However, alcohol and other mood-altering drugs popular among a broader range of people may be just as likely to influence high-risk sexual behaviors, although the evidence of this is mixed (Bolton et al., 1992; Leigh and Stall, 1993).

The biological variables that determine HIV infectivity (the tendency to spread from host to host) and susceptibility (the tendency for a host to become infected) are incompletely understood. HIV has been isolated from the semen of infected men, and it appears that it may be harbored in the cells of pre-ejaculate fluids or sequestered in inflammatory lesions (Fischl et al., 1987). Furthermore, there is evidence that women can harbor HIV in vaginal and cervical secretions in varying concentrations at different phases of the menstrual cycle (Vogt et al., 1986, 1987; Wofsy et al., 1986). Also, there are a number of concurrent or prior infections that represent potential cofactors, particularly those infections associated with sexually transmitted diseases, such as syphilis, gonorrhea, anal and genital warts, and herpes. These cofactors may operate to enhance HIV susceptibility during either anal, vaginal, or oral sex.

A number of studies have suggested that cofactors affect the likelihood of vaginal (heterosexual) transmission of HIV. For example, in one study, despite repeated sexual exposure, an average of only 15 percent of women who were steady partners of HIV-infected men acquired the infection (European Study Group, 1989; Johnson, 1988). These and other studies suggest that the risk of contracting HIV through a single sexual exposure is not particularly high in the great majority of instances (Hearst and Stephen, 1988; Holmberg et al., 1989). However, there is evidence that, although some people remain uninfected after hundreds of episodes of unprotected sex, others have become infected after only one or just a few sexual encounters (Padian, Wiley, and Glass, 1988).

Three groups of factors influencing the probability of acquiring HIV through vaginal contact have been suggested: (1) sexual behavior and risk duration; (2) infectiousness of the HIV-positive partner; and (3) host susceptibility (Johnson and Laga, 1988). Surprisingly, a majority of early studies of heterosexual transmission failed to show a relationship between risk of infection and either the frequency of sexual intercourse or the duration of a relationship with an infected partner (Goedert et al., 1988; Johnson, Petherick, Davidson, et al., 1989; Laga et al., 1988; Peterman et al., 1988). These results were counterintuitive, and may have been the result of measurement error, improper statistical analysis, and the failure to account for other factors. More recent investigations have found that the number of exposures to an infected partner is indeed associated with transmission. Important findings in this regard came from the California Partners' Study, an investigation that surveyed the opposite-sex partners of individuals infected with HIV or diagnosed with AIDS (Padian et al., 1990). Of 150 female partners of infected men recruited for the study during the second half of the 1980s, 48 percent were partners of bisexual men, 15 percent were partners of injection drug users, 23 percent were partners of hemophiliacs, 5 percent were partners of men infected through contaminated blood transfusions, 5 percent were partners of men in multiple risk groups, and 4 percent were partners of men in unidentified risk groups. Of the 85 women who had 0 to 200 sexual contacts with their infected partners, 13 percent were HIV positive; of the 65 women who had 201 to 2,170 sexual contacts with their infected partners, 37 percent were HIV positive.

With regard to the infectiousness of the seropositive partner, a higher rate of infection among the female partners of men in advanced clinical stages of HIV disease has been well documented (Laga et al., 1989). This is probably due to the fact that declining immune function enhances infectivity in an HIV-positive individual, and as such, bodily fluids such as blood and semen contain higher concentrations of HIV. One factor in this regard is a history of sexually transmitted diseases (CDC, 1987).

One of the more comprehensive studies of heterosexual transmission to examine the full range of risk behaviors was conducted by the Italian Study Group on HIV Heterosexual Transmission (Lazzarin et al., 1991). The sample included 368 women whose only potential exposure to HIV was having a male sex partner who was HIV positive, and 27.7 percent of these women were seropositive. The findings of the study documented risk duration, type and frequency of sexual intercourse, the man's infectiousness, and the woman's susceptibility as the key factors. With respect to risk duration, for example, women having a relationship with an infected male for 1 to 5 years had the highest prevalence of seropositivity, and a frequency of sexual intercourse more than twice a week was associated with a twofold increased risk of infection. Seropositive women reported anal intercourse twice as frequently as seronegative women, but condom use had a clear association with reduced rates of heterosexual transmission. In addition, infected women were more frequently those whose partners' disease had progressed to AIDS. Finally, seropositive women also reported histories of syphilis, genital warts, or genital herpes more so than seronegative women.

All of these studies document that, although the transmission of HIV from an infected male to a female partner is not always certain with any amount of exposure, considerable risk is always present. Such risk can increase dramatically depending on the type and frequency of the sexual contacts and the immunological state of the partners.

Female-to-male sexual transmission of HIV is supported by biological plausibility, equal numbers of male and female AIDS cases in African and Asian countries, case reports of males with no risk factors other than heterosexual intercourse, and seroconversion of male sex partners of infected women that occurred while the couples were being studied prospectively. With respect to the biological plausibility of female-to-male transmission, it has been argued that since other sexually transmitted diseases are bidirectional in nature, it is not unreasonable to assume that HIV can spread in the same manner. A number of studies have documented that African and Indian men who have multiple female sex partners or sexual contact with commercial sex workers are at high risk for becoming infected with HIV (Cameron, Plummer, and Simonsen, 1987; Carswell, Lloyd, and Howells, 1989; Clumeck et al., 1985; Kreiss, Koech, and Plummer, 1986). The most persuasive case reports of female-to-male transmission have been those in which (1) the female acquired the infection from a transfusion or organ transplant and her male partner (without other known risk factors) subsequently seroconverted (L'Age-Stehr, Schwarz, and Offermann, 1985) and (2) a sequential chain of male-to-female-to-male transmission was observed (Calabrese and Gopalakrishna, 1986).

Although significant numbers of female-to-male infections have been documented in Africa (Barnett and Blaikie, 1992; Panos Institute, 1988; Shannon, Pyle, and Bashshur, 1991), such a mode of transmission has been reported only infrequently in the United States, and the majority of the more recent case reports have come from investigators in Europe (Beck et al., 1989; European Study Group, 1992; Johnson, Petherick, Davidson, et al., 1989; Lefrere et al., 1988). Several explanations have been offered for the differences in female-to-male transmission rates between the United States and certain countries in Africa. A number of researchers have suggested that the documentation of infrequent heterosexual transmission from women to men in this country may be a function of the history of the epidemic, since the initial phase was largely confined to men who have sex with men and injection drug users, so that during that time the number of infected women was low, and the possibility of female-to-male transmission was small. Because the majority of AIDS cases occurring today reflect infections that were acquired during the early years of the epidemic, most heterosexually acquired infections among men may still be in the asymptomatic or latent stage (Friedland and Klein, 1987; Osmond, 1990). Also, the fact that the infectivity of an HIV carrier increases over time may magnify the effects alluded to above. Following this line of reasoning, it has been argued that virus concentration in genital secretions may also increase over the course of the infection (Burke and Redfield, 1988). Researchers from NIDA recently have argued that the relative frequency of female-to-male transmission has been underestimated (primarily as a result of the way that cases are classified), suggesting that it represents a more significant public health concern than is generally believed (Haverkos and Battjes, 1992).

In sum, although many high-risk practices and cofactors have been observed most predominantly among men who have sex with men, they are not limited to that population. Nor are they the only behaviors linked to sexual risk. As the AIDS epidemic spreads more widely among women and heterosexual men, a broader range of sexual practices must be considered for their potential in transmitting HIV, including the possibility of female-to-female sexual transmission, which has been notably understudied. Although lesbians and bisexual women have been considered to be a low-risk group for contracting and transmitting HIV, the fact that women can transmit STDs such as chlamydia, herpes, and genital warts to one another makes it likely that they could similarly transmit HIV. There is some evidence that among injection drug users, women who have sex with women are at particular risk for HIV (Friedman, Des Jarlais, Deren, et al., 1992; Jose et al., 1993; Reardon et al., 1992).

HIV RISK AND INJECTION DRUG USE

The sharing of hypodermic needles, syringes, and other injection paraphernalia is the most likely route of HIV transmission among intravenous and other injection drug users. When the blood of the previous user is lodged in the needle, the syringe, or some other part of the *works* (drug paraphernalia), that blood serves as the vector for transmission. Levels of risk may vary depending on the particular injection practice, but this has not been well studied. One practice is *skin-popping*—the subcutaneous or intramuscular injection of cocaine, narcotics, and other drugs. Skin-popping (or simply *popping*) is a common method of heroin use by experimenters and novice and casual users who mistakenly believe that addiction cannot occur through this route (Baden, 1975; Kaplan, 1983). Skin-popping also is done by long-term injectors who can no longer find veins into which they can inject.

Another injection method is *booting*, also known as *kicking*, a process that uses a syringe to draw blood from the user's arm, mixes the drawn blood with the drug already taken into the syringe, and injects the blood-drug mixture into the vein. Booting leaves traces of blood in the needle and syringe, thus placing subsequent users of the injection equipment at risk (Inciardi, 1990a). There are three reasons for booting. First, most injectors draw blood into the syringe for the sake of vein registration, that is, to ensure that the needle is properly placed in the vein. Second, many injectors draw large amounts of blood into the syringe, pumping it in and out several times to mix the blood with the drug solution, believing that this practice potentiates a drug's effects. Third, many users wish to test the strength or effect of the drug before injecting the entire amount (Greenfield, Bigelow, and Brooner, 1992).

Jacking is another technique used by drug injectors. It is a practice more common to cocaine injectors than users of other injection drugs. Jacking is staged shooting, in which the user injects a portion of the dissolved cocaine, pulls blood back into the syringe, and waits for the rush to subside. The user then repeats this process with a larger amount of the drug until all of the drug is mixed with blood and injected and no cocaine is left in the syringe (Ouellet et al., 1991).

Although most injection drug users are generally aware of the risks associated with booting, jacking, and needle sharing, they may be less aware of risks associated with other aspects of the injection process. Shared water used in the injection process represents a potential reservoir for disease. Virological studies have indicated that HIV can survive in ordinary tap water for extended periods of time. In a series of experiments conducted at the Laboratory of Tumor Cell Biology at NIH, infectious cell-free virus was recovered from dried material after up to three days at room temperature, and in an aqueous environment virus survived longer than 15 days at room temperature (Resnick et al., 1986). Similar results were found in complementary studies conducted at the Institut Pasteur in Paris (Barre-Sinoussi, Nugeyre, and Chermann, 1985; Martin, McDougal, and Lsokoski, 1985).

Injection drug users require water both to rinse their syringes and to mix with their drugs to liquify them for injection. Rinsing is not done for hygienic purposes, but to make sure a syringe does not become clogged with blood and drug residue, so that it can be used again. Rinse water is often shared. As such, water contaminated through the rinsing of a syringe is used for rinsing other syringes and for mixing the drug. Similarly, spoons, cookers, and cottons—components of the injection kit—also represent potential reservoirs of disease. *Spoons* and *cookers* are the bottle caps, spoons, baby food jars, and other small containers used for mixing the drug, and *cottons* are any materials placed in the spoon to filter out undissolved drug particles. Filtering is considered necessary since undissolved particles tend to clog injection equipment. Spoons and cottons are frequently shared, even by drug users who carry their own syringes, thus increasing the risk of HIV transmission.

Viral contamination may also result from *frontloading* and *backloading*, techniques for distributing a drug solution among a drug-injecting group (Grund et al., 1989, 1990). In frontloading, the drug is transferred from the syringe used for measuring by removing the needle from the receiving syringe and squirting the solution directly into its hub. Common in many *shooting galleries* (places where injection equipment is rented and shared and drugs are injected, discussed below) is the intercontamination of drug doses through the mixing and frontloading of *speedball* (a heroin and cocaine combination). Since heroin is *cooked* (heated in an aqueous solution) during its preparation for injecting, whereas cocaine is not, separate containers are used for the mixing process. Those who share speedball draw the heroin into one syringe and the cocaine into another, remove the needle from the cocaine syringe and discharge the heroin into it through its hub, and return half the speedball mixture back into the syringe that originally contained the heroin. If either syringe contains virus at the start of such an operation, both are likely to contain it afterward (Inciardi and Page, 1991).

The backloading of speedball has also been observed in shooting galleries. Backloading involves essentially the same process, but the plunger, rather than the needle, is removed from the receiving syringe. Backloading has been found to be a risk factor for HIV transmission among injection drug users in New York City (Jose et al., 1993). Frontloading seems to be the preferred mixing/sharing method; backloading is substituted when syringes with detachable needles are unavailable. An alternative method of drug sharing is referred to by some drug injectors as *shooting back and drawing up*. This practice has been observed in instances when every member of the drug-sharing group has a syringe. After the heroin, cocaine, or speedball is thoroughly mixed, it is discharged from the mixing syringe into a common spoon, cap, or container. Each member of the sharing group then draws a specific amount.

All forms of needle sharing tend to occur among *running partners*—drug users who are lovers, good friends, crime partners, or who live together. They serve as lookouts for one another—one watching for police and other intruders while the other purchases, prepares, or injects the drug. Running partners also provide other elements of safety, such as monitoring each other's responses to the drugs in order to prevent overdoses or other acute reactions (Des Jarlais, Friedman, and Strug, 1986).

HIV risk is associated not only with certain drug-using practices, but also with certain locations where drug use occurs. In most urban locales where rates of injection drug use are high, common sites for injecting (and sometimes purchasing) drugs are the neighborhood *shooting galleries*, typically referred to in some settings as *safe houses* or *get-off houses*. After purchasing heroin, cocaine, amphetamines, or other injectable substances in a local drug-selling area, users are faced with three logistical problems: how to get off the street quickly to avoid arrest for possession of drugs, where to obtain a set of works with which to administer the drugs, and where to find a safe place to *get off* (inject and then experience the effects of the drugs). Shooting galleries occupy a functional niche in the world of injection drug use, where for a fee of two or three dollars users can rent an injection kit and relax while getting off. After using a syringe and needle, the user generally returns them to a central storage place in the gallery where they are held until someone else rents them. On many occasions, however, these works are simply passed to another user in the gallery.

Shooting galleries have not been systematically studied. However, based on the observations of a number of investigators combined with reports from a variety of ethnographic and other research studies in drug communities in several parts of the United States (Agar, 1973; Fiddle, 1967; Gould et al., 1974; Hanson et al., 1985; Johnson et al., 1985; Murphy and Waldorf, 1991; Rettig, Torres, and Garrett, 1977), their more obvious roles and characteristics can be described. Reports suggest many similarities from city to city. Most shooting galleries are situated in basements and back rooms, apartments and hotel rooms, and even house trailers in the rundown sections of cities where drug use rates are high. Other galleries are in abandoned buildings, darkened hallways, alleys, and under railroad bridges and highway ramps. Characterized by the stench of urine and littered with trash, human feces, garbage, and discarded injection paraphernalia, shooting galleries are typically unfurnished and extremely unsanitary. Rarely is there heat, running water, or functional plumbing.

Most galleries are run by drug users, drug dealers, or people who are both. Neighborhood heroin and/or cocaine sellers may operate galleries as a service to customers—providing them with a convenient location to inject for a slight charge. More often, however, gallery operators are drug users themselves who provide a service for a small fee or a sample of someone else's drugs.

For the majority of injection drug users, shooting galleries are considered to be the least desirable places to patronize. Most prefer to use their own homes or apartments or those of drug-using friends, since these are considered safer than galleries. Few users truly relish having to pay a fee to use someone else's drug paraphernalia. Some hard-core injectors do consider personal hygiene a priority. For many drug injectors, however, the use of shooting galleries is routine and commonplace. Moreover, there are repeated occasions in the lives of all injection drug users, including the most hygienically fastidious, when galleries become necessary. If they have no works of their own, or if friends or other running partners have no works, then a neighborhood gallery is the only recourse. Similarly, users who purchase drugs far from home also gravitate toward galleries. This tendency is based on the heightened risk of arrest when carrying drugs and drug paraphernalia over long stretches. In addition, for the heroin or cocaine user undergoing withdrawal, going somewhere close by to inject after purchasing drugs is imperative. Moreover, the gallery operator often serves as a middleman between drug user and drug dealer, thus making the get-off house the locus of exchange.

Because of the way that injection equipment is cleaned and distributed in galleries, the potential for coming in contact with an HIV-infected needle and syringe is high (Marmor et al., 1987; Schoenbaum et al., 1989). As the user has paid his or her fee to use the gallery, a needle/syringe is taken from those available on a table or in a container. In some galleries, the user has no choice in the selection of a syringe, but is merely given one by the gallery operator. Regardless of who selects the syringe, the equipment is not usually scrutinized for traces of blood, but rather for dull or clogged needles. Should such an impairment be evident, only then will the user return it for a substitute. Moreover, needles are generally not cleaned prior to use. Shooting up as quickly as possible is of primary importance. After injecting and before returning the needle and syringe to the common container, the user is expected to rinse them—again, not necessarily for the sake of decontamination, but to prevent any drug or blood residue from hardening and causing an obstruction. Sometimes the paraphernalia are indeed rinsed, but with water, which does not deactivate HIV. And sometimes they are rinsed with infected water taken from a container used to rinse other needles.

While systematic research and clinical observation suggest that the use of shooting galleries, the sharing of needles and other drug paraphernalia, and the practices of booting and jacking combine to explain the increasing proportion of injection drug users infected with HIV, little is known about the prevalence of HIV antibodies in needle and syringe combinations utilized by drug injectors. To address this question, samples of needle and syringe combinations from major shooting galleries in Dade County (Miami) Florida were collected and their contents analyzed for the presence of HIV antibodies (Chitwood, McCoy, Inciardi, et al., 1990). All needle and syringe combinations were labeled and visually graded by their condition—"clean" if they contained no visible dirt, stains, or blood; "dirty" if they contained dirt or stains but no visible blood; and "visible blood" if they appeared to contain any liquid or dried blood. Of a total of 212 needle and syringe combinations collected, 62 could not be analyzed for the presence of HIV antibodies because of clogging, broken plungers, or other physical damage, leaving 150 available for laboratory analysis. Of the 150 needles tested, 15 were found to be seropositive—133 were seronegative, and in two cases serostatus was indeterminate. The overall seropositivity rate was 10.1 percent with no significant differences between sites. In addition, although the number of customers frequenting these galleries tended to vary from one day to the next, further analysis demonstrated that there were no apparent changes in seropositivity rates by day of the week. However, a strong relationship was found to exist between the graded condition of needle and syringe combinations and the presence of HIV antibodies. Of the 55 combinations graded as "clean" through visual inspection, only 5.5 percent were found to be seropositive, with a similar rate (4.7 percent) for "dirty" needles and syringes. By contrast, 20 percent of the needle and syringe combinations containing visible blood were found to be HIV positive. This study indicated a clearly significant relationship between the appearance of a needle and syringe and the presence of HIV antibodies. A "clean" needle/syringe had a significantly lesser chance of containing HIV antibodies. Conversely, 1 out of 5 needle/syringe combinations containing visible blood also contained HIV antibodies. Moreover, the data were indicative of the high rate of seropositivity among users of the three shooting galleries selected for this study and the high risk a user has in choosing a needle/syringe containing blood. Thus, it would appear that shooting galleries represent a significant health problem as far as the spread of the HIV infection is concerned.

CRACK COCAINE AND HIV RISK:
THE INTERSECTION OF DRUG USE AND SEXUAL BEHAVIOR

Although the potential for viral transmission is considerable in shooting galleries as a result of the multiple use of injection equipment, exchanges of sex for drugs are not particularly common. They occur, but not with great frequency. By contrast, however, sex-for-drugs exchanges are commonplace in many *crack houses*—places where crack cocaine is sold and smoked.

Crack is a variety of cocaine base, produced by cooking cocaine hydrochloride in boiling water and baking soda. It has been called the "fast-food" variety of cocaine, and is popular in the United States because it is cheap, it is easy to conceal, it vaporizes with practically no odor, and the gratification is swift: a short-lived (up to five minutes) but nevertheless intense, almost sexual euphoria. Smoking cocaine as opposed to snorting it results in more immediate and direct absorption of the drug, producing a quicker and more compelling high, which greatly increases the potential for dependence (Inciardi, 1987, 1992; Wallace, 1991). For many users, once crack is tried it is not long before it becomes a daily habit.

Users typically smoke for as long as they have crack or the means to purchase it—money, personal belongings, sexual services, stolen goods, or other drugs. It is rare that smokers have only a single "hit" of crack. More likely they spend $50 to $500 during a three-or four-day binge, smoking almost constantly. During these cyclical binges, crack users neglect food, sleep, and basic hygiene, severely compromising their physical health. In addition, mouth ulcerations and burned lips and tongues from the hot stems of the pipes are not uncommon, and many smokers have reported and have been observed to have untreated STDs (Inciardi, Tims, and Fletcher, 1993; McCoy and Miles, 1992; Ratner, 1993).

The use of crack first became popular in many inner-city communities in the United States during the mid-1980s, and shortly after the drug was noticed by the media, press and television reports began describing crack use as an "epidemic" and a "plague" that was devastating entire communities (Inciardi, 1987). Considerable focus was placed on how the high addiction liability of the drug instigated users to commit crimes to support their habits, how crack engendered a so-called hypersexuality among users, and how the drug was contributing to the further spread of HIV and AIDS (Gross, 1985; Hackett and Lerner, 1987; Kerr, 1986a,b, 1988; Lawlor, 1986; Lee, 1988; Minebrook, 1989; Morganthau and McKillop, 1986; Raab and Selwyn, 1988; Seligman, 1986; *Time*, 1988).

Since the beginnings of the crack epidemic, the drug has been viewed as a sexual stimulant and enhancer, as well as the cause of excessive sexual behavior in many users. Reports from the field and in the media have indicated that crack is the "ultimate turn-on"; that crack users readily engage in a variety of sexual activities, at any time and under any circumstances, and with an abundance of partners; that crack use has initiated a "new prostitution" and the crack house has become the "new brothel"; and that the numerous rates of sex-for-crack exchanges in some locales are increasing the spread of HIV infection (Chiasson et al., 1991; Fullilove and Fullilove, 1989; Grant, 1988; Greve, 1989; Inciardi, 1989). The association between crack use and apparent excessive sexual behavior has been evident in numerous ethnographic analyses of the crack scene (Ratner, 1993). Indeed, the tendency of crack users to engage in high-frequency sex with numerous, anonymous partners is a feature of crack dependence and crack house life in many locales (Bourgois, 1989; Hamid, 1990; Inciardi, 1992, 1993; Treaster, 1991; Williams, 1992). Much of the sexual activity associated with crack houses occurs in a separate bedroom specifically provided for sexual activities. However, sex acts also occur in the more public smoking rooms as well. Although many street prostitutes who barter sex for money to purchase drugs often insist that their customers use condoms, this is not usually the case with crack house sex. In fact, condoms are rarely seen in crack houses. Given the health status of crack users (including a high likelihood of compromised immune systems), the incidence of STDs (many of which go untreated), and general lack of condom use, many of the conditions that have contributed to the heterosexual transmission of HIV in Africa exist in crack houses in Miami, New York, Philadelphia, and other urban areas across the United States. In addition, given the frequency of sex and the large number of partners associated with crack house sex, the potential for coming into contact with HIV through heterosexual sex is even greater.

To understand this situation, one must consider a few things about cocaine and crack. First, cocaine's (and hence crack's) potent psychic dependence has been well documented (Washton and Gold, 1987). Compulsive users seek the extreme mood elevation, elation, and grandiose feelings of heightened mental and physical prowess induced by the drug. When these sensations begin to wane, a corresponding deep depression is felt, which strongly motivates users to repeat the dose and restore their euphoria. Thus, when chronic users try to stop using crack, they often are plunged into a severe depression from which only the drug can arouse them.

Second, cocaine is problematic as an aphrodisiac, in either its powdered or its base form. Researchers have found considerable differences in sexual responses to the same dosage level of cocaine, depending primarily on the setting of the use and the background experiences of the user. Among male recreational users, cocaine not only helps to prevent premature ejaculation, but at the same time permits prolonged intercourse before orgasm. Among female recreational users, achieving a climax under the influence of cocaine is often quite difficult. For both, however, when an orgasm finally occurs, it is quite intense. Medical accounts generally conclude that because of the disinhibiting effects of cocaine, its use among new users does indeed enhance sexual enjoyment and improve sexual functioning, including more intense orgasms (Grinspoon and Bakalar, 1985; Weiss and Mirin, 1987). These same reports maintain, however, that among long-term addicts, cocaine decreases both sexual desire and sexual performance (MacDonald et al., 1988).

The association between crack and sex appears to be both pharmacological and sociocultural in nature. The pharmacological explanation begins with psychopharmacology: one effect of all forms of cocaine, including crack, is the release of normal inhibitions on behavior, including sexual behavior. The disinhibiting effect of cocaine is markedly stronger than that of depressants such as alcohol, Valium, or heroin. While the latter drugs typically cause a release from worry and an accompanying increase in self-confidence, cocaine typically causes elation and an accompanying gross overestimation of one's capabilities. Moreover, because the effects of cocaine have a rapid onset, so too does the related release of inhibitions.

Often, the association between crack and sex results from the need of female crack addicts to pay for their drugs. This connection has a pharmacological component—crack's rapid onset, extremely short duration of effects, release of inhibitions, and high addiction liability combine to result in compulsive use and in a willingness to obtain the drug through any means. In addition, although overdose is a constant threat, crack use does not pose the kind of physiological limit on the maximum needed (or possible) daily dosage that other drugs do. Whereas the heroin addict typically needs four doses per day, and an alcoholic commonly passes out after reaching a certain stage of intoxication, the heavy crack user typically uses until the supply is gone—be that minutes, hours, or days. The consequent financial burden can be staggering. Other parts of the economic relationship between crack and sex, however, are strictly sociocultural. As in the legal job market, women's access to income in the illegal, street subcultures is typically more limited than men's. Prostitution has been the easiest, most lucrative, and most reliable means for women to finance drug use (Goldstein, 1979).

Because crack makes its users ecstatic and yet is so short-acting, it has an extremely high addiction potential. Use rapidly becomes compulsive use. Crack acquisition thus becomes enormously more important than family, work, social responsibility, health, or personal values. This makes sex-for-crack exchanges psychologically tolerable as an economic necessity. Furthermore, the disinhibiting effects of crack enable users to engage in sexual acts they might not otherwise even consider.

Although the bartering of sex for crack was mentioned in the popular media at the very beginnings of the crack epidemic (Gross, 1985; Lamar, 1986; Lawlor, 1986), the first empirical study of the phenomenon did not appear in the scientific literature until 1989. In that analysis, drawn from a larger study of drug use and street crime among serious delinquents in Miami, the potential for HIV acquisition and transmission through sex-for-crack exchanges was addressed (Inciardi, 1989). Of 100 girls ranging in age from 14 to 17 years, 27 had bartered sex for crack during the one-year period prior to interview. Of these, 11 had traded sex for drugs on fewer than six occasions, but had nevertheless exchanged sex for money on an aggregate of 6,850 occasions.

At about the same time that this research was being reported, several observers began to notice rising rates of syphilis and other STDs among crack users (Bowser, 1989; Fullilove and Fullilove, 1989; Fullilove, Fullilove, Bowser, et al., 1990; Kerr, 1989; Knopf, 1989a,b). Shortly thereafter, sex-for-crack exchanges were targeted for systematic study by CDC and NIDA. However, one of the difficulties in assessing the nature of HIV risks associated with crack use remained the fact that most crack users engage in multiple risk behaviors.

A study of risk factors for HIV infection was conducted at an STD clinic in an area of New York City where the cumulative incidence of AIDS among adults through mid-1990 was 9.1 per 1,000 population and where the use of illicit drugs, including crack smoking, was common (Chiasson et al., 1991). Overall seroprevalence among the 3,084 volunteer subjects was 12 percent, with 80 percent of those reporting risk behaviors associated with HIV infection, including male-to-male sexual contact, intravenous drug use, and heterosexual contact with an injection drug user. The seroprevalence rate in individuals denying these risks was 3.6 percent in men (50 of 1,389) and 4.2 percent in women (22 of 522). Among women, the behaviors associated with infection were prostitution and the use of crack, and among men, a history of syphilis, crack use, and sexual contact with a crack-using sex worker were associated with HIV infection.

The potential for a male in sex-for-crack exchanges to come into contact with an HIV-positive female partner was demonstrated in a study of 87 New York City women who had been admitted to a municipal hospital with a diagnosis of pelvic inflammatory disease (Des Jarlais, Abdul-Quader, and Minkoff, 1991). Crack use was reported by 56 percent of the subjects (n = 49), and of these, 20 percent were HIV positive. Crack use was significantly related to both traditional AIDS risk behaviors (injecting drugs and having sex with an injection drug user) and other unsafe sexual behaviors (exchanging sex for money or drugs and having casual sex partners).

Given the potential for sex-for-crack exchanges to spread HIV to new populations, in 1989 NIDA began supporting ethnographic studies of the phenomenon in eight cities—Chicago, Denver, Los Angeles, Miami, Newark, New York, Philadelphia, and San Francisco (Ratner, 1993). A total of 340 crack users (69 percent of whom were women) were interviewed in depth. Of the 233 women, 108 had participated in sex-for-crack exchanges, as had 69 of the men. HIV testing was done with 168 of the subjects, and a total of 14 percent were found to be positive for HIV antibodies. Of the 24 males who were non-injectors and who had engaged in heterosexual sex-for-crack exchanges, 3 were HIV positive.

ALCOHOL USE AND SEXUAL TRANSMISSION

Only very recently has the possible link between alcohol consumption and risky sexual behavior been explored in the context of HIV transmission. This is somewhat surprising, given that it is a fairly common belief that alcohol use and risky sexual behavior are causally linked. Alcohol is perceived to reduce inhibitions, causing impulsive or out-of-control behavior and thereby increasing the likelihood of risky sexual activity. Nevertheless, despite this widespread—and intuitively appealing—belief, direct *causality* of alcohol use and risky sexual behavior has not been established.

Recent research on the relationship between alcohol and risky sexual behavior has produced contradictory findings. For example, a study of a group of 461 gay and bisexual men in England and Wales found no statistically significant difference in rates of risky sexual behaviors between sexual encounters that involved alcohol use and those that did not. Furthermore, for those men who engaged in sexual behavior while under the influence of alcohol, the quantity of alcohol consumed had no effect on sexual behavior (Weatherburn et al., 1993). Studies of gay men in two cities in Australia found that in Melbourne drinking was not significantly associated with unsafe sex, but in Sydney it was (Leigh and Stall, 1993). Additionally, a study of gay and bisexual men in San Francisco discovered higher rates of risky sexual behavior among men in an outpatient alcohol and drug abuse treatment program than among gay and bisexual men who were not in the program and who were not identified as having a substance abuse problem (Paul, Stall, and Davies, 1993). At the same time, however, a study of 2,174 students in England found that those students who drank more also had higher rates of unsafe sex. The respondents themselves associated alcohol with sexual risk taking, reporting, for example, that when drinking they were more likely to have sex without contraceptives or with someone they know has had many previous sexual partners (McEwan et al., 1992).

In a recent study of HIV seroprevalence rates among heterosexual alcoholics in treatment, researchers in San Francisco found that, after controlling for injection drug use, the rate of HIV infection was 3 percent in men and 4 percent in women (it was 5 percent overall, including injection drug users). People in this study also had a high prevalence of unsafe sexual behaviors (Avins et al., 1994).

The reasons for the mixed results from the studies cited above are not yet understood, but taken together, the studies suggest that it is premature to assume a causal relationship between alcohol use and risky sexual behaviors. Indeed, much of the research to date could be consistent with a number of explanations, including causality, correlation, and coincidence (Leigh and Stall, 1993). The lack of consistent findings may be due in part to the variety of methodologies and measures used in studying the relationship between alcohol and risky behaviors. A great variety of research foci, methods, study populations, variables and measures, sampling and weighting issues, and definitions of "risky sex" and "alcohol use" has negated the possibility of reliable synthesis of research results. Some studies, for example, only compare behavioral extremes, which distorts their generalizability. Other studies are conducted with populations for which the overall patterns of alcohol use or sexual behavior have changed over time. This variability of study design and purpose has made comprehensive synthesis difficult. But it is also complicated by a difference among researchers in the conceptualization of the issue. Some focus on the individual, proposing that the links among alcohol, risky sexual behavior, and HIV may be a result of a certain personality type—that is, one who may be predisposed both to drink and to engage in risky sexual behavior (and thereby put himself or herself at risk of HIV). Others view the link between alcohol and sexual risk as a contextual phenomenon, that is, alcohol may be related to unsafe sex because sexual encounters often begin in drinking establishments or contexts (e.g., parties) where people drink to subconsciously rationalize or facilitate their subsequent risky behavior.

It has been argued elsewhere (Leigh and Stall, 1993) that, given the lack of certainty resulting from research to date on the links between alcohol, risky sexual behavior, and HIV/AIDS, causality need not be established for additional research and public policy efforts to be undertaken. Future research to assess the alcohol-HIV link should include alternative approaches such as correlational studies designed to identify other variables that are relevant (e.g., determining the usefulness of the concept of a risk-taking personality, examining other psychosocial variables). This approach would provide more information on causality by characterizing the nature and relevant weight of the variables involved in risky sexual behaviors. Observational studies of the association of alcohol use and risky sex might determine if there is indeed an association between the two, in which case reducing the levels of substance abuse might lower the levels of risky sex. Finally, using excessive drinking as a marker for risky sexual behavior, even in the absence of any causal relationship between the two behaviors, would provide a useful shorthand for a complex set of social and psychological variables that result in higher risk. For all markers, there is no claim that such characteristics cause risky sexual behaviors, only that the correlation is useful in designing public health and information efforts (Leigh and Stall, 1993; Stall and Leigh, 1994).

Because HIV infection is transmitted by intimate acts, the epidemic spread of the virus through social and sexual networks has illuminated the personal connections that link the disparate parts of the world together. HIV infection occurs because individuals are socially and sexually engaged with each other. These intimate acts take place between specific people, acting in specific places. The central problem in AIDS epidemiology, from the perspective of the social and behavioral sciences, is to describe the connections between individual acts and social settings that lead to the spread of infection. On the basis of the careful delineation of the social structure of viral transmission, scientists can develop targeted strategies for prevention campaigns.

MONITORING THE EPIDEMIC

Epidemic surveillance—numbers of AIDS cases and HIV infection—is an essential first element for delineating the social and geographic structure of the epidemic. Those basic data provide the framework for more detailed analysis of the specific social settings and interpersonal interactions that will promote or contain further spread of infection, and have been useful for estimating the magnitude of the AIDS epidemic. As with all estimates, however, the number of AIDS cases is an imperfect reflection of the magnitude of the epidemic. AIDS cases reflect only the numbers of people with advanced illness. AIDS is characteristic of the end stage of HIV disease, and may follow a period of latency or milder illness lasting, on average, about 10 years. AIDS cases thus reflect the patterns of transmission and infection that occurred at some time in the past. The criteria for AIDS, originally established in 1981, have been altered in 1985, 1987, and 1993 to reflect the information accumulated about the natural history of HIV disease. Finally, AIDS case reporting is incomplete. Although in the United States a vast majority of cases are reported, this is not true in many parts of the world. Despite these limitations, AIDS case reporting has been a central tool for examining the epidemic, and has revealed much about its spread over the past 13 years.

In the United States, the epidemic has disproportionately affected men, who constituted more than 85 percent of the adults diagnosed with AIDS as of December, 1993. Early in the epidemic, the predominance of cases among men who had sex with men gave rise to the stereotype that AIDS was a "gay" disease. However, this stereotype has been challenged as the list of groups at risk for contracting HIV has expanded to include injection drug users, their sexual partners, infants born to mothers infected with HIV and, in very rare cases, those exposed to blood or blood products by occupational activities or transfusion.

AIDS cases have also been disproportionately reported among African Americans and Hispanics/Latinos (Selik, Castro, and Pappaioanou, 1988), and this excess risk for AIDS has increased as the epidemic has progressed. African Americans and Hispanics/Latinos compose approximately 20 percent of the U.S. population. Early in the epidemic, 42 percent of those with AIDS were African American or Hispanic/Latino; by 1993, that proportion had reached 48 percent. The analysis of this excess risk for AIDS has required that researchers develop specific hypotheses regarding the role of race and ethnicity as explanatory factors in HIV infection (Osborne and Feit, 1992). Little support has emerged for biological explanations of excess risk for infection. More support has emerged for social hypotheses that examine race/ethnicity and socioeconomic status as factors in the organization of interpersonal networks within which people have sex or use drugs (Neaigus, Friedman, Curtis et al., 1994; Potterat et al., 1985; Wallace, 1988).

The number of AIDS cases reported in the United States has grown rapidly, surpassing 100,000 in 1988, 200,000 in 1990, and 300,000 in 1992. A comparison of the second 100,000 cases with the first demonstrated some of the trends of the epidemic. For example, while the first set of cases were reported between 1981 and 1988, the second set of cases were reported in the two-year period from 1988 to 1990. There was a larger proportion of cases attributable to heterosexual transmission in the second 100,000 than there was in the first 100,000. The proportion of cases among African American and Hispanics/Latinos increased from 42 percent to 48 percent of cases. Among the first 100,000 people with AIDS, 9 percent were women, while women represented 12 percent of the second 100,000 (CDC, 1992a).

Sixty percent of adults and 53 percent of children diagnosed with AIDS have died. In November 1993, the Centers for Disease Control and Prevention reported that by 1992 HIV infection had become the leading cause of death for men aged 25 to 44 and the fourth leading cause of death for women in this age group. AIDS is the cause of 19.9 percent of deaths among men and 7.3 percent of deaths among women in this age group (Figure 2.1). Factors such as socioeconomic status and access to health care are thought to affect length of survival and quality of life after diagnosis (Curtis and Patrick, 1993).

As AIDS has spread in numbers and through risk groups, it has also spread geographically. From the major urban centers where it was first identified, AIDS was disseminated through hierarchi-

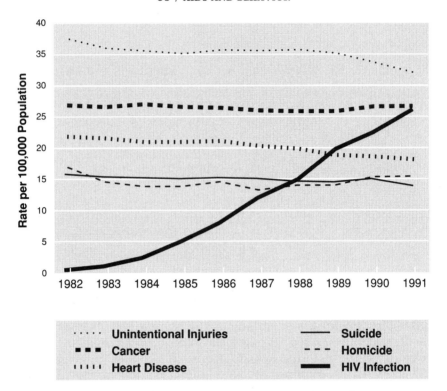

FIGURE 2.1 Death Rates for Leading Causes and HIV Infection for Persons Aged 25-44, 1982-1991. Note: 1991 rates are provisional. Data are from NVSS, NCHS, DVS. Source: National Vital Statistics System, CDC, NCHS.

cal diffusion, spatial contagion, and social diffusion. AIDS spread from major cities to smaller cities connected to them by transportation routes (hierarchical diffusion). AIDS also spread within the commuting field of each of the affected cities, extending outward from local epicenters (spatial contagion). Within a particular area, AIDS has been transmitted within the social and sexual networks of infected people (social diffusion). The characteristics of these networks, including the frequency and density of high-risk intimate interactions among individuals within them, appear to determine the rate and extent of spread both within and between local networks. Networks are placed at risk because individual members of one network may have connections to other networks. This spread of infection into new populations has characterized the AIDS pandemic worldwide.

PREVALENCE AND INCIDENCE OF HIV INFECTION

Measuring HIV prevalence (the number of infections at a point in time) and incidence (the number of new infections over time) is critical for monitoring the course of the epidemic. Descriptions of prevalence and incidence of HIV infection provide a more complete picture of the magnitude of the epidemic than do AIDS case reports, because they do not rely on presentation of end-stage disease. Efforts to determine HIV prevalence have been based on a range of seroprevalence studies—small cross-sectional studies and large-scale surveys. The most difficult challenge in conducting seroprevalence studies is the selection of the sample. Samples drawn from the general population, such as household surveys, will include many at low risk for infection, but few at high risk for infection. Conversely, samples chosen to select those at higher risk cannot be generalized to the population at large. As a partial solution to this problem, surveys have been conducted among high-risk subgroups as well as in the general population. The combined insights provided by this "family of surveys" have guided estimates of seroprevalence.

CDC has conducted seroprevalence surveys of sex workers, drug users (in and out of treatment), patients in STD clinics and sentinel hospitals, childbearing women, and newborn infants. The surveys have been of two types: blinded surveys, in which the serum cannot be connected to the donor, and unblinded surveys, in which people provide consent for their blood to be tested and the results can be linked to the donor. All branches of the military have conducted HIV testing on new recruits as well as enlisted personnel. The Jobs Corps has conducted HIV testing of its applicants. The National Center for Health Statistics has conducted a national household study of seroprevalence. Local studies of the general population have been conducted in Dallas, San Francisco, and Chicago. Studies of special populations, such as psychiatric patients, homeless psychiatric patients, runaway adolescents, and prisoners, have been conducted in localities throughout the United States.

These seroprevalence studies demonstrate that HIV infection spread rapidly through the large, tightly knit, geographically concentrated networks of gay men and injection drug users that occurred in certain cities. The San Francisco Cohort, a study that began in the 1970s as a study of the hepatitis vaccine, was able to document retrospectively that substantial spread of HIV had transpired before the first cases were officially recognized in 1981.

Aside from hemophiliacs, the highest seroprevalence rates have been documented among drug users in the New York metropolitan area: as early as 1984, rates of infection as high as 50 percent were reported in some studies (Marmor et al., 1987). However, alarming HIV seroprevalence rates also have recently been observed among other groups, including female Job Corps students, young gay men, alcoholics in treatment, and psychiatric patients.

While there is some evidence that HIV rates among gay males in some cities have plateaued (San Francisco Department of Public Health, 1994), other trends give cause for alarm. For example, the overall prevalence of HIV among Job Corps students, at 3 per 1,000 is high given their youth (Conway et al., 1993). Among female Job Corps students, the HIV rate rose from 2.1 per 1,000 in 1988 to 4.2 per 1,000 in 1992. The rate among male students decreased during this time from 3.6 to 2.2 per 1,000.

One indicator of trouble is the relapse to unsafe sex by men who had adopted safer practices (Stall et al., 1990; Stall et al., 1992). A second indicator of possible negative future trends is the high rate of unsafe behavior reported by the low-risk population (Catania et al., 1992; Tanfer et al., 1993). In fact, rates of risk behavior may provide a more accurate window to the future than that offered by AIDS case rates or HIV seroprevalence.

With respect to injection drug users, numerous HIV seroprevalence studies have been conducted in many cities around the world, and have generated prevalence estimates ranging from 0 percent to greater than 50 percent of the relevant populations. A number of these cities have seroprevalence rates of 30 percent or higher among drug injectors, and several have seen the rapid spread of HIV among drug injectors soon after the introduction of HIV into the drug-using population (Brown and Beschner, 1993; CDC, 1990, 1993b; Des Jarlais et al., 1989; Des Jarlais, Friedman, Choopanya, et al., 1992; Hahn et al., 1989).

Although most seroprevalence studies have been performed among convenience samples, and most have involved prevalent rather than incident HIV infections, they have generated useful information regarding the levels of HIV infection within these defined population groups. HIV incidence can be an important predictor for the future course of the epidemic. Although some studies have measured incidence among various high-risk groups (including gay men and injection drug users), there is a need for additional data on HIV incidence (Metzger et al., 1993; Moss et al., 1994; Rezza et al., 1990; van Ameijden et al., 1992; Vlahov et al., 1990; Vlahov, 1994). Such data provide insight into the spread of

HIV infection among various populations, and may ultimately provide the basis for intervention programs aimed at curtailing further transmission.

Among injection drug users, in particular, it is also critical to develop effective epidemiologic surveillance mechanisms for identifying new drug injectors within populations, to be able to track trends in drug injection over time. Due in part to difficulties in identifying and gaining access to the population groups initiating or relapsing into drug injection, most of the HIV epidemiologic studies among drug users to date have focused on long-term, chronic injectors. While older injectors have generally had higher documented levels of prevalent HIV infection, the group of younger, new injectors may be at particularly high risk of acquiring and transmitting HIV infection, and thus may be an important group for preventive interventions in the future.

Another population at potentially high risk for HIV infection, but one that has been neglected in the research until very recently, is the seriously mentally ill (Box 2.1). Recent seroprevalence studies among the seriously mentally ill reveal rates of HIV infection higher than the general population. Because risk among this group relates to comorbidity of mental illness, substance abuse, and unprotected sex, the seriously mentally ill are an important population for monitoring concurrent epidemics.

FACTORS INFLUENCING THE EPIDEMIC'S COURSE:
RISKY ACTS, SOCIAL NETWORKS, AND UNSAFE PLACES

As has been noted, HIV infection is spread through specific behaviors, particularly sexual intercourse without barrier protection and the sharing of contaminated drug injection paraphernalia. In order to understand the potential course of the epidemic, social and behavioral research has focused on determining the likelihood that infected individuals in one group will have contact with uninfected individuals in the other; identifying the contexts that influence risk taking; investigating whether people in high- and low-risk groups are adopting recommended preventive behaviors; and examining how the spread of HIV infection will be altered by changing patterns in concurrent epidemics of drug use and infectious diseases.

The risk posed by unprotected sexual intercourse is linked to the probability that the sexual partner is HIV infected. Several studies have examined the risk status of sex partners of people who are neither homosexually active men nor intravenous drug

Box 2.1
HIV Risk Among the Seriously Mentally Ill

It is estimated that 2.8 million Americans suffer from a serious mental illness, yet little is known about their sexual and drug-using behavior, or about the incidence and prevalence of HIV/AIDS among them. A series of recent studies conducted in facilities in New York City show HIV seroprevalence rates among the seriously mentally ill ranging from 4.0 percent to 19.4 percent (Cournos et al., 1991; Sacks et al., 1992; Susser, Valencia, and Conover, 1993; Volavka et al., 1991; Zamperetti et al., 1990). In all cases, these rates are higher than for the general population. These data suggest that people with severe mental illness may constitute a significant high-risk group for HIV infection. Only very recently has the seriously mentally ill population been considered a group of people at risk of contracting or transmitting HIV, even though it is generally assumed that cognitive impairments, problems in judgment, affective instability, and impulsivity increase the likelihood that people will engage in unsafe sexual behavior and drug use (Brady and Carmen, 1990). Indeed, comorbidity of substance abuse and psychiatric illness has been recognized for quite some time (Cournos et al., 1991), and recently the "triple diagnosis" of HIV, substance abuse, and psychiatric disorder has been identified (Batki, 1990a).

With respect to sexual risk, contrary to the longstanding stereotype of the mentally ill population as asexual, recent studies suggest that one-half to two-thirds of seriously mentally ill patients have been sexually active within the previous year, and among those approximately one-half to two-thirds have had more than one sex partner during that time (Cournos et al., 1994; Kalichman et al., 1994). Chronically mentally ill women are more sexually active than are their male counterparts (Lyketsos et al., 1993; Test and Berlin, 1981). Moreover, many mentally ill persons engage in homosexual or bisexual activities, even though they may not identify themselves as homosexual or bisexual (Brady and Carmen, 1990; Cournos et al., 1994; Kalichman et al., 1994). Psychiatric symptoms may impede the ability of these individuals to perceive their own sexual risk for HIV or to employ necessary prevention measures, such as using condoms (Cournos et al., 1991; Cournos et al., 1994; Kalichman et al., 1994).

users. CDC's study of HIV infection in Belle Glade, Florida, interviewed residents of the community at home and in clinic settings. Those with HIV infection were significantly more likely than those who were HIV negative to report a high-risk sex partner (Castro et al., 1988). Castro and colleagues suggested that the lessons of Belle Glade might be relevant to other cities.

Box 2.1 Continued

The seriously mentally ill also are at risk for HIV because of their aggregate high rates of comorbidity with substance abuse. Data from the Epidemiological Catchment Area Survey sponsored by NIMH indicate that the rate of alcohol and drug abuse is 47 percent among schizophrenic patients and 61 percent among patients with bipolar disorder (Grinspoon, 1994). Moreover, substance abuse often is a cofactor in risky sexual behavior among the mentally ill (as well as other populations).

Two recent studies, in New York and Milwaukee, found that a majority of sexually active psychiatric patients used alcohol or drugs in conjunction with sex—more commonly alcohol than other substances (Cournos et al., 1994; Kalichman et al., 1994). Approximately 50 percent of these patients also exchanged sex for money, drugs, or other goods. Women were more likely to sell sex and men were more likely to buy it (Cournos et al., 1994; Kalichman et al., 1994).

While these studies provide important information about HIV risk and prevalence among the seriously mentally ill, they are limited in a number of ways. First, and most obviously, nearly all research has been conducted in one place—New York City—and may not, therefore, be generalizable. The particular demographic characteristics of that city's seriously mentally ill population—for example, the overrepresentation of racial/ethnic minorities—may not be common to the rest of America. Second, except for one study of mentally ill homeless men in a shelter (Susser, Valencia, and Conover, 1993), all research has taken place among psychiatric patients in hospitals or clinics. The population of seriously mentally ill who have not undergone treatment has not been adequately examined. Third, a number of researchers report that relating serostatus to specific risk behaviors among the mentally ill has been made difficult by the fact that hospitals and clinics often do not take sexual and drug-using histories from patients upon arrival (Cournos et al., 1991). Moreover, many inpatients are released without a record of their serostatus, suggesting a lack of testing and reporting of HIV status on their charts (Mahler et al., 1994). HIV testing and reporting among the mentally ill raise significant ethical issues, which undoubtedly contribute to this situation. (For a discussion of some of the ethical issues of testing in this population, see Satriano and Karp, 1993.)

The AIDS in Multiethnic Neighborhoods (AMEN) Study was designed to examine the possibility that similar risky sexual networks existed in an urban setting. The AMEN Study interviewed single adults residing in high-risk neighborhoods adjacent to the Castro district, the AIDS epicenter of San Francisco. Among the 1,573 heterosexually active people who did not inject drugs interviewed in that study, the prevalence of risk behaviors (sex with an HIV-infected person or homosexually active man or injection drug user, unprotected sexual intercourse with more than 4 partners, and having a sexually transmitted disease) was 12 percent overall, with specific race-gender estimates ranging from 5 percent among Hispanic/Latina women to 21 percent among white women (Fullilove et al., 1992). Similar findings were reported from a study of two high-risk neighborhoods in Chicago (Wiebel et al., 1993). The behavioral bridge between low-risk and high-risk populations is the potential pathway for further spread of HIV infection.

That spread may be addressed by examining the interaction between social and individual risk taking. Unstable communities created by war, social upheaval, or social marginalization have been called "risky situations," contexts in which people are predisposed to engage in risky behavior and thus are at greater risk of HIV infection and other diseases (Obbo, 1993; Wallace, 1988; Zwi and Cabral, 1991). For example, sharing of drug injection equipment is concentrated among those who use illicit drugs, particularly heroin, cocaine, and amphetamines. Because of the illegal nature of drug use, drug users are forced to live in hidden subcultures, mostly located in poor communities in urban centers (Drucker, 1991). One such setting is the South Bronx section of New York City. This section of New York was partially destroyed by a program of "planned shrinkage," which curtailed city fire services in the 1970s. A substantial portion of the housing in the area—up to 80 percent of some blocks—was burned down. The social networks of poor people, including those of intravenous drug users, were greatly disrupted by this process. It has been argued that the social disruption of the 1970s, which occurred just as HIV infection was established in that neighborhood, contributed to subsequent high rates of HIV seroprevalence (Wallace, 1988).

A 1990 study of the social setting and kinship networks of women heroin addicts in the Bronx demonstrated the social character of drug use that has evolved in that community (Pivnick et al., 1994). Drug use was rare among the parents of the 126 women studied. However, of the 589 siblings of the subjects, 31 percent were reported to have a history of drug abuse, and 6 percent had a history of alcohol abuse. Drug use patterns were influenced by the drug use of the women's sex partners. In addition, half of the women lived with one or more of their children, supporting a perception of drug use as normative. The drug-using social networks, located in a distressed social setting, create a risky situation in which the likelihood of HIV infection is greatly increased for anyone having unprotected sexual intercourse or using needles for drug injection.

Social settings and networks are also implicated in efforts to reduce HIV risk. In a recent study of injection drug users in Brooklyn, consistent condom use was shown to be a characteristic of social relationships rather than an individual attribute (Friedman et al., 1994). Condom use by an individual varied from relationship to relationship. Relationship characteristics, as well as peer norms, influenced the extent of consistent condom use. Overall, condoms were consistently used in about two-thirds of the relationships between HIV positive injection drug users and their non-drug using partners.

The HIV epidemic is tightly linked to a complex set of diseases whose prevalence in the community will change over time. The progression of the other, concurrent epidemics—infectious disease epidemics such as STDs and behavioral epidemics such as drug use—can be expected to influence either the incidence and prevalence of HIV infection or the course of HIV disease. Several examples may serve to highlight this process.

New drug use epidemics can alter the patterns of needle use or sexual behavior, increasing the prevalence of risk behavior in the community. An increase in the number of people practicing risky behaviors implies an increase in the risk for spread of infection. The crack epidemic has demonstrated the increased spread of HIV infection through the confluence of new epidemics. As discussed earlier, the risk for HIV infection among crack users is thought to be attributable to the widespread practice of risky sex-for-drugs exchanges.

Some diseases will influence the course of HIV disease, rather than the spread of new infections. HIV-infected people are more likely to move rapidly from tuberculosis infection to active tuberculosis disease. The prognosis for tuberculosis in the HIV-infected person appears to be poor and requires early diagnosis and aggressive treatment. Thus, infection with tuberculosis may shorten the course of HIV disease for those dually infected.

CONCLUSION AND RECOMMENDATIONS

CONCLUSION

The AIDS epidemic in the United States, while still predominantly affecting the gay male community, has spread through sexual contact and injection drug use to other communities and populations. Epidemiological and social research have contributed much to an understanding of the primary modes and conditions of HIV transmission, which is important both for charting and for predicting the course of HIV/AIDS and concurrent epidemics of other infectious diseases and drug use. Qualitative research has played a particularly important role in explicating the specific activities, conditions, and meanings of sexual and substance-using behaviors among the people engaged in them. Knowledge of this sort is essential for designing effective prevention and treatment interventions, especially among hard-to-reach populations.

At the same time, serious gaps remain in the information available on the prevalence of behaviors that put people at risk for HIV. Nationally representative data on sexual and substance-using behaviors are still unavailable, so it is impossible to estimate with any accuracy how many people are indeed at risk for HIV infection from any particular behaviors. Nor is it known to what extent individuals engage in multiple risk behaviors. Until these kinds of data exist, it will be difficult to monitor the epidemic and to design and target truly effective HIV interventions.

RECOMMENDATIONS FOR UNDERSTANDING HIV TRANSMISSION

2.1 The committee recommends that a national survey be undertaken to determine the prevalence and correlates of HIV risk-taking behavior. NIAAA, NIDA, and NIMH should collaborate to sponsor such a survey.

2.2 The committee recommends that NIAAA, NIDA, and NIMH support studies of the social, psychological, and biological determinants of HIV risk-taking behavior using a variety of methods complementing the national survey. These studies would allow an understanding of the detailed mechanisms of such behavior, the social dynamics within which they occur, the differing conceptualization and terminology in specific communities, and the role of concurrent health events.

2.3 The committee recommends that NIAAA, NIDA, and NIMH develop studies of the high-risk settings, such as shooting galleries and crack houses, that may contribute to epidemic spread and implement prevention efforts in those settings.

2.4 The committee recommends that NIAAA, NIDA, and NIMH support research that integrates basic biological, epi-

demiological, psychological, and social research to better understand transmission of HIV through sex and drug use.

2.5 The committee recommends that NIAAA, NIDA, and NIMH support research on AIDS risk and behavior change among seriously mentally ill men and women and people with other cognitive impairments, including those not in psychiatric treatment. Such research should be conducted in a range of geographic locations.

2.6 The committee recommends that the Public Health Service coordinate interagency efforts to monitor and respond to concurrent epidemics (such as drug use, violence, and infectious diseases) that will alter the course of the HIV epidemic.

3

Understanding the Determinants of HIV Risk Behavior

Human behavior is determined by multiple factors in individuals and the environment. These factors occur at the micro-level (molecular and biological) and the macro-level (social and environmental) and often interact in mutually reciprocal relationships. The behaviors most closely linked with the epidemiology of AIDS—sexual contact and the injection of addictive drugs—are intense, intimate, and strongly driven. Approaching them requires a cross-disciplinary effort that should include refined knowledge of their neurobiological, psychological, and social bases, and the manners in which they interact.

This chapter presents an overview of findings and gaps in research on the determinants of HIV risk behavior and the application of that research to AIDS preventive interventions. This research constitutes a significant portion of the AIDS programs at NIAAA, NIDA, and NIMH.

NEUROBIOLOGICAL DETERMINANTS OF RISK BEHAVIOR

As reviewed later in this chapter, much has been learned from research on the psychosocial determinants of AIDS-related sexual and drug-using behaviors. However, research on the brain biology of sexuality and drug addiction has rarely been integrated into these studies, even though it may be critical for understanding and preventing high-risk behavior. Even to begin approaching the putative biology of high-risk behavior, including certain sexual behaviors and drug use, requires an expanded basic knowledge base. With respect to sexuality, characterization of sexual dimorphism at the genomic, molecular, cellular, and behavioral levels is still in its early stages. Whether and how it may relate to the drive to engage in specific, high-risk sexual behavior is not known, but it should at least be explored. Similarly, although much has been learned about the biology of substance abuse, further elucidation of molecular and cellular mechanisms underlying addictive behavior may assist in the development of new therapeutic approaches to addiction, which in turn may profoundly alter the AIDS epidemic.

Recent neuroscience investigations have contributed to knowledge about the biology of sexuality. However, to date most research has focused on the sexually dimorphic nature of the brain (e.g., how aspects of synaptic architecture differ in males and females) (Raisman and Field, 1971) and on potential neuroanatomical correlates of homosexuality in men (Gorski et al., 1978; LeVay, 1991). Extensive studies using experimental animals have identified specific pathways and centers in the brain and spinal cord involved in sexual responses among both males and females (Gorski, 1988; Gorski et al., 1978; Johnson, Coirini, Ball, et al., 1989; Johnson, Coirini, McEwen, et al., 1989; McEwen, Luine, and Fischette, 1988; Meisel and Pfaff, 1985; Parsons et al., 1982; Pfaff and Reiner, 1973; Pfaff and Sakuma, 1979; Pfaff and Schwartz-Giblin, 1988; Sar and Stumpf, 1975). Experimental animal studies have provided a rather detailed account of the neural and hormonal bases of a spectrum of sexual behaviors. However, it remains unknown if and how neuroanatomical and genetic factors in sexuality translate into sexual risk behavior.

Indeed, the biology of sexual risk taking is a missing element in basic biomedical and neurobiological AIDS research. Some outstanding issues include: identifying the neurochemical molecular substrates, if any, associated with sexual risk taking; determining how insights from the studies of the neurobiology of sexuality would relate to high-risk sexual behavior and to sexually transmitted diseases, including AIDS; and determining how society might best integrate the study of the biology of sexuality and sexual risk taking into the broader context of sexuality, sexual behavior, and sexually transmitted diseases.

NEUROBIOLOGICAL BASIS OF DRUG-USING BEHAVIOR

Understanding the biological basis of drug addiction is an important link to understanding drug abuse behaviors, and unlike the biology of sexuality has been the object of a great deal of research. (However, it may be less useful in understanding high-risk drug use such as sharing injection equipment.) The possible link between alcohol and high-risk sexual behaviors has also become a subject of more intense research in recent years. The addiction syndrome consists of physical dependence, psychic dependence, and tolerance (Koob and Bloom, 1988). *Physical dependence* is considered to be an adaptive state resulting in profound physiological disturbances upon withdrawal of drug administration. *Psychic dependence* has been associated with the behaviorally reinforcing properties of the drug, resulting in a sense of satisfaction and a drive requiring continued administration to produce pleasure and avoid discomfort (Koob and Bloom, 1988). *Tolerance* is the requirement for progressively higher drug doses for a given effect with chronic use and appears to have a major learned component (Chen, 1979; LeBlanc, Gibbins, and Kalant, 1973; Schuster, Dockens, and Woods, 1966; Siegel, 1976, 1978; Siegel and Sdao-Jarvie, 1986; Wenger et al., 1981). Recent studies on the cellular and molecular basis of dependence and tolerance suggest that the processes are separate and distinct and are mediated by different brain systems (Koob and Bloom, 1988).

Traditional models of addiction suggest that one set of unspecified brain mechanisms mediate the primary, reinforcing, hedonic (pleasure-seeking) aspects of drug abuse and that, with time, a second "adaptive" set of brain mechanisms antagonizes the first, necessitating higher doses to get the same subjective effect. The brain's adaptive response, however, also leads to a physiological reaction if the drug is withdrawn (Collier, 1980; Himmelsbach, 1943; Jaffe and Sharpless, 1968; Martin and Sloan, 1977; Solomon, 1977; Tabakoff and Hoffman, 1988). Contemporary studies are beginning to define the molecular and cellular bases of some of these well-known clinical phenomena.

Identification of opioid peptides (short proteins produced by nerve cells that bind to the same receptors as heroin and other opiate drugs) and mapping of their pathways in the brain have contributed an enormous amount of new data about the biology of opiates, including heroin (Bjorklund and Lindvall, 1984; Bloom, 1983; Khachaturian et al., 1985; Merchenthaler and Maderdrut, 1985). Some of the structures associated with addiction are now being defined at the molecular level. Decades of clinical research on opiate addiction have recently been augmented by the molecular cloning of opioid receptor molecules. There are three major categories of receptors (mu, kappa, and delta), each of which has at least two subtypes. Molecular genetics has begun to separate the various classes and subclasses of opioid receptors, and their structures can be used to identify and perhaps even to deliberately design drugs to further improve the treatment of opiate addiction (IOM, 1994). Cocaine addiction is less well understood than opiate addiction, but here too progress has been dramatic in recent years. It has been apparent for some time, for example, that dopamine-containing neurons are required for the primary reinforcing effects of psychostimulants such as cocaine and amphetamines (Goeders and Smith, 1983; Lyness, Friedle, and Moore, 1979; Roberts, Corcoran, and Fibiger, 1977; Roberts and Koob, 1982; Roberts et al., 1980; Routtenberg, 1972). Details of biologic mechanisms may be illustrated by focusing on cocaine, which, along with heroin, plays a pivotal role in the AIDS epidemic.

Dopaminergic neurons of the ventral tegmentum and their pathways that innervate limbic and frontal cortex are essential for the acute reinforcing actions of cocaine (Goeders and Smith, 1983; Lyness, Friedle, and Moore, 1979; Pickens, Meisch, and Dougherty, 1968; Roberts, Corcoran, and Fibiger, 1977; Roberts and Koob, 1982; Roberts et al., 1980; Routtenberg, 1972; Yokel and Wise, 1975, 1976). Considerable evidence suggests that cocaine acts by inhibiting the reuptake of dopamine by nerve cells (Ritz et al., 1987). That is, dopamine is normally released by one nerve cell and binds to its nearby neighbor. The nerve cell that releases the dopamine also has a molecular pumping system that recovers a fraction of the dopamine released. Cocaine inhibits this molecular pump, thereby increasing the amount of dopamine available to bind to the second nerve cell and also keeping levels high for longer periods. Inhibition of reuptake thus prolongs and intensifies dopamine actions. Inhibition of reuptake has been documented in the limbic nucleus accumbens and produces reinforcing actions. The increased available dopamine appears to elicit reinforcement by specifically stimulating D1 and D2 dopamine receptor subtypes (Koob, Le, and Creese, 1987; Woolverton, 1986). In sum, the specific transmitter (dopamine), the molecular reuptake transporter (the molecular "pump"), and the specific receptors involved (subtyped D1 and D2) have been associated with cocaine addiction. Each of these molecules constitutes a potential target for new therapeutic agents.

The actual anatomical circuits in the brain that participate in the addictive process have been identified in some detail, although the story is not yet complete. Ventral tegmental dopaminergic nerve cells lead to the nucleus accumbens, which in turn projects to the ventral pallidum. Pallidal fibers innervate the pedunculopontine nucleus and dorsal medial thalamus, which are thought to mediate motor activation in experimental animals (Koob and Bloom, 1988). These pathways appear to play critical roles in cocaine-induced arousal-reinforcement.

The neuroanatomic and molecular bases of the withdrawal syndrome are less clearly understood (see Koob and Bloom, 1988, for review). Chronic drug use is presumed to result in compensatory, adaptive responses that antagonize the positive, reinforcing drug actions, but details of this adaptive response are not yet clear. Drug withdrawal presumably leads to the unopposed actions of the antagonistic mechanisms resulting in adverse effects, including malaise, dysphoria, and anhedonia. Additional studies are required to define the biology of the withdrawal syndrome and associated behaviors.

Neuroscience has now presented an opportunity to begin approaching the treatment of addictive drugs, including those used by injection and thus associated with HIV transmission such as heroin and injectable cocaine. Methadone has long been a successful treatment that can prevent injection of opiate drugs. Indeed, one of the principal rationales for developing new antiaddictive medications is the high mortality associated with both opiate and cocaine addiction, to which the risk of AIDS is an important contributor. In 1993, the Food and Drug Administration also approved levo-alpha-acetylmethadol (LAAM) to treat opiate addiction, and several other compounds are in clinical testing (IOM, 1994). The isolation of dopamine transporter and receptor molecules also will provide specific targets for drug development, although it is not yet clear whether or not affecting these molecular pathways will address the craving associated with cocaine addiction, and so an effective medication to combat cocaine may require substantial further advances in basic neuroscience (IOM, 1994). It may be some time before an antiaddictive medication to treat cocaine addiction, similar to methadone and LAAM in effectiveness against opiate addiction, can be found. In the long run, however, the combined efforts of neuroscientists studying the molecular, anatomic, and behavioral aspects of cocaine will very likely produce promising leads with direct treatment implications.

These new molecular insights now allow entirely new approaches to the biology of addiction. The scientific community faces a remarkable opportunity to combine biological and psychosocial approaches to treat addiction, reduce the factors that initially encourage abuse, and help to address a critical mode of HIV transmission. Prevention of transmission through a reduction in drug abuse is a potentially realistic goal best achieved through cross-disciplinary research.

PSYCHOSOCIAL DETERMINANTS OF RISK BEHAVIOR

More than a decade into the AIDS epidemic, efforts to change sex and drug using behaviors to reduce transmission of HIV have met with limited success. Sexual risk taking in the general population assessed in a limited number of studies appears to be substantial, and there is evidence that preventive behaviors have not generally been adopted. For example, a national probability study of the general heterosexual population of the United States found that condom use was low. Only 17 percent of those with multiple sex partners, 12.6 percent of those with risky sex partners, and 10.8 percent of untested transfusion recipients used condoms all the time (Catania et al., 1992). These data also suggest that the U.S. population as a whole has failed to incorporate prevention messages into sexual behavior. In fact, a consistent observation from many studies is that many of those at risk for HIV infection—whether through sex or drug use—do not recognize the danger they face (Brunswick et al., 1993; Klepinger et al., 1993; Kline and Strickler, 1993) and that, even when they do, knowledge alone is not enough to effect behavior change to reduce their risks. Understanding the resistance to as well as the motivation for behavior change is essential for designing effective AIDS prevention interventions. Basic and applied psychological and social research have contributed much to an understanding of the psychosocial and cultural determinants of HIV risk behavior.

PSYCHOSOCIAL PERSPECTIVES ON RISK BEHAVIOR

Theoretical models (primarily psychological) that dominate studies of HIV risk behavior fall into two major groups: those that predict risk behavior and those that predict behavior change. Models that predict risk behavior attempt to identify variables that explain, for example, why some members of a given population perform a given behavior at a given time while others do not (Fishbein et al., 1991). Models that predict behavior change focus on stages through which the individual may proceed while attempting to change behavior (Fishbein et al., 1991). A third set of theoretical issues is raised by the maintenance of safe behavior once such behavior has been initiated.

Early in the HIV/AIDS epidemic the Health Belief Model (Becker, 1974; Maiman and Becker, 1974; Rosenstock, 1974) and the Theory of Reasoned Action (Ajzen and Fishbein, 1977), which had been developed to explain health behaviors, were widely used to identify determinants of HIV risk behavior. The application of these models focuses on perceived susceptibility, perceived benefits, constraints to behavior, and intentions to behave in particular ways, such as using condoms, in the context of HIV risk.

Social Cognitive Learning Theory (Bandura, 1977), which in its early years was used to help people overcome phobias, also has been applied to HIV risk behavior. Its central concepts are those of "modeling" and "efficacy beliefs." Modeling is the process by which people are influenced by observing others. Efficacy beliefs include outcome (or response) efficacy, which is the belief that a given behavior will result in a given outcome (e.g., a belief that wearing a condom will prevent HIV transmission), and self-efficacy, which is the individual's belief that he or she can effectively carry out a desired behavior in a particular setting (e.g., successfully negotiate the use of a condom during a sexual encounter). In recent years self-efficacy has been viewed as the key social cognitive learning variable in predicting risk behavior.

By the mid-1980s most models of behavioral performance included an amalgam of variables from health belief models and social cognitive learning theory. This amalgamated theory tends to assume that individuals who formulate an intention to behave in a particular way and have the skills and self-efficacy beliefs to do so are likely to carry out the intended behavior. Many of the intervention studies reviewed below are influenced by these models and use variables from this amalgamation, especially variables assessing susceptibility, skills, and efficacy.

PSYCHOLOGICAL THEORIES OF BEHAVIOR CHANGE

Behavior change is a process, and as such we need models that can describe the process and identify benchmarks along its way. Stage theories of behavioral change provide researchers with tools for identifying these benchmarks so that interventions can be tailored to the place in the process that a group or community has attained with the goal of advancing them from that place. A successful intervention, therefore, might not result in the elimination of a risk behavior. Instead, a successful intervention is one that advances an individual or group from one stage to another. Two stage models of change have been adapted for use with HIV risk behavior: the AIDS Risk Reduction Model and the Stages of Change Model.

The AIDS Risk Reduction Model (ARRM) (Catania, Kegeles, and Coates, 1990) incorporates elements of the health belief and social cognitive learning models to describe the process through which individuals change their behavior. A goal of this model is to understand why people fail to progress over the change process. ARRM highlights three stages in the change process: Stage One is labeling high-risk behavior as problematic, which incorporates the notion of susceptibility from the health belief models. This involves knowing which sexual activities are associated with HIV transmission, believing that one is personally susceptible to contracting HIV, and believing that having AIDS is undesirable. Stage Two is making a commitment to changing high-risk behaviors, which includes weighing costs and benefits, and evaluating response efficacy, incorporating the efficacy concept from social cognitive learning theory. Stage Three is seeking and enacting solutions, that is, taking steps to actually perform the new behavior and then performing it. This enactment is influenced by social norms and problem-solving options, and it may include seeking help.

The Stages of Change Model (Prochaska, in press; Prochaska and DiClemente, 1983; Prochaska, DiClemente, and Norcross, 1992), formally called the Transtheoretical Model, was developed in the context of psychotherapy and has only recently been applied to HIV risk behavior. The Centers for Disease Control and Prevention, for example, is using the model in its AIDS Community Demonstration Projects, which target hard-to-reach groups at risk for HIV infection (O'Reilly and Higgins, 1991). This model posits four stages of change: *Precontemplation*, in which the individual does not intend to change behavior within the next six months; *Contemplation*, in which the individual intends to change behavior within the next six months; *Preparation*, in which the individual is seriously planning behavior change within the next 30 days, has made some attempt to modify behavior, but has not yet met a specific criterion (such as always using condoms); and *Action*, in which the individual has modified a behavior and met a specific criterion for less than six months. *Maintenance* is used to describe the period in which the individual continues the behavior change beyond six months. Movement through these stages does not always occur in a linear manner. Individuals often must make several attempts at behavior change before they achieve their goals. The efficacy of an intervention program to change behavior requires a good fit between the stage the individual is in and the stage that the intervention targets.

The model specifies ten cognitive, affective, and behavioral strategies and techniques people use as they progress through the stages of change over time. These strategies and techniques include consciousness raising, in which the individual's level of awareness is heightened; self-reevaluation, which is the individual's reappraisal of his or her problem; social reevaluation, which focuses on the impact of a problem on others; self-liberation, which acknowledges the role of choice in behavioral change; social liberation, which involves changes in the environment that lead to more options for the individual; counter-conditioning, which changes the conditional stimuli that control responses; stimulus control, which restructures the environment to reduce the probability of a particular conditional stimulus; contingency management; dramatic relief, as through catharsis; and support relationships (Prochaska and DiClemente, 1983).

An alternative to stage models is Diffusion Theory (Rogers, 1983) which describes the process by which an innovation is communicated through certain channels over time among members of a social system. Diffusion Theory informs interventions that involve entire communities rather than individuals. As such, it takes into account sociocultural influences that might inhibit or encourage particular behaviors, and it has been applied successfully in community-level interventions that will be described later (e.g., Kelly, Winett, Roffman, et al., 1993). One of the key channels for communicating new ideas is through opinion leaders. In any system, there may be innovative opinion leaders whose influence can accelerate the rate at which innovations are adopted through the social system. The interpersonal networks of opinion leaders allow them to disseminate information and to serve as social models whose behavior may be imitated by other members of the system.

Interventions based on Diffusion Theory have focused on the training or persuasion of peer opinion leaders who may or may not be the same as community leaders. Diffusion Theory indirectly addresses sustainability of the intervention; a successful diffusion intervention changes the community such that the new (safer) behavior becomes normative. Additional intervention is not needed once a critical portion of the targeted community has adopted the new behavior.

Stage models of behavior change are helpful in that they provide diagnostic tools for determining where in the behavior change process a given group or community finds itself. For example, given the history of the AIDS epidemic in the United States, gay men as a group may recognize that unprotected sexual intercourse is a behavior that places them or their partners at risk of HIV infection. In contrast, Hispanic/Latina women as a group may not yet recognize this behavior as potentially harmful (Gómez and Marin, 1993). These two groups being at different stages of behavior change would thus require different kinds of interventions.

Despite their conceptual contributions, current theoretical models are limited in their ability to predict risk behavior for two main reasons. First, with respect to sexual behavior, the models are based on the assumption that sexual encounters are regulated by self-formulated plans of action, and that individuals are acting in an intentional and volitional manner when engaging in sexual activity. However, sexual behavior is often impulsive and, at least in part, physiologically motivated. A well-formulated plan of action that is the product of a careful weighing of potential harms and benefits can be dismissed in the context of a passionate sexual encounter when competing proximal goals (i.e., sexual gratification) offset well-informed intentions (i.e., to use a condom).

Second, the dominant theoretical models of behavior do not easily accommodate contextual personal and sociocultural variables such as gender and racial/ethnic culture. Gender roles and cultural values and norms influence the behavior of women and men and the nature of the relationships in which sexual activity occurs. Unsafe sexual practices often are not the result of a deficit of knowledge, motivation, or skill, but instead have meaning within a given personal and sociocultural context. With the exception of Diffusion Theory, which takes gender and culture into account, current theoretical models of HIV risk behavior do not easily accommodate contextual personal and sociocultural variables. A great deal of work remains to be done in this area.

One theory that some think has potential application to understanding the context of HIV risk for women is the Self in Relation Theory of women's development. This theory suggests that the "relational self" is the core of self-structure in women and the basis for growth and development (Miller, 1986). Furthermore, this theory argues, women are basically oriented to others, and as a consequence their relationships and the maintenance of these relationships are highly charged with meaning. When applied to HIV, the Self in Relation Theory would suggest that the risk involved in initiating changes in intimate relationships (i.e., changes related to risk reduction) is greater for women than for men and may undermine women's intentions and their attempts to adopt safer sex behaviors. According to this theory, within women's ascribed roles as unequals, giving to others is a central aspect of women's identity, and sex becomes something that women "give" to men. There is little room for women's realization of their own sexuality (Miller, 1986). Stepping out of the traditional role, as required by safer sex negotiation, therefore potentially places women in direct conflict with men (Miller, 1986).

To date, models designed to explain or predict risk behavior tend to treat the social and environmental variables as independent variables, without considering that they may be interactive or mutually reciprocal. The models also tend to focus only on one level of analysis—the individual—without regard for other levels, such as the culture and community to which an individual belongs.

SOCIAL SCIENCE PERSPECTIVES ON BEHAVIOR AND BEHAVIOR CHANGE

Social science perspectives have only recently been applied broadly to AIDS research (Adam, 1992), but their potential for productively refocusing the investigation of AIDS is evidenced in some of the more recently completed ethnographies, social network analyses, and community outreach interventions and evaluations. Social science research has the capability to reveal the complex and important linkages between social structure and individual behavior and to suggest how specific social changes can inspire individual changes (Friedman, Des Jarlais, and Ward, 1994).

Several social science researchers contend that an overemphasis on behavioral change at the individual level has weakened attempts to reduce the spread of HIV and is in part to blame for the limited success of behavioral interventions to date (Friedman, 1993; Kayal, 1993). Individual behavior occurs in a complex social and cultural context, and analysis that removes that behavior from its broader setting ignores essential determinants. Current theory and research, dominated by psychological models that examine rational factors and cognitive processes that shape the isolated individual's decision-making patterns, have obscured the social and relational factors involved in behavior, such as the role of

peer pressure, emotions, cultural beliefs, and organizational structures of communities at risk (Friedman, 1993; Wermuth, Ham,
and Robbins, 1992).

A number of factors have contributed to the focus on the individual as the unit of analysis in AIDS research. First, some have
argued, prevailing public perceptions of the AIDS epidemic as just
punishment for the immoral and dangerous behaviors practiced
among devalued and stigmatized groups (gays, injection drug users, people with low-income, and racial/ethnic minorities) result
in a "blame the victim" mentality. From this viewpoint AIDS
patients are held personally responsible for contracting the disease (Albert, 1986; Crystal and Schiller, 1993). A distinction is
made in the public eye between "innocent" AIDS victims (infants, hemophiliacs) and "guilty" AIDS victims (gays, injection
drug users). AIDS is thus a disease inextricably bound up with
moral judgments. Unfortunately, such judgments and lack of interest in trying to fully understand the disease and its victims are
not confined to the lay public. Patient reports of hostile and
dismissive treatment by medical personnel are further corrobo-
rated by studies that show physicians' lack of sympathy for AIDS
patients (Sosnowitz and Kovacs, 1992). Second, an individualistic
emphasis is further fueled when the groups hardest hit by the
AIDS epidemic are frequently represented as problem populations
and socially distanced as "not like the rest of us" (NRC, 1993).
Third, because of the representation of AIDS as punishment for
sins and the portrayal of those most affected as outside of normal
society, different standards of success and failure are used to judge
their attempts at behavior change. Individuals are held responsible for the exertion of self-control during sex and drug activities, situations notorious for their uncontrollable and spontane-
ous nature (Schensul and Schensul, 1990). Finally, government
policies predominant during the 1980s were structured to place
responsibility for prevention of the disease at the local level; funds
cut from urban programs, including health programs, did little to
shift primary responsibility for AIDS prevention from the individual to the community or to government. Taken together, it is
not difficult to see why an individualistic focus has prevailed and
why the incorporation of a broader social science perspective on
the spread of HIV has been slow in coming (Adam, 1992).

Several levels of social arrangements can affect behaviors related to the transmission of HIV—ranging from couples to social
networks to the community to society as a whole. Each level of
analysis reveals different factors that shape behavior, and demon-

strates that individual behavior cannot be accurately analyzed apart from the social and cultural structures in which it is embedded.

At the broadest level, social conditions, such as the lack of universal access to health care, racial and ethnic discrimination, unemployment, and lack of public monies to promote AIDS prevention, contribute to a social context in which HIV transmission is prone to occur. For example, the continuing high unemployment rate among African American men (45 percent) fuels the appeal of the illegal drug trade as an alternate means of support, which in turn creates an environment that fosters drug use. Yet unemployment is not often represented as integral to the high rate of injection drug use among African American men and the subsequent transmission of HIV (Schneider, 1992). Similarly, the lack of access to health care among many low-income and racial and ethnic groups means that many cases of HIV infection never reach the attention of the medical community for diagnosis and treatment, thereby ensuring both an underestimation of the AIDS epidemic in certain populations, and its spread to other group members. Unfortunately, then, current health care arrangements make it likely that those populations most affected by HIV are those least likely to receive the preventive care needed to stem its spread. To effect change in the social arrangements at this level requires federal policy initiatives of broad scope as well as changes in the public's prevailing attitudes and mores. Both of these can be influenced by better knowledge about the structures of social life that affect the transmission and prevention of HIV. One important structure in this regard is the social network.

Social Networks

A social network is composed of an individual's relationships in the immediate social world; the number and type of relationships and the degree of closeness among those relationships are part of the structure of that network. Thus, networks are an indicator of social integration—how extensively and how tightly one is woven into the fabric of social life. Social networks are a source of emotional and instrumental support, providing companionship, information, and reference groups. Both the *content* (e.g., friendship, professional) of the interactions in the network and the *form* or structure of the network itself (e.g., close knit or loose; extensive or limited) can affect behavior profoundly. Recent research using network analysis suggests that the social network may be highly amenable to specific intervention efforts.

Contained within one's network is the smallest unit of social interaction, the dyad—or couple—which has been studied in research on relations between sex partners and drug-using partners. However, social influence does not begin and end with a partner; intimate partner relationships, though important, are just one small unit of an individual's larger social network. The scope and character of one's broader social network—the array of contacts upon whom one relies for support, who serve as reference groups, and who establish group standards of conduct (social norms) and sanction behavior—is central to understanding the behavior that puts one at risk for HIV infection (Klovdahl, 1985; Klovdahl et el., 1994; Neaigus et al., 1994). It is at this level that the operation of social norms can best be observed and understood, and where intervention may be feasible. For example, in a study subsequently replicated, peer opinion leaders ("trendsetters") in gay communities in three different cities were identified, recruited, and trained in the active encouragement of safe sex practices among their peers. Pre- and post-intervention measures, while imperfect, showed significant self-reported changes in safer sex practices among the target population (Kelly, St. Lawrence, Stevenson, et al., 1992). This manipulation of the network to reinforce safe sex behaviors was a direct attempt to change the norms of the group to support the practice of safe sex.

Research on the social networks of injection drug users has also yielded some provocative results. These studies directly contradict prevailing views of the injection drug user as socially isolated from all influences other than those of other injection drug users. Negative stereotypes of injection drug users foster the notion that, motivated solely by the overwhelming need to obtain a fix, injection drug users inevitably sever all social ties. However, recent research reveals that injection drug users with AIDS receive instrumental and (less often) emotional support from family members, particularly mothers or other female relatives (Crystal and Schiller, 1993). In addition, a number of male injection drug users engage in sustained relationships with women who do not inject drugs, tying the men (if loosely) to a broader social network not composed exclusively of other drug addicts (Wermuth, Ham, and Robbins, 1992). The extent of such ties with non-injectors is related to the extent of high-risk behavior (Neaigus et al., 1994).

Social network analysis has also been used to examine whether alcohol use among injection drug users increases the likelihood of unsafe sex practices. In one study for example, researchers found that injection drug users who had loose ties to extensive networks were more likely to engage in unsafe sex while using alcohol (Latkin et al., 1993).

Finally, network analysis has also been employed as a technique to better estimate the actual number of AIDS cases in a population. The current reporting system contains weaknesses that result in the underreporting of AIDS cases, including: loss of information forwarded by individual doctors to local health authorities who then pass information on to CDC; delays of two or more months from the time an AIDS death is recorded to the time it is reported to local authorities; and the apparent reluctance of some physicians to report AIDS as the cause of death for married men. By asking a nationally representative sample for the characteristics of people they knew who died of AIDS, researchers in one large-scale study were able to obtain an ostensibly more reliable count of AIDS deaths than would have come from the CDC (Laumann et al., 1993).

Social Norms

Social norms are rules or standards of conduct that are generated and enforced by the members of a group. It is within the context of social networks that norms of behavior can be clearly identified and observed and that peer influences and social pressures upon individuals to engage in seemingly irrational behaviors can be seen in context and become more comprehensible. If the norms specific to HIV-related behaviors are reinforced and sanctioned within social networks, then the hope of behavioral change may reside at this same level.

Drug use, for example, is presented to initiates as a social and romantic act among friends. Introduction to injection drugs is accomplished by an experienced user injecting the novice with the user's needle. Needle sharing is thus represented as an act of trust and friendship in a subculture otherwise characterized by mistrust. Sharing needles is seen as integral to the maintenance of the subculture. Refusal to share needles is seen as implying distance, hostility, and mistrust, something that injection drug users can ill afford to engender in their partners, who are needed for material support (Des Jarlais, Friedman, and Strug, 1986). Promotion of the use of clean needles and the avoidance of sharing needles must be understood in this context.

Similarly, using a condom can be seen as an act of distrust and suspicion, rather than an act of caring, respect, and mutuality. Traditional norms of sexual behavior, supported by gender differentials in power, dictate that women should not initiate discussion of sexual practices or try to change their male partner's sexual behavior. Thus, under these conditions, programs that highlight the importance of open communication between women and their partners in order to promote condom use may be of limited value (Wermuth, Ham, and Robbins, 1992).

Community

Through social networks, individuals are linked to neighborhoods and communities both geographic and cultural. The overlap of disparate sociocultural communities in a single geographic space is a feature of most areas in the United States. Geographic co-location creates important linkages between distinct subgroups, but it does not overcome all factors that create social distance. This fact has implications for the spread of AIDS in local sexual networks. Such networks may be based in a particular social group, but they likely include individuals from other groups as well. For example, strong sexual connections exist between members of drug-using networks and others in the non-drug-using community. As described in Chapter 2, this is a major source of HIV infection; and reaching the non-drug-using partners of injection drug users has constituted one of the most difficult challenges for HIV prevention.

Communities defined culturally often traverse geographic boundaries. In the context of AIDS, the most obvious example is the gay community, whose national political organization was instrumental in the dissemination of critical information and provision of social support and health care to gay men at a time when lethargy characterized the response of the medical community to the spread of HIV among them. The organized gay community succeeded in getting members of the larger gay community to practice safer sex. For example, the Gay Men's Health Crisis (GMHC) created support groups and dispensed needed information about HIV transmission. Thus, social organization and social context were shown to be critical factors in the reduction of risky behaviors (Schneider, 1992). Effective lobbying and media campaigns by groups such as ACT-UP convinced the government and research community to accelerate the distribution of experimental AIDS drugs, prompted the establishment of needle exchanges in many cities, and served to change the nature of public discourse about AIDS, by bringing an informed discussion of the AIDS epidemic "out of the closet."

In addition to the dissemination of essential information about the HIV virus, provision of health care and support services, and changes in government practices regarding access to experimental drugs, other equally important but relatively uninvestigated effects that result from such successful community organization include greater recognition of responsibility for one's behavior and identification with and pride in one's community (Kayal, 1993). Thus, community organization may not only be an efficient conduit for the provision of information to a broader group, but may also serve as an agent of change and a source of inspiration, pride, and identification for individual members.

Cultural Sensitivity

The greatest rate of increase of AIDS cases is among racial and ethnic groups and women—HIV is spreading fastest among African American and Hispanic/Latina heterosexual women and African American and Hispanic/Latino injection drug users (Singer, 1991). It is a commonly held belief that HIV informational campaigns and prevention and treatment services will not be effective unless they are carefully tailored to take into account the beliefs and practices of diverse cultural groups. This is especially so because the behaviors involved in HIV transmission are of such a highly sensitive, private, and potentially controversial nature. Communities differ in such things as their ability to organize, the extent of financial and other resources available to them to support HIV prevention efforts, and other dimensions such as religiosity, literacy, and privacy needs. This means that the skills, resources, personnel, and procedures needed to organize African American and Hispanic/Latino injection drug users may differ markedly from those employed successfully among the predominantly white gay community (Friedman et al., 1992). This leads many to believe that community leaders must be carefully identified and intimately involved, and that members of the target population must be consulted in the formulation and organization of any informational campaign or intervention strategy.

However, others argue that, as important as it is in crafting meaningful community messages and programs, cultural sensitivity itself may be inherently problematic for HIV prevention. As Bayer (1994) points out, modification of those behaviors responsible for HIV transmission often entails endorsement of a political and moral agenda unacceptable to the communities involved. For example, racial/ethnic community leaders in New

York and other cities where needle exchange programs have been proposed protest vehemently against their implementation, contending that the supply of clean needles actively encourages and perpetuates the very drug trade and drug addiction that community leaders are trying to eradicate among the local population. In this instance, observance of cultural sensitivity to one group may prevent implementation of proven HIV reduction measures for another. Balancing concern for cultural sensitivity with concern for HIV prevention is a delicate act.

The issue of cultural sensitivity in HIV prevention is also bound up with a larger social-structural problem affecting the ability to design effective interventions: the problematic dynamics of race and ethnicity in American culture and society. Just as it is important to understand stigma and antipathy against gays and lesbians in the HIV context, it also is important to understand racial and ethnic bigotry and the ways in which these may be institutionalized. Some scholars contend that continued inattention to the legacy of racism in governmental health research, particularly with regard to the infamous Tuskegee study, will necessarily undermine HIV prevention efforts directed to the African American community (Dalton, 1989; Thomas and Quinn, 1991). The deep suspicion engendered by this and other negative experiences, such as CDC's announcement in the early 1980s that AIDS came from Haiti and that Haitians were a high-risk group (Farmer, 1992) and past practices of sterilization of poor, African American, Hispanic/Latina, and Native American women without their knowledge or consent, has fueled the way in which racial/ethnic communities perceive the representation of the HIV epidemic. Until and unless these concerns are directly addressed—at least by open discussion—efforts at HIV related behavioral change in racial/ethnic communities likely will be met with continued resistance.

Women and Gender Dynamics

A growing number of investigators are recognizing that gender differences influence HIV risk factors and barriers to behavior change (Fullilove, Fullilove, Haynes, et al., 1990; Gomez and Marin, 1993; Grinstead et al., 1993; Icovics and Rodin, 1992; Mondanaro, 1990; Schilling, El-Bassel, and Gilbert, 1993; Schneider, 1992; Seidman, Mosher, and Aral, 1992; Solomon et al., 1993; Soskolne, Aral, Magder, et al., 1991; Weinstock et al., 1993). However, these studies have been based on theoretical models that do not provide an explanation for expected and observed gender differences.

It would be useful to explore how theoretical work might help to conceptualize the meaning of gender in HIV risk reduction and potentially improve understanding of the psychosocial context of HIV risk in a gender-specific manner. A gender-specific approach to prevention would take into account the broader social context of women's "permanent inequality" (Miller, 1986) in status and power relative to men, gender differences in psychosocial development, and gender role socialization. Investigating women's risk of HIV within this gender-specific framework is especially relevant because sexual and drug-using behaviors often occur within the context of relationships with men (Amaro, 1993).

Male partners play a critical role in women's initiation and progression of drug use, and in involvement in drug-related criminal activities such as prostitution (Anglin, Hser, and McGlothlin, 1987; Hser, Anglin, and McGlothlin, 1987; Rosenbaum, 1981; Worth and Rodriguez, 1987). For men, introduction and progression in drug use and related criminal activity occurs primarily through a same-sex friend. For women this occurs most often in the context of love or a sexual relationship or friendship with someone of the opposite sex. Thus, for women, addiction is often closely tied to love and sexual relationships with men, which brings a different dynamic into disengaging from drug use.

The impact of the male partner in women's drug use begins at an early age. Research indicates that adolescent girls with a male partner who uses marijuana and/or cocaine are three times more likely to use drugs during pregnancy and six time more likely to use drugs a year after delivery than girls whose partners did not use drugs (Amaro, Zuckerman, and Cabral, 1989). Having a male partner who uses drugs—especially heavier drug use—places girls at risk of drug use themselves (Amaro, Zuckerman, and Cabral, 1989), a finding that is consistent with reports among women addicts (Anglin, Hser, and McGlothlin, 1987) and women alcoholics (Lisansky Gomberg and Lisansky, 1984).

Some suggest that research that places women at the center of analysis should investigate women's efforts to transform sexual relationships, among other topics (Schneider, 1992). Research is needed to understand power relations between women and men and how these play out in the negotiation of safer sex, as well as the role of physical and sexual abuse and its impact on HIV risk reduction. Violence and abuse are a daily reality in the lives of many addicted women and among women with male partners who are addicted (Amaro et al., 1990; Fullilove, Fullilove, Kennedy, et al., 1992); but research is needed to document the extent to which fear of abuse or experience of abuse deter women from discussing condom use with male partners, as well as how women cope with such fear. The work of Gomez and Marin (1993) for example, suggests that fear of the partner's anger in response to requests to use condoms is an important predictor of condom use among Hispanic/Latina women.

Motherhood is another gender-specific issue to consider. Many women in the United States who are HIV positive are both African American or Hispanic/Latina and mothers. It is thus essential to recognize the centrality that motherhood plays in the lives of these women. For many African American and Hispanic/Latina women, the role of mother is the primary pathway to greater social status and respect in their communities. Particularly for those women devalued because of their drug-using status, the role of mother takes on added importance (Wermuth, Ham, and Robbins, 1992). Inconsistent use of birth control and condoms and ambivalence about abortion may contribute to difficult and problematic decision making about pregnancy. Many women are torn between the value placed on children and motherhood and the possibility that the child may be born HIV positive. In addition, many who are taught to place the care of others before their own needs do not take the steps necessary to foster their own well-being, a problem exacerbated by the fact that they are also less likely to have the support of a mate once they become infected with HIV. As a consequence, the support network of HIV-positive women may be more constricted than that of other AIDS patients. Their unfavorable financial position bars them from obtaining the expensive drugs needed to treat AIDS and prevents them from traveling long distances for the limited amount of care that may be available to them. They are also consumed by worry over the care of their children after they die, given that foster care systems are already overwhelmed and given the likelihood that children who are HIV positive may suffer even greater discrimination in placement.

In sum, in the collective effort to prevent HIV infection, strategies employed without an understanding of the social conditions that facilitate HIV infection—such as poverty, discrimination, and inequality between women and men—may ultimately be ineffective. Increasingly, it will be important to investigate the interactions of such social conditions with psychological and neurobiological factors that possibly together influence the behavior of individuals.

INTERVENTIONS TO CHANGE BEHAVIOR

The theoretical models and constructs described above (notwithstanding their limitations) have been applied to the design of preventive interventions and behavior change strategies in an attempt to prevent further transmission of HIV. AIDS preventive intervention research typically focuses on identifying and modifying behaviors—usually those related to drug use and sex—known to be associated with HIV infection and targets both infected and uninfected persons in a range of populations and settings. Although, as noted above, most studies targeted individuals, some recently have begun to focus on the community as the target for intervention, recognizing the importance of socially created norms as determinants of behavior.

AIDS intervention studies employ a range of methodologies. Although experimental studies that randomize subjects into control and experimental groups have been considered to be the "gold standard," most studies do not adhere to this rigid design because of the difficulties associated with maintaining experimental conditions in the settings involved. (For a critique of the randomized controlled trial, see Oakley, 1989.) Rather, simple pre-post comparison studies are the most common means of assessing the effects of prevention programs, and specific changes (such as increased condom use) and mediating variables (such as demonstrated self-efficacy) have been the standard outcome measures for determining whether or not a particular intervention has been successful.

This theoretically based intervention research has identified some significant predictors of changes in sexual and drug-using behaviors among gay men, adolescents, and heterosexual adults, including: perceived social norms or social supports that favor behavior change, self-efficacy, accurate estimation of personal risk, alcohol and other drug-use patterns, HIV serostatus knowledge, and removal of structural barriers (for example, the provision of clean needles through needle exchange programs).

Table 3.1 displays a sample of AIDS preventive intervention studies funded by the institutes discussed in this report. The sample is limited to those studies that are reported in published articles or abstracts from international AIDS meetings. The following discussion, however, also refers to findings from studies funded by other sources as well as intervention studies that may not have been published. Most HIV interventions utilize strategies to reduce either high-risk sexual or drug-using behaviors, although some target both. Additionally, while most interventions focus on the individual, a few have targeted the community as the context in which individual behavioral choices are made.

INDIVIDUAL-FOCUSED INTERVENTIONS

Sexual Behavior

HIV intervention studies targeting sexual behavior have been conducted in a variety of settings for a variety of groups, including men who have sex with men, adolescents, young adults, and heterosexual adult men and women (including drug users). Some researchers have conducted controlled studies on modifying the risk behaviors of men who have sex with men and have shown that interventions focused on individuals and small groups can produce behavior changes, at least in the short term. Some techniques found to be effective in modifying risk behavior include: audiovisual presentation that eroticized safer sex materials (D'Emaro et al., 1988), brief training on how to negotiate safer sex (Valdiserri, Lyter, Leviton, et al., 1989), training on how to reduce stress (Coates et al., 1989), and intensive group counseling (Kelly et al., 1989; Kelly et al., 1990). Group counseling of a brief nature also has resulted in sustained behavior change. In one study, for example, researchers found that one year after the counseling intervention, condom use during insertive anal intercourse had increased at a higher rate among subjects in the experimental group (36 percent at baseline to 80 percent) than among those in the control group (44 percent at baseline to 55 percent) (Valdiserri, Lyter, Leviton, et al., 1989).

Short-term behavior change has been achieved among adolescents as a result of AIDS education, but this varies by sexual experience. For example, studies that have assessed the long-term effects on risk behavior reduction of interventions focusing on high school students have demonstrated that intensive sex education delays the onset of intercourse among high school students who have never had sex. However, among sexually experienced teenagers, even this intense sex education seems to produce no effect in reducing sexual risk taking (Eisen, Zellman, and McAlister, 1990; Howard and McCabe, 1990; Kirby, et al., 1991).

Some adolescents, such as runaway youth, are particularly hard to reach with AIDS behavioral interventions. As part of an effort to reduce HIV risky sexual behaviors among such adolescents, one group of researchers engaged runaway youths in residential shelters in intensive small-group AIDS education and coping skills training combined with individual risk reduction counseling. Fol-

TABLE 3.1 A Sample of AIDS Preventive Intervention Research

Investigator	Title	Institute	Participants
Allen, Serufilira, Bogaerts, Van de Perre, Nsengumuremyi, Lindan, Carael, Wolf, Coates, Hulley (1992)	Confidential HIV testing and condom promotion in Africa: Impact on HIV and gonorrhea rates	NIMH	Women of childbearing age [N = 1,458), outpatient research clinic, Rwanda
Calsyn, Meinecke, Saxon, Stanton (1992)	Risk reduction in sexual behavior: A condom giveaway program in a drug abuse treatment clinic	NIDA	Men attending outpatient drug abuse treatment clinic (N = 103), Seattle, WA
Calsyn, Saxon, Freeman, Whittaker (1992)	Ineffectiveness of AIDS education and HIV antibody testing in reducing high-risk behaviors among injection drug users	NIDA	Female and male IDUs receiving or seeking treatment (N = 313), Seattle, WA
Calsyn, Saxon, Wells, Greenberg (1992)	Longitudinal sexual behavior changes in injecting drug users	NIDA	Female and male IDUs receiving or seeking treatment (N = 313), Seattle, WA
Colon, Robles, Freeman, Matos (1993)	Effects of a HIV risk reduction education program among injection drug users in Puerto Rico	NIDA	Female and male IDUs not in treatment [N = 2,144), San Juan, Puerto Rico

Projects Funded by NIAAA, NIDA, and NIMH

Objective of Intervention	Study Design	Key Findings
To evaluate the impact of HIV testing and counseling on self-reported condom and spermicide use, gonorrhea rates, and HIV seroconversion.	Prospective design (questionnaire; observed STD incidence)	At l-year follow-up, condom use increased, HIV seroconversion and prevalence of gonorrhea decreased.
To determine whether condom availability would increase condom use. Condom-filled jars were placed throughout the clinic (in offices, rest rooms, waiting room, and therapy room).	Pretest-posttest design (questionnaire)	At 4-month follow-up, condom possession increased and use of condoms for vaginal intercourse increased.
To determine effectiveness of AIDS education in reducing high-risk sexual and drug-using behaviors. Random assignment was made to one of three conditions: (1) AIDS education, (2) AIDS education with optional HIV testing, and (3) wait list.	Multiple group, randomized, controlled design (structured interview)	At 4-month follow-up, drug use, needle sharing, and risky sexual behavior decreased among all three groups. Educational effects were absent.
To determine whether injection drug users maintained positive changes in sexual behavior over an 18-month period.	Repeated measures design (structured interview)	At 18-month follow-up, fewer men and women had multiple sex partners. Condom use increased for the men. Women did not report significant increases in condom use.
To measure the effect of adding an educational component to a community outreach program for reducing high-risk drug-using and sexual behaviors among IDUs.	Randomized, controlled design (structured interview)	Although substantial reduction in risk behaviors was measured, there were no significant group differences at 7-month follow-up. Educational enhancement effects were absent.

continued on next page

TABLE 3.1 Continued

Investigator	Title	Institute	Participants
El-Bassel, Schilling (1992)	Fifteen-month follow-up of women methadone patients taught skills to reduce heterosexual HIV transmission	NIDA	Female methadone patients (N = 62), New York City
Feucht, Stephens, Gibbs (1991)	Knowledge about AIDS among intravenous drug users: An evaluation of an education program	NIDA	Female and male IDUs [N = 657], Cleveland, OH
Friedman, Jose, Neaigus, Sufian et al. (1991)	Peer mobilization and widespread condom use by drug injectors	NIDA	Female and male sexually active IDUs (N = 243), New York
Hays, Kegeles, Coates (1993)	Community mobilization promotes safer sex among young gay and bisexual men	NIMH	Young gay and bisexual men (N = 303), Santa Barbara, CA and Eugene, OR
Jemmott, Jemmott (1992)	Increasing condom-use intentions among sexually active black adolescent women	NIMH	Inner-city black female adolescents (N = 109)
Kaplan, O'Keefe (1993)	Let the needles do the talking! Evaluating the New Haven needle exchange	NIDA	Needles used by IDUs in New Haven, CT

Objective of Intervention	Study Design	Key Findings
Follow-up of original study participants (see Schilling) to determine any differences in maintenance of changes in risk behavior.	Follow-up evaluation of randomized, controlled study	At 15-month follow-up, skills training group members were more likely to use condoms and were more comfortable talking about safe sex.
To assess the effect of a one-on-one AIDS educational session, which included a film, a discussion about AIDS risk behaviors and how to change them, and voluntary AIDS testing.	Pretest-posttest design (structured interview)	There were significant increases in AIDS knowledge following the education session.
To evaluate whether mobilizing peer pressure during group meetings, one-on-one counseling, and while distributing condoms, bleach, and other supplies increases condom use among drug injectors.	Pretest-posttest design (structured interview/ ethnography)	Both consistent condom use and the proportion of sexual acts in which a condom was used increased at follow-up.
To develop and evaluate a community intervention to reduce high-risk sexual behaviors. The intervention community received peer outreach, peer-designed safer sex promotional materials, and a workshop. The other community was wait listed.	Sequential stepwise lagged controlled design (mail surveys)	Rates of unprotected anal intercourse decreased at the intervention site while remaining stable at the control site.
To evaluate whether social cognitive theory intervention (Urban League AIDS prevention program) would increase intentions to use condoms. The intervention included factual information, outcome expectancies about condom use, and self-efficacy training.	Pretest-posttest design (questionnaire)	Program participation was associated with increased AIDS knowledge and intentions and self-efficacy to use condoms.
To evaluate the effectiveness of the New Haven Needle Exchange Program for reducing needle sharing and HIV infection.	Mathematical and statistical modeling using data from a syringe tracking and testing system (STT)	Incidence of HIV infection among needle exchange participants was estimated to have decreased by 33 percent as a result of the needle exchange program.

continued on next page

TABLE 3.1 Continued

Investigator	Title	Institute	Participants
Kelly, St. Lawrence, Diaz, Stevenson, Hauth, Brasfield, Kalichman, Smith, Andrew (1991)	HIV risk behavior reduction following intervention with key opinion leaders of population: An experimental analysis	NIMH	Male patrons of gay bars in small U.S. cities (N = 659 surveys), Biloxi, MS, Hattiesburg, MS Monroe, LA
Kelly, St. Lawrence, Hood, Brasfield (1989)	Behavioral intervention to reduce AIDS risk activities	NIMH	Gay men engaging in unsafe sexual practices (N = 104)
Kelly, St. Lawrence, Stevenson, Hauth, Kalichman, Diaz, Brasfield, Koob, Morgan (1992)	Community AIDS/HIV risk reduction: The effects of endorsements by popular people in three cities	NIMH	Male patrons of gay bars in small U.S. cities (N = 1,469 surveys), Biloxi, MS, Hattiesburg, MS, Monroe, LA
Magura, Siddiqi, Shapiro, Grossman, Lipton (1991)	Outcomes of an AIDS prevention program for methadone patients	NIDA	Female and male methadone patients (N = 289), New York City
McCusker, Stoddard, Zapka, Morrison, Zorn, Lewis (1992)	AIDS education for drug abusers: Evaluation of short-term effectiveness	NIDA	Clients of an inpatient drug detoxification program (N = 567), Worcester, MA

Objective of Intervention	Study Design	Key Findings
To evaluate the effectiveness of a community intervention using one experimental city and two control cities. Trained opinion leaders in experimental city delivered AIDS risk reduction intervention to their peers to reduce high-risk sexual behaviors.	Quasi-experimental field study (repeated survey)	Repeated surveys of the men in each city found larger reductions in unprotected anal intercourse in the experimental city.
To evaluate a 12-session group intervention program with AIDS risk education, skills training, and reinforcement for reducing unsafe sexual behavior.	Randomized, controlled design	At 4-month follow-up, AIDS knowledge, sexual assertiveness, and condom use increased, whereas unprotected anal intercourse decreased.
To evaluate effectiveness of a mass-level community intervention in three cities. Trained opinion leaders provided AIDS risk reduction messages to reduce high-risk sexual behaviors.	Sequential stepwise lagged controlled design	Intervention consistently produced systematic reductions in unprotected anal intercourse.
To evaluate effects of a voluntary AIDS prevention program with didactic AIDS education, HIV antibody counseling/testing, and facilitated peer support groups to reduce risky IV drug use and sexual behavior.	Comparative design (self-administered questionnaires)	AIDS education was associated with increased knowledge of AIDS risks and improved attitudes toward condom use. Peer group participation was associated with increased use of condoms.
To compare effects of two AIDS interventions (basic vs. enhanced) on reducing risky drug use and sexual behavior. The basic intervention included two group educational sessions, whereas the enhanced program included one individual and six group sessions.	Multiple group, randomized design	Immediately following intervention, enhanced-group members reported greater self-efficacy; other knowledge and attitudes did not differ by intervention. At 6-month follow-up, enhanced group reduced frequency of injection.

continued on next page

TABLE 3.1 Continued

Investigator	Title	Institute	Participants
Nyamathi, Leake, Flaskerud, Lewis, Bennett (1993)	Outcomes of specialized and traditional AIDS counseling programs for impoverished women of color	NIDA	Impoverished African-American and Latina women (N = 858), Los Angeles, CA
Rhodes, Wolitski, Thornton-Johnson (1992)	An experiential program to reduce AIDS risk among female sex partners of injection-drug users	NIDA	Female sex partners of male IDUs (N = 93), Long Beach, CA
Rolf, Baldwin, Trotter, Alexander et al. (1991)	AIDS prevention for youth of rural Native American tribes	NIAAA	Rural Native American youth (N = 180)
Rotheram-Borus, Koopman, Haignere. Davies (1991)	Reducing HIV sexual risk behaviors among runaway adolescents	NIMH	Runaway female and male youth; mostly African American and Hispanic (N = 145), New York City
Schilling, El-Bassel. Schinke, Gordon, Nichols (1991)	Building skills of recovering women drug users to reduce heterosexual AIDS transmission	NIDA	Female methadone patients (N = 91), New York City
Stephens, Feucht, Roman (1991)	Effects of an intervention program on AIDS-related drug and needle behavior among intravenous drug users	NIDA	Female and male IDUs (N = 322), Cleveland, OH

Objective of Intervention	Study Design	Key Findings
To compare differential effects of two AIDS education programs for reducing risky drug use and sexual behavior. The standard intervention lasted one hour. A specialized two-hour intervention was individualized to the expressed concerns of the women.	Pretest-posttest comparative design	There were significant improvements for both interventions. The specialized program was not more effective than the standard one.
Education and counseling to motivate personal risk reduction, provide participants with cognitive and behavioral skills, and enhance participants' ability to make positive changes in their lives.	Pretest-posttest design	Ninety-one percent of program participants reported positive behavioral changes; 98 percent reported a greater sense of control.
Multi-component, community outreach program conducted in school, focusing on HIV/AIDS and alcohol and other drug abuse. Intention was to change high-risk sexual and drug-using behaviors and local norms of attitudes and behaviors.	Quasi-experimental design (surveys)	Data from pilot studies of two schools indicate that intervention increased knowledge about AIDS and alcohol and other drugs, and intentions to reduce high-risk behaviors.
Intensive intervention to provide risk education about HIV/AIDS, training in coping skills for high-risk situations, counseling to address individual barriers to safer sex and access to health care and other services.	Non-randomized controlled design	At 3- and 6-month follow-ups, consistent condom use increased and reports of high-risk sexual behavior decreased among youth receiving intervention.
To compare information-only control group and skills-building intervention group for reducing high-risk sexual behavior and increasing condom use.	Multiple group, randomized design (structured interview)	Skills-building intervention was associated with increased condom use and comfort with discussion of sexual issues. Intervention had no impact on drug use.
To evaluate the impact of an AIDS educational intervention for reducing HIV risk behaviors. The intervention included individual risk reduction counseling. Each participant received condoms, bleach, and brochures.	Quasi-experimental pretest-posttest design (interviews)	Intravenous drug use and syringe sharing decreased. Effects of intervention endured for up to one year.

continued on next page

TABLE 3.1 Continued

Investigator	Title	Institute	Participants
Walter, Vaughan (1993)	AIDS risk reduction among a multiethnic sample of urban high school students	NIMH	Female and male high school students (N = 1,316), four New York City schools
Watters, Estilo, Clark, Lorvick (1994)	Syringe and needle exchange as HIV/AIDS prevention for injection drug users	NIDA	Female and male IDUs (N = 5,644), San Francisco, CA
Wiebel, Jimenez, Johnson, Ouellet et al. (1993)	Positive effect on HIV seroconversion of street outreach intervention with IDUs in Chicago: 1988-1992	NIDA	IDUs not in drug treatment (N = 641), Chicago, IL

lowing up both three and six months later, researchers found a higher increase in condom use and safer sex among those who attended the intervention site than among those at the control site (Rotheram-Borus et al., 1991). The long-term efficacy of this shelter-based intervention is yet to be assessed; however, the results of this study suggest that, at least on a short-term basis, adolescents with multiple risks in their lives, including vulnerability for HIV infection, can modify their sexual risk taking.

Most HIV prevention efforts targeting sexual behavior among young adults have focused on college students. Of those efforts, none on record has demonstrated measurable behavioral change as an outcome. These prevention programs have spanned a great variety of interventions, from a single audiovisual presentation of AIDS information (Gilliam and Seltzer, 1989; Rhodes and Wolitski, 1989), to a human reproduction course covering AIDS (Gerrard and Reis, 1989), to a full semester course specifically on AIDS

Objective of Intervention	Study Design	Key Findings
To evaluate effectiveness of a teacher-delivered curriculum geared toward increasing knowledge about AIDS, increasing self-efficacy related to AIDS-prevention, and reducing AIDS risk behaviors. Control groups received no formal AIDS education.	Experimental field study (surveys)	At 3-month follow-up, modest favorable effects of the intervention were observed: increases in knowledge, beliefs, and self-efficacy, and reductions in risky sexual behavior.
To evaluate the effects of an all-volunteer syringe exchange program on risky injection drug use. Community outreach workers provided AIDS education, bleach, and referral to drug treatment.	Serial, cross-sectional design (surveys)	The intervention resulted in increased condom use, use of bleach to clean needles, and decreased syringe sharing.
To evaluate the effectiveness of street outreach for out-of-treatment drug users on drug-using behavior and HIV seroconversion.	Prospective design	Intervention reduced HIV seroconversion and sharing of unsterile injection equipment. Sexual risks were somewhat resistant to the intervention.

(Abramson, Sekler, and Cloud, 1989), to a week-long AIDS awareness program for the whole campus (Dommeyer et al., 1989). Of all these programs stressing education and awareness, only one examined the behavioral outcomes of its intervention (Abramson, Sekler, and Cloud, 1989). Moreover, that study, which found an increase in carrying and using condoms following a semester-long intervention, also reported a high attrition rate (37 percent of experimental subjects, 69 percent in the control group), so it is possible that the behavior change may not be attributable to the intervention.

University students in three skills training programs demonstrated improved skill in negotiating safer sex and in developing positive attitudes toward condoms, at least in the short term (Franzini et al., 1990; Kyes, 1990; Tanner and Pollack, 1988). However, it is not known how these improved skills and attitudes will affect sexual risk-taking behavior over time. Design of these programs varied. One randomized study compared an experimental group that participated both in an AIDS education lecture and in a three-session sexual assertiveness training course with a control group that only received the AIDS education lecture (Franzini et al., 1990). Two other studies eroticized safer sex messages in order to change attitudes toward condom use (Kyes, 1990; Tanner and Pollack, 1988). Because they did not assess long-term behavior change, no resulting behavior change can be attributed to the interventions.

Studies designed for adult heterosexual women and men have reported short-term behavior change as a result of interventions. In one study, four 90-minute skills training sessions combined with two follow-ups were given to patients at an urban primary health care clinic (Kelly et al., in press). After three months, researchers found a higher rate of condom use among experimental subjects relative to control subjects. In another study, in this case, among blood donors, the number of men and women who practiced unsafe sex was reduced by an intervention consisting of HIV status notification and post-notification counseling (Cleary et al., 1991).

Prospective cohort studies that focus on couples with discordant HIV status (one partner seronegative and the other seropositive) have in some cases demonstrated long-term program effectiveness. A study in Zaire involving intensive couples counseling after notification of HIV test results found that condom use had increased dramatically—from less than 5 percent at baseline to 71 percent after one month. After 18 months, 77 percent of the couples reported still using condoms during all sexual encounters. The rate of HIV seroconversion during the follow-up was 3 per 100 person-years (Kamenga et al., 1991). A study in Rwanda that offered HIV antibody posttest counseling combined with AIDS education group counseling to cohabiting discordant couples produced similar results: condom use increased from 3 percent at baseline to 57 percent at follow-up one year later; the rate of HIV seroconversion was 4 per 100 person-years among men and 9 per 100 person-years among women during follow-up (Allen, Tice, and Van de Perre, et al. 1992).

The efficacy of HIV counseling and testing among commercial sex workers has been evaluated in a few studies (Corby, Barchi, and Wolitski, 1990; Ngugi et al., 1988; Papaevangelou et al., 1988). In one prospective study, condom use increased among female sex workers in Kenya who received HIV counseling, testing, and AIDS education relative to those who did not (Ngugi et al., 1988). A subsequent evaluation of the program estimated that such health education interventions could prevent between 6,000 and 10,000 new HIV infections annually (Moses et al., 1991).

All of the studies targeting sexual behavior and condom use have focused on the acceptance and regular use of male condoms. However, there may be woman-controlled methods of sexual risk reduction that may be more appropriate or useful in some instances. As illustrated in Box 3.1, the new "female condom" has potential in this regard, but data on its acceptability and efficacy are still preliminary.

Injection Drug Use

Some prospective studies report that methadone maintenance treatment may prevent the spread of HIV. The treatment itself has been found to have a significant impact both on decreasing the use of injection drugs (Ball et al., 1988) and on HIV seroconversion (Metzger et al., 1993; Moss et al., 1994). Moss et al. (1994) found that those who stayed in methadone maintenance for one or more years had lower HIV seroconversion rates (1 percent) than those who had been in the program for less than one year (3.8 percent). Yancovitz et al. (1991) found in their experimental study that among patients waiting for comprehensive methadone maintenance treatment, far fewer in the experimental group injected heroin (63 percent at intake to 29 percent at one-month follow-up) than those in the control group (62 percent to 60 percent). However, it has not been determined that limited services to injection drug users will have lasting effects on modifying such AIDS-related risk behaviors as needle sharing and unsafe sex.

Researchers have found mixed results from controlled clinical trials of individual and group counseling that provide skills training for people who inject drugs. Some studies found skills training to be effective in changing behavior in certain areas: use of condoms had increased at 2-week follow-up in one study (Schilling, El-Bassel, Schinke, et al., 1991) and drug injection had decreased at 6-month follow-up in two others (Des Jarlais, Casriel, Friedman, et al., 1992; McCusker et al., 1992). However, other studies demonstrated no measurable risk reduction as a result of skills training (Colon et al., 1992; Sorensen et al., in press), brief AIDS information counseling (Calsyn, Saxon, Freeman, et al., 1992; Dengelegi, Weber, and Torquato, 1990; Gibson et al., 1991), and HIV counseling and testing (Gibson, Young, and Lovelle-Drache, 1993). Because in these studies control group subjects modified their be-

Box 3.1 The Female Condom

An estimated 3 million women worldwide have HIV infection, and AIDS has become the leading cause of death among women between the ages of 20 and 40 years in major cities throughout sub-Saharan Africa, Western Europe, and the Americas (Chin, 1990; Hankins and Handley, 1992). In the United States, women still represent a small percentage of all AIDS cases; however, their proportion is growing (CDC, 1993a). While the sharing of injection equipment had been the primary risk factor for HIV infection among women in the United States, current epidemiologic data indicate that sexual activity has now surpassed needle sharing as the leading risk factor for AIDS among women. There are indications that many of the traditional HIV prevention and intervention programs have not had a major impact in reducing high-risk sexual behavior among women (Sorensen et al., 1991; Weissman and National AIDS Research Consortium, 1991). To date, the most common and effective risk reduction method is condom use. But many woman at risk report not using them, a situation resulting from a variety of factors, including socioeconomic circumstances, sex roles in the street drug culture, and fear that mistrust, rejection, and even violence will result if they suggest that their partners use condoms (Padian, 1988; Schilling, El-Bassel, Gilbert, et al., 1991; Valdiserri, Arena, Proctor, et al., 1989).

There are few woman-controlled methods of sexual risk reduction, and what is available is not effective in preventing HIV infection. For example, both the effectiveness and the side effects of spermicides have raised questions about their feasibility as an HIV risk reduction technique (Stein, 1992). Sponges and diaphragms are promoted as HIV risk reduction mechanisms because they reduce the incidence of sexually transmitted diseases (Rosenberg and Gollub, 1992), but neither has actually been tested to determine whether it reduces risk of HIV infection.

However, a new device called the "female condom," may potentially address this need. The first female condom, made of rubber with a steel coil rim, was introduced in the 1920s (British Journal of Family Planning, 1992). It was not until the late 1980s, however, that a more acceptable device was developed—the Femidom™ female condom, which has been commercially available in the United Kingdom since September 1992 and received FDA approval in the United States in 1993. In the United States, the female condom has been marketed since January 2, 1994 by Wisconsin Pharmacal Company under the name of Reality™. The design combines features of the male condom and the diaphragm (Bounds, 1989). The Reality™ female condom is a polyurethane sheath with a flexible inner ring that secures the condom against the cervix and an outer ring that prevents the condom from entering the vaginal canal. Various tests

Box 3.1 Continued

have shown that there is no viral leakage from the female condom (Leeper, 1990; Voeller, 1991).

The female condom has several advantages over the male condom, both as a contraceptive and as an STD prevention method. First, since it is woman-controlled, women are not as dependent on the cooperation of sex partners to protect themselves from HIV and other sexually transmitted diseases. Second, the female condom is inserted before intercourse, providing additional protection against infections from pre-ejaculated fluids. Third, the female condom protects a greater proportion of the vagina, providing additional protection against STDs. Fourth, the Reality™ condom is less likely to rupture than the male condom (Bounds et al., 1988; Gollub and Stein, 1993; Leeper and Conrardy, 1989). Also, because of its loose fit, it causes less loss of sensitivity, permits penetration before complete erection of the penis, and permits continued intimacy in the resolution phase of intercourse, since it need not be removed immediately.

Several small-scale studies have tested the acceptability of Reality™ among both women and men, but only two studies to date have been conducted among women at high risk of HIV infection—commercial sex workers. In one such study, participants claimed that female condoms were more protective against HIV and STD infection and were more feasible to use than male condoms. Many used them with their regular sex partners, who also found them acceptable (Hernandez-Avila, 1992). In the other study, 90 percent of the women said they would recommend the female condom to friends (Sakondhavat, 1990). In all acceptability studies, although the samples have been small, a majority of women and men have felt that the female condom was easy to use and was an acceptable method of both contraception and HIV/STD prevention (Schilling, El-Bassel, Leeper, et al., 1991).

This preliminary research suggests promising results for the female condom, including acceptability among female populations with varying sexual histories and practices. However, studies so far have been based on very small samples, and additional data are needed to further test the acceptability and efficacy of female condom use. Moreover, no studies have been conducted in the United States among women at high risk for HIV infection, such as commercial sex workers, injection drug users, or those who exchange sex for drugs. In addition, the female condom is not readily accessible in the United States. How the new female condom will fare among high-risk populations, and in the general population, remains to be seen.

havior to the same extent as did subjects participating in inter-ventions, it is impossible to tell whether behavior actually changed in both groups or if other factors influenced reports of behavior. Such factors might include informal communication between subjects, intensive and repeated interviews, and general societal trends (Calsyn, Saxon, Freeman, et al., 1992; Gibson, Young, and Lovelle-Drache, 1993; McCusker et al., 1992).

Even though many of these individual-focused intervention studies have demonstrated sexual and drug-use behavior change, they may be limited in a few ways: (1) most rely solely on self-reported data; (2) for the most part they have not yet demonstrated long-term behavior change (beyond 6 months); (3) it is not yet known whether they work with populations outside of their target groups; (4) many interventions may not be cost-effective to implement on a larger scale; and (5) with few exceptions, they do not measure HIV transmission and do not necessarily indicate that HIV infec-tion has been averted.

COMMUNITY-FOCUSED INTERVENTIONS

Sexual Behavior

Intervention research at the community level has employed peer-led AIDS education to reach people at high risk for HIV infection who may not be willing to participate in small-group/programs (Kegeles et al., 1993) and to change norms in the community as a whole (Kelly, St. Lawrence, Stevenson, et al., 1992; Kelly, Winett, Roffman, et al., 1993). In one intervention study mentioned pre-viously, gay men who served as popular opinion leaders were trained to deliver AIDS risk reduction messages to other gay men who frequented gay bars. The result of this intervention was that after three months, the number of gay men in the study who practiced unprotected sex was reduced in the range of 15 to 24 percent from baseline levels (Kelly, St. Lawrence, Stevenson, et al., 1992). When this community-based intervention was replicated in other small cities in Wisconsin, Washington, West Virginia, and New York, similar results were found at 9-month follow-up (Kelly, Winett, Roffman, et al., 1993). The goal of attracting socially isolated men into participating in safer sex educational activities was ac-complished by an intervention designed by and for young gay men aged 18 to 29. This intervention reduced unprotected anal inter-course among its subjects, from 33 percent at baseline to 25 per-cent at 9-month follow-up in one experimental city; however, little change was observed at follow-up in control cities (Kegeles et al., 1993). Although these experiments effected short-term behavioral change among gay men as a result of community-level peer education, both long-term impact and generalizability to other risk groups remain to be demonstrated.

In a number of African countries, a combination of peer-led education with free condom distribution has been used to attempt to change behaviors among commercial sex workers and their clients (Lamptey, 1991; Welsh et al., 1992); however, so far, only a few programs have been evaluated for their effectiveness (Asamoah-Adu et al., 1994; Williams et al., 1992; Wilson et al., 1993). In the Nigerian state of Cross River, community-based interventions trained commercial sex workers, clients, and brothel owners and managers as peer educators, initiated community outreach by peer educators, and distributed condoms at brothels (Williams et al., 1992). A follow-up evaluation one year later found that consistent condom use had increased from 12 percent to 24 percent and, among clients, AIDS knowledge had improved and attitudes toward condom efficacy were more favorable. In Zimbabwe a similar community-level peer education and condom distribution program resulted in increased consistent condom use among sex workers (8.6 percent at baseline to 58.3 percent at 1-year follow-up) and clients (25.4 percent at baseline to 44.7 percent at follow-up) (Wilson et al., 1993). Consistent condom use by sex workers and their clients in Ghana rose from 6 percent in 1987 to 71 percent in 1988 and then fell back to 64 percent in 1991 (Asamoah-Adu et al., 1994). Condom distribution strategies have been widely used, but more careful study should be initiated to determine their efficacy in reducing HIV infections. Also, interventions should target steady partners of sex workers, since it appears that sex workers use condoms less frequently in their personal relationships than in their interactions with clients (Dorfman, Derish, and Cohen, 1992; NRC, 1990b).

The impact of AIDS education on other adult heterosexuals has mostly come from mass media campaigns directed at the general public. Several studies have found evidence that these campaigns have had an impact on AIDS knowledge, attitudes, and behavior (Hausser et al., 1988; Izazola, Valdespino, and Sepulveda, 1988; Lehmann et al., 1987; Mills, Campbell, and Waters, 1986; Moatti et al., 1992; Wober, 1988). For example, media campaigns in Switzerland that included mail distribution of an AIDS informational booklet and multimedia advertisements promoting condom use, nonsharing of syringes, and monogamy resulted in a demonstrated increase in AIDS knowledge, condom sales, and condom use (Hausser et al., 1988; Lehmann et al., 1987).

Injection Drug Use

Research results from evaluations of needle exchange programs have been highly promising in showing reductions in risky drug using behavior, despite the fact that none of the evaluation studies was a randomized, controlled trial (due to the extreme difficulty of conducting such a trial in this context). In a 1993 report prepared for CDC, Lurie and Reingold (1993) reviewed sixteen such studies and found that among the 14 that evaluated the impact of needle exchange programs on the sharing of syringes, 10 demonstrated decreases in sharing and 4 showed no change. Of the 8 studies that evaluated the impact of needle exchange programs on frequency of drug injection, 3 showed a decrease, 4 showed no change, and one found that needle exchange clients were less likely to stop using drugs than a comparison group. Because these studies did not specifically address the interaction of needle exchange programs and risky sexual behavior, no firm conclusions were made in this regard (see Lurie and Reingold, 1993, for details).

In the NIDA-sponsored National AIDS Demonstration Research Program (NADR), (see Box 6.1 in Chapter 6), street outreach projects that recruited out-of-treatment injection drug users into HIV prevention services contributed to a substantial reduction in the percentage of injection drug users who shared needles—from 48 percent at baseline to 24 percent at follow-up 6 months later (Stephens et al., 1993). Drug users and their sex partners also increased their consistent use of condoms by 9 percent as a result of this program (see Stephens et al., 1993, for details). Social networks of injection drug users were also targeted for peer-led street outreach in the NADR program. In one study in Chicago, 86 percent of subjects stopped sharing injection equipment and HIV seroconversion rates dropped substantially as a result of the network-approach intervention, from 5 percent at baseline to less than 1 percent at the follow-up four years later (Wiebel et al., 1993).

MAINTAINING BEHAVIOR CHANGE AND PREVENTING RELAPSE

Initiating change in risky behavior is only the first step in controlling the spread of HIV/AIDS. Maintaining behavior change over time is a much more significant challenge. Because many years may elapse between a person's initial infection with HIV and the onset of serious AIDS symptoms, people infected with

HIV must consistently restrict their sexual expression and drug use to only those acts that are safe if they are to avoid transmission of HIV to their sex and drug-using partners. Also, because HIV infection is highly concentrated within some well-defined subpopulations, each unsafe act within those groups conveys far greater risk for HIV transmission. Broad, if not universal, efforts to initiate and maintain risk reduction are necessary for avoiding continued high HIV seroconversion levels, especially among communities at higher risk. Research on sustained behavioral risk reductions has primarily focused on gay men. Although it should broaden to other groups, findings from this research may significantly contribute to all HIV prevention efforts.

Using longitudinal data from the San Francisco Men's Health Study, Ekstrand and Coates (1990) discovered that after a period of engaging only in safer sex, 16 percent of participants reinitiated unprotected insertive anal intercourse and 12 percent reinitiated unprotected receptive anal intercourse. A replication study—also among gay men in San Francisco—similarly found that it was more common for men to return to unsafe sexual practices after a period of exclusively safer sex than to engage consistently in high-risk sex (Stall et al., 1990). Given the fact that HIV prevention efforts for gay men have traditionally focused almost exclusively on initiation of safer sex techniques, these findings as well as those of other longitudinal studies (Hart et al., in press; Kippax et al., 1991; O'Reilly et al., 1990) clearly indicate that ensuring consistent maintenance of safer sex over long periods of time is a challenge.

The variability in rates of maintenance of safer sexual practices reported in such studies might reflect differences in sampling methods, measurement of sexual risk, observation, time periods, number of observations, the effect of loss due to follow-up bias, and prevalence of risk-taking behaviors across different populations of gay men. However, one finding that is clear from all the studies, despite these important methodological differences is that some portion of gay men reinitiate riskier sexual behaviors after a period of safer sexual behaviors, and that this behavioral pattern could be the source of continuing HIV seroconversions.

The research described above relies exclusively on self-reported data, the validity of which have been discussed at length elsewhere (NRC, 1991). While self-reporting remains the best available methodology for obtaining information about AIDS risk behaviors in diverse populations, it is useful to supplement and validate these data with a reliable biological outcome measure of seroconversion where possible.

One study that did so (Kingsley et al., 1991) used data from the Multicenter AIDS Cohort Study (MACS), a four-city study of gay-identified men, and found that declines in HIV seroconversion observed during the first three years of the study were reversed by the fifth year, by which time 11.3 percent of the men who were initially HIV negative were estimated to have seroconverted. Based on the health education offered to study participants (including HIV testing) and based on the fact that the cohort defined by the study is aging, the researchers believed that this estimate of new seroconversions was conservative when applied to the community at large.

Correlates of nonmaintenance of safer sex techniques have been empirically detected from several longitudinal research projects. These correlates include low self-efficacy, heavy drug or alcohol use, having sex under the influence of drugs or alcohol, having larger numbers of sex partners, having had sex before 1984 with someone diagnosed with AIDS, relative youth, and depression (Kelly, St. Lawrence, and Brasfield, 1991; O'Reilly et al., 1990; Stall et al., 1990). In addition to individual behavioral factors, certain social factors may influence nonmaintenance of safer sex behaviors, such as lack of community support for risk reduction, social support or pressure to take health risks, high reinforcement value for unprotected sex, and identification of unprotected anal intercourse as a favorite sexual act (Kelly, St. Lawrence, and Brasfield, 1991; O'Reilly et al., 1990; Stall et al., 1990). Identifying and understanding these correlates may have more significant impact on HIV prevention than does measuring the rates of long-term behavior maintenance.

Identifying the characteristics of gay men who have seroconverted may also provide useful information about nonmaintenance of behavioral risk reduction over time. Racial/ethnic minority status, youth, lower education levels, lower socioeconomic status, and higher likelihood of cocaine or amphetamine use have been identified as correlates of HIV seroconversion in several independent studies (Kingsley et al., 1991; Waight and Miller, 1991; Willoughby et al., 1990). However, because these analyses were conducted using data sets that were not specifically designed to study nonmaintenance of safer sex techniques over time, and because many of the earlier study cohorts are aging, new cohorts of men who have sex with men should be formed in order to specifically study safer sex behavioral maintenance issues. Also, most of the analyses conducted so far have not had the benefit of a theoretical model of HIV risk behavior lapse. In order to develop both basic and applied research in this area, exploratory, inductive, retrospective research designs should be employed to identify conditions under which maintenance of safer sex techniques is attenuated.

That reductions in risk behavior among men who have sex with men have been maintained at all is a tribute to the successful interventions employed within these communities. However, successful HIV prevention requires long-term, community-wide maintenance of risk reduction which in turn calls for the development of new intervention models, especially those that target multiple risk behaviors.

EVALUATING THE EFFECTS OF AIDS INTERVENTIONS

Although identifying behavioral changes is an important outcome measure for AIDS preventive interventions, these changes do not automatically translate into reductions in HIV transmission in ways that are immediately obvious. Moreover, although modifying risky behavior is key to reducing HIV transmission, behavior change alone may not be sufficient for evaluating prevention efforts. However, with few exceptions, an attempt to estimate the number of infections averted has not been included in the design or evaluation of behavior change interventions. While it would not be possible to employ such an analysis to every prevention project, its utility as an approach should be further assessed.

An ideal experimental design would be to compare direct measurement of seroconversions in populations targeted by intervention programs to those of similar populations not receiving the intervention (preferably with random assignment to treatment and control groups). There are difficulties in mounting such large-scale social experiments. For example, interventions targeting entire communities (such as needle exchange programs or making condoms available in schools) do not allow for the easy formation of treatment and control groups, while randomization is virtually impossible in such environments.

Even if one could achieve such experimental setups, the incidence rate of new infections is low even in many populations at relatively high risk for HIV. This means that unless the number of persons involved in an intervention study is extremely large, it would take many years before conventional statistical methods could prove that a highly successful program is in fact highly successful.

For example, consider an intervention (with 100 in the control group and 100 in the intervention group) that cuts the infection rate in half for a population of injection drug users experiencing an incidence rate of 4 infections per 100 per year. After two years the study would detect on average 7.7 new infections in the control group (incidence of .04) and 3.9 new infections in the intervention group (reduced incidence of .02). Although reducing an infection rate in half is effective, conventional statistical methods would fail to find this difference statistically significant. (Precisely this same issue currently plagues the planning and design of HIV preventive vaccine trials.)

This very issue led a previous National Research Council panel to recommend using behavior change as the primary approach to evaluating AIDS preventive intervention research (NRC, 1991). However, focusing solely on behavior change outcome measures leaves unanswered the fundamental question of how many infections are really averted as a result of prevention programs.

An intermediate course between solely measuring changes in behavior on the one hand, and insisting on lengthy field studies with enormous numbers of subjects on the other is the use of mathematical modeling to provide evidence for how a given prevention activity may reduce infection. The mathematical theory of epidemics is well established, and numerous researchers have applied modeling techniques to gain insights into various aspects of the AIDS epidemic (Anderson and May, 1991; Brookmeyer and Gail, 1993; Castillo-Chavez, 1989; Jager and Ruitenberg, 1992; Kaplan and Brandeau, 1994). These models mathematically integrate the key features of risky behavior (i.e., numbers of unprotected sex partners per person per unit time, number of needle-sharing occasions per person per unit time), epidemiology (i.e., the probability of HIV transmission per potentially infectious exposure, progression of HIV infection through AIDS, AIDS-induced mortality), and demography (i.e., population immigration, birth, and non-AIDS mortality rates). In addition to incorporating behavioral variables, the models allow for incorporation of prevention program operations as demonstrated by studies of needle exchange (Kaplan and O'Keefe, 1993), bleach distribution to injection drug users (Siegel, Weinstein, and Fineberg, 1991), HIV counseling and testing (Brandeau et al., 1993; Gail, Preston, and Piantadosi, 1989), and self-deferral from blood donation (Kaplan and Novick, 1990). Thus, modeling provides an attractive approach to thinking about how prevention programs effect change in HIV transmission, assuming the models are structured to include all relevant parameters.

For example, the evaluation of a needle exchange program in New Haven, Connecticut employs a mathematical model to estimate the impact of the program on HIV transmission among the participants of the needle exchange. The evaluation uses a syringe tracking and testing (STT) system to collect data on needles distributed and returned to the program by using anonymous code names for participants, tracking numbers for needles, and a technique that is capable of detecting HIV in the traces of blood remaining in the syringes. The data derived from the STT have revealed a significant drop in the portion of needles testing positive for HIV, and it is estimated that HIV incidence among needle exchange participants has fallen by 33 percent (Kaplan, 1994; Kaplan and O'Keefe, 1993).

The ability to estimate the impact of an intervention on HIV transmission also contributes to the possibility of conducting a cost-effectiveness assessment of that intervention. In a time of shrinking federal budgets and increasing research costs, the scientific community faces greater pressure to demonstrate the social value of taxpayer-supported research. One measure of value is the cost-to-benefit ratio. In the context of HIV intervention research, dollar costs are both the costs of conducting the intervention itself and the costs of medical care for a person with AIDS. Assuming one could use the methods described above for estimating the number of HIV infections averted by the implementation of an intervention, one could then compare dollars saved in medical costs affiliated with those infections with dollars spent on conducting the intervention. One could then make an assessment about the value of investing in that particular intervention.

CONCLUSION AND RECOMMENDATIONS

Conclusion

Basic science research in the neurobiological, psychological, and social sciences has uncovered a great deal of information about the range of factors underlying the behavior of individuals and groups, information that has been influential in the design of HIV preventive interventions. Theoretical models from psychology have played a particularly significant role. Yet, the mixed results of interventions informed by this basic research suggest that much remains to be learned—in particular, how the biological, psychological, and social dimensions of behavior interact to encourage or prevent risky behavior and to initiate and maintain positive behavior change. Cross-disciplinary research in this regard will play an important role in improving the design and application of HIV preventive interventions.

The efficacy and value of such interventions may be measured by demonstrated, sustained, positive behavior change; but with respect to AIDS prevention, it also is important to show that new infections have been averted by such change. Epidemiological and mathematical methods now exist to assess the efficacy of interventions in this regard—and their cost-to-benefit ratio—and their employment should be considered wherever appropriate.

RECOMMENDATIONS FOR UNDERSTANDING THE DETERMINANTS OF HIV RISK BEHAVIOR

3.1 The committee recommends that NIAAA, NIDA, and NIMH expand basic research on the biology of sexuality as it potentially relates to high-risk sexual behaviors. This might include research on the central nervous system (CNS) sexual systems that mediate sexual behaviors, the CNS neural systems underlying sexual behavior, and the molecular genetics of sexual behaviors.

3.2 The committee recommends that NIAAA, NIDA, and NIMH expand research on the biology of substance abuse to provide additional knowledge for approaching high-risk behaviors. This might include research to define structure-activity relationships in the function of dopamine systems; the role of noradrenergic systems and molecular mechanisms in the components of addiction (including euphoria, tolerance, sensitization, and withdrawal); the role of opiate peptide receptor subtypes in components of the addiction-abuse syndrome; as well as research to identify mechanisms of cocaine addiction.

3.3 The committee recommends that, where appropriate, NIAAA, NIDA, and NIMH coordinate their efforts with other relevant federal agencies (e.g., other NIH institutes, the National Science Foundation) that are also attempting to integrate biological, behavioral, and social research to define high-risk behaviors.

3.4 The committee recommends that NIAAA, NIDA, and NIMH support AIDS research that integrates theories of gen-

der (identity, development, and dynamics) and behavior change models.

3.5 The committee recommends that NIAAA, NIDA, and NIMH expand the research effort examining social and structural factors (such as class, race/ethnicity, gender relations, and community) that increase risk for AIDS, affect progression of disease, and provide points of intervention. This might require research that takes as the unit of analysis the social context and relationship (e.g., dyads, families, communities) in which HIV occurs—as opposed to the individual at risk of or who has HIV.

3.6 The committee recommends that NIAAA, NIDA, and NIMH, in conjunction with other NIH institutes, develop new and existing woman-controlled HIV/STD prevention methods (e.g., female condoms and microbicides) and examine the social and behavioral issues related to their use.

3.7 The committee recommends that NIAAA, NIDA, and NIMH support basic and applied research on the maintenance of behavior change, for example, risky sexual behavior and alcohol and other drug-using behavior, including the prevention of relapse. (The committee notes that this has been recommended in previous NRC reports—*AIDS: The Second Decade,* 1990; *AIDS, Sexual Behavior, and Intravenous Drug Use,* 1989—but has not been attended to adequately.)

3.8 The committee recommends that NIAAA, NIDA, and NIMH expand funding for HIV intervention research initiatives, particularly those that: (1) have rigorous evaluation components; (2) investigate motivations, intentions, and barriers in addition to behavior change; (3) include outcome measures in addition to behavior change, such as HIV seroprevalence, STD rates, and pregnancy rates; and (4) target a full range of racial/ethnic, gender, and cultural groups for the purpose of assessing between-group differences.

3.9 The committee recommends that NIAAA, NIDA, and NIMH support research that estimates the number of HIV infections averted by current prevention efforts and that includes cost estimates for these efforts.

4

Disease Progression and Intervention

Although every effort must be made to prevent new transmission of HIV, it is equally important to diagnose, treat, and care adequately for people who already are infected. This chapter presents an overview of findings from research on the pathogenesis and disease progression of HIV/AIDS relevant to mental health and substance abuse and on possible interventions to control the infection's effects. This research, which has developed quickly over the past decade, ranges from basic molecular and cellular biology to clinical pathology to social psychology, and has recently provided some important clues about the relationships between HIV, the brain, and behavior, and most importantly, about their *interactive* nature. In so doing, this research demonstrates the need for cross-disciplinary approaches to HIV prevention and intervention.

Chief interactions reviewed here include: (1) HIV infection of the brain and the effects HIV has on the central nervous system; (2) effects of interactions among HIV infection, substance use, and mental illness and the unique medical care and treatment issues associated with such interactions; and (3) the relationship between psychosocial factors and HIV infection for individuals with the disease, as well as for their loved ones and caregivers.

THE RELATIONSHIP BETWEEN HIV AND
THE CENTRAL NERVOUS SYSTEM

EFFECTS OF HIV ON THE CENTRAL NERVOUS SYSTEM:
DEFINING THE ISSUES

A group of organic nervous system disorders may complicate the course of HIV infection and may result directly from HIV infection. HIV-associated conditions affecting both the central nervous system (CNS) and peripheral nervous system (PNS) are common and result in considerable morbidity and mortality. They can be classified in a number of ways. Many can be considered *secondary* complications of HIV infection, resulting from opportunistic infections or systemic organ dysfunction that follows from immune deficiency induced by HIV infection. Among the major CNS complications of AIDS are cerebral toxoplasmosis, primary CNS lymphoma (an opportunistic neoplasm associated with B-lymphocyte infection by Epstein-Barr virus), cryptococcal meningitis, and progressive multifocal leukoencephalopathy (PML) caused by the JC virus (for reviews, see Brew et al., 1988; Johnson, 1994; Koppel, 1992; Price, 1994; Price and Worley, 1994; Snider et al., 1983).

Other conditions likely relate more directly to HIV infection itself, rather than to an additional opportunistic infection or systemic organ dysfunction. These can be considered *primary* nervous system complications of HIV. While their pathogenesis is not yet clearly understood, they are thought to be sequelae of interactions among HIV, the immune system, and various components of the nervous system. These include some unusual disorders complicating the early phases of HIV infection as well as common conditions occurring later. In the earliest phase of infection, a number of syndromes have been described, including mild meningitis with headache. However, while these syndromes are usually absent or mild, it is likely that in the course of spreading throughout the lymphatic system, HIV also reaches the brain at this time within infected lymphocytes, but without causing any clinical symptoms or signs.

Later in the course of systemic HIV infection, patients may develop so-called "aseptic" meningitis that presumably is caused by HIV infection of the membranes surrounding the brain. They also may experience a peripheral neuropathy causing pain in the feet. However, of particular relevance to the issues of this report, HIV-infected persons also are susceptible late in the course of systemic infection to an affliction that impairs brain function in a stereotyped manner. This syndrome, referred to as AIDS dementia complex (ADC), as well as by a variety of other terms (HIV dementia, HIV-associated cognitive-motor complex), likely is caused by HIV itself and is mediated either by toxic effects of certain molecules coded by the viral genome or by cell-coded products, principally cytokines (American Academy of Neurology AIDS Task Force, 1991; Price, 1994; Price and Perry, 1994).

ADC can be a source of protracted and severe disability, modifying and markedly diminishing the quality of remaining life, reducing enjoyment of work and daily life, depriving the patient of social and intellectual pleasures, and requiring emotionally and financially costly care needs. In its mild form, ADC syndrome slows intellectual processing, blunts concentration, and impairs rapid and fine motor control. When more severe, it causes truly devastating dementia that reduces the patient to a shell of his or her former self—dulling the personality, impairing walking, and eventually leaving the victim bedridden, incontinent, and mute (Navia, Cho, Petito, et al., 1986; Navia, Jordan, and Price, 1986; Price and Sidtis, 1992). This neurological syndrome was in fact recognized early in the course of the AIDS epidemic by U.S. clinicians in the epicenters of the disease on both the east and west coasts. However, because ADC was first noted in the setting of a novel infection, it took some time to recognize and refine its clinical features, to describe precisely its natural history and pathogenesis, and subsequently to approach and evaluate its prevention and treatment. Eventually, a clearer picture began to emerge, with speculation focusing on a possible relationship between AIDS and human cytomegalovirus (CMV) opportunistic infection of the CNS (Snider et al., 1983). However, after further clarification of the features of the syndrome, with its pathology and the clinical-pathological correlations, CMV infection no longer seemed to provide an adequate explanation (Navia, Cho, Petito, et al., 1986). Because this syndrome was unlike any known complications of immunosuppression previously described in other populations, such as cancer and transplant patients, speculation turned to the same putative agent that caused AIDS itself; and when HIV was then identified (as LAV and HTLV-III) research began to test whether this virus might not only cause immunosuppression, but might more directly cause the AIDS dementia complex (Price et al., 1988).

The search for the virus in the brains of ADC patients soon revealed evidence of high amounts of proviral DNA in some (Shaw et al., 1985). At the same time, molecular studies of HIV showed that it was related to visna virus, a prototype slow or lentivirus type of retrovirus well known to cause CNS infection and disease in sheep (Gonda et al., 1985). Further reports documented early exposure of the brain (or at least cerebrospinal fluid, or CSF) to HIV and also identified active infection of the brain late in the disease (Brenneman et al., 1988; Dreyer et al., 1990; Gabuzda et al., 1986; Koenig et al., 1986; Wiley et al., 1986). These rapid developments led to the initial concept that ADC was the result of CNS HIV infection and thus that the virus infected not only the immune system but the brain as well. However, more detailed subsequent work indicated that the cause and pathogenesis of ADC are not so straightforward, but rather involve a complex interaction among the virus, the immune system, and the CNS (Epstein and Gendelman, 1993; Price et al., 1988; Price, 1994; Spencer and Price, 1993).

STAGING AND CELLULAR SITES OF CENTRAL NERVOUS SYSTEM INFECTION IN AIDS DEMENTIA COMPLEX

The core features of the AIDS dementia complex have now been well characterized, and a descriptive staging system, useful to provide a common vocabulary for both clinical practice and clinical investigation, has been developed (see Price, 1994; Sidtis, 1994). Nonetheless, more precise defining characteristics still must be developed in order to standardize clinical trials. Likewise, evaluation methodologies have been developed, but more precise definition of abnormalities is still needed. Standard measures are needed to interpret and quantify neuroimaging studies (MRI and CT scanning), CSF profiles, and neuropsychological test results (Price and Sidtis, 1990; Sidtis, 1994). Defining markers for the degree of viral infection will also be important. Together these will aid the more precise characterization of the natural history and epidemiology of ADC. Likewise, these methods should improve evaluation of the efficacy of prevention and treatment, as new agents to reduce the viral burden and to interrupt neurotoxic processes are brought into the clinic. These are all important clinical issues in reducing the disease burden associated with established HIV infection.

The character of HIV infection of the CNS is not yet fully understood. It appears to vary in its profile during the course of systemic HIV infection. This variability relates to the importance of the immune system in suppressing HIV replication early and then failing to suppress replication late in infection. Additionally, changes in the virus, both with respect to predominant cell tropism and virulence may be important. Thus, from the very early period of infection, the CNS is exposed to HIV presumably through the traffic of infected cells from the bloodstream. This traffic may continue throughout infection, perhaps with diminished intensity during the phase of clinical latency, but increasing again in the later (AIDS) phase of infection (Spencer and Price, 1993). Thus, a number of studies have shown early invasion of the CNS and early local host immune responses in the CSF. A critical question remaining to be answered is whether the virus then persists in the CNS in latent form or as an indolent infection that is asymptomatic. If it can remain latent, then research must discover which cells might harbor the proviral DNA: microglia, astrocytes, or other CNS cells.

If the virus is latent in, for example, astrocytes, is that important for the subsequent course of infection in the CNS and for disease production? Or is the course of later infection dominated not by the *opportunity* for infection, but rather by the factors that control replication? Thus, the later stage of systemic infection is dominated by high-titer viremia with enhanced probability of viral entry into the CNS; this late entry might far overshadow earlier events. Subsequent replication of HIV within the CNS appears to relate to loss of immune control, determined by the effects of systemic infection on the immune system (O'Brien, 1994).

MECHANISMS FOR CAUSING SYMPTOMS

The characteristic symptoms and signs of ADC have led to classification of this syndrome among the *subcortical dementias*, a group that includes Parkinson's disease, progressive supranuclear palsy, hydrocephalus, and other conditions in which cognitive dysfunction is associated with damage to nerve cell nuclei and white matter in the diencephalon rather than cerebral cortex. AIDS dementia complex shares with these disorders a slowing of thinking and concentration along with motor dysfunction, in contrast to the *cortical dementias* such as Alzheimer's disease and Creutzfeldt-Jacob disease, in which amnesia, aphasia, apraxia, and the like are more characteristic. Understanding the nature and physiology of brain dysfunction in AIDS patients has both practical and theoretical importance. A clear characterization of ADC should capture its salient features and set it off from other conditions. The lack of such a distinction, and the unfortunate evolving usage of the term *dementia*, which is most often applied to Alzheimer's disease and multi-infarct dementia, has already resulted in some confusion in both the definition of AIDS dementia complex and the criteria for diagnosis, with an inappropriate effort to apply criteria that relate more to those other dementing conditions than to ADC itself (American Academy of Neurology AIDS Task Force, 1991). The emphasis on symptoms of cognitive decline, as opposed to motor slowing and other features more prominent in subcortical diseases, also has confused efforts to develop neuropsychological test batteries for ADC and other subcortical syndromes.

Understanding why patients develop the changes in thinking and behavior characteristic of ADC holds lessons for cortical-subcortical relations and for the abnormalities noted in other subcortical dementias. Positron emission tomography (PET) studies of brain glucose metabolism have shown a curious enhanced metabolism of diencephalic regions compared with cortex (Rottenberg et al., 1987). The reason for this seemingly paradoxical finding remains to be explained (paradoxical because *reduced* metabolism might have been anticipated on the basis of symptoms, and because these structures appear to be more susceptible to HIV infection than cortex).

MECHANISMS OF CENTRAL NERVOUS SYSTEM INJURY

A complex picture emerges from pathological studies indicating that productive HIV infection in the brain occurs in cells of bone marrow origin (monocyte-macrophages and microglia) rather than in the neuroectodermal cells (nerve cells and other supporting cells in the brain such as oligodendrocytes and astrocytes) that perform the specialized work of the CNS. The extent of infection often appears greater than the degree of brain dysfunction, at least until the later stages of ADC, suggesting that the pathological effects of infection are somehow attenuated despite high levels of CNS infection. Early studies of CSF, and more recent studies of brains taken at autopsy, indicate better correlation between CNS dysfunction and markers of immune activation than with infection. Taken together, these observations suggest that the virus *indirectly* injures the brain rather than directly killing or infecting nerve cells. This distinguishes HIV from other viral infections of the brain caused by poliovirus or herpes simplex virus. Poliovirus, the most intensely studied human virus of an earlier era, directly infects motor neurons and causes the death of these cells, producing paralysis. By contrast, in the case of

HIV, the link between the viral genome and CNS dysfunction is far less direct. The virus itself does not appear to kill nerve cells, and its presence in the CNS early in infection appears to be benign. Later neuronal dysfunction bears an uncertain relationship to the CNS virus load (Masliah et al., 1994; Price, 1994).

Gradually, a coherent picture is emerging of initiation of brain injury by HIV infection, which is mediated by immunopathological processes in which cell-coded signals result in brain injury. Such processes might be involved in many infectious diseases, but are less prominent because they are overshadowed by the direct neurotoxic effects of the foreign organism and because they are short-lived. HIV infection differs because the virus is not, in itself, capable of damaging neuroectodermal cells directly, and because infection is so protracted. The regulation and profile of immune responses are also profoundly disturbed, with alterations or loss of normal feedback inhibition loops.

In particular, interest has recently focused on the neurotoxic properties of gene products from the HIV virus itself, and from HIV-infected immune cells. The HIV coat glycoprotein, gp120, allows HIV to bind to macrophages and may in turn be released by infected cells, resulting in neuronal damage and death (Giulian, Vaca, and Noonan, 1990; Pulliam et al., 1991). Extremely low concentrations of gp120 increase intraneuronal calcium, which causes injury and death in cell and tissue culture systems (Brenneman et al., 1988; Dreyer et al., 1990). Moreover, injection of gp120 into the brain ventricles of rats induces misshapen hippocampal pyramidal cell processes associated with behavioral abnormalities (Hill and Brenneman, 1990; Panlilio et al., 1990; Pert et al., 1989). The HIV nuclear protein *tat* was found to be neurotoxic for glioma and neuroblastoma cell lines (derived from brain support cells) in culture and to mice *in vivo* (Sabatier et al., 1991). The significance of these observations is being explored.

Recent experiments have raised other possibilities to account for HIV-elicited neurotoxicity. Astrocytes, another critical class of supporting cells in the nervous system, produce growth and survival factors that are essential for normal brain function (see Lu et al., 1991). In a culture of hippocampal cells, the peptide neuromodulator VIP (vasoactive intestinal peptide) prevents gp120-induced neuronal toxicity (Brenneman et al., 1988). VIP is known to act on astrocytes, releasing factors necessary for neuronal survival and neurite outgrowth (Festoff, Rao, and Brenneman, 1990; Russell et al., 1990).

Parallel studies focusing on immune system cells, including

macrophages and microglia, suggest that these infected cells in the nervous system release unidentified toxic factors that kill chick, rodent, and human neurons *in vitro* (Giulian, Vaca, and Noonan, 1990; Pulliam et al., 1991). The toxic agents may represent gp120 itself, a fragment thereof, or other molecules released in response to gp120. The precise relationships between HIV, immune cells, toxic factors, and neuronal damage remain to be elucidated.

While causal mechanisms have not been traced, some final common pathways of neuronal damage are being explored. Activation of calcium channels (both those that respond to voltage and to so-called NMDA receptors, which respond to excitatory amino acids) appears necessary for HIV-induced neuronal injury. Extensive study suggests that gp120 sensitizes neurons to the toxic effects of NMDA receptor stimulation (for review, see Lipton, 1992). In aggregate, studies suggest that agents blocking gp120 or NMDA receptors might ameliorate the neuropathological effects of HIV infection. Consequently, pharmacologic agents that have little influence on HIV itself may nevertheless represent important therapeutic adjuncts in the treatment of HIV-induced neurologic disease. It may be possible to treat symptoms of ADC with a different class of agents that block virus replication itself.

The activation of certain immune reactions late in infection has likewise led to studies of the mechanisms of damage to the immune system. These have centered principally around effects of cytokine upregulation. Some putative cell-coded neurotoxins are quinolinic acid (an endogenous excitatory amino acid), nitric oxide, Tumor Necrosis Factor, NMDA agonists, and arachidonic acid metabolites (Benos et al., 1994, Brenneman et al., 1988; Dawson et al., 1993; Epstein and Gendelman, 1993; Garry and Koch, 1992; Guilian, Vaca, and Noonan, 1990; Heyes et al., 1991; Heyes, Saito, Crowley, et al., 1992; Kaiser, Offerman, and Lipton, 1990; Lipton, 1991, 1992, 1994; Masliah et al., 1994; Pulliam et al., 1991; Toggas et al., 1994; Wahl et al., 1989; Werner et al., 1991; Wesselingh et al., 1993). A picture is emerging of multiple toxins acting in concert as part of dysregulated cytokine cascades triggered by immune responses or by viral signals, together disrupting or destroying neuronal function in selected brain regions. However, these processes are only beginning to come into focus and require considerable investigation to clarify both relevance and mechanisms.

Understanding these pathogenic mechanisms has great potential for treating ADC patients, using not only methods that interfere with the virus, but also employing strategies directed at interrupting some of these toxic processes. Indeed, these considerations underlie some of the approaches now being taken to treat the AIDS dementia complex, including treatment protocols using nimodipine, a calcium channel blocker that can prevent gp120-induced neuronal death *in vitro,* and pentoxyphilline, an antagonist of Tumor Necrosis Factor.

Some of the critical areas regarding the pathogenesis of the ADC and others that remain to be addressed include: identifying the precise molecular and cellular cascades through which gp120, *tat,* and other HIV peptides contribute to AIDS neuropathology; identifying which peptides or receptors constitute appropriate pharmacologic targets; determining if such new agents can be safely combined with antiviral therapy to enhance clinical efficacy; identifying the mechanisms through which monocytoid cells, including macrophages and microglia, elicit neuropathology; revealing the identity of the mediating molecules and how they are regulated at the transcriptional, translational, and post-translational levels; determining how HIV infection itself evokes monocytoid-induced neuropathology; determining whether inhibition of astrocyte growth and trophic factors mediates AIDS neuropathology; identifying the mechanisms through which gp120 and VIP putatively interact; defining a monocytoid-astrocyte-neuron cascade in AIDS brain pathology; determining whether elevated intracellular calcium accounts for all the neuropathology in AIDS; characterizing the relationship of voltage-gated and NMDA-receptor-channel calcium influx in causing nerve cell damage; and determining whether gp120 and NMDA receptors directly interact and, if so, what the mechanisms are that foster calcium influx. Based on the foregoing, the next step is to see if new agents to prevent the neurologic sequelae of AIDS can be designed and tested in culture models, experimental animals, and the clinic, and to determine if there are any animal models of predictive value, other than non-human primates.

These questions may seem daunting, but studies on the AIDS dementia complex have evolved in a short period of time from a primitive state of empirical observations to experiments with possible direct therapeutic implications, not only for ADC, but also for other neurological and psychiatric diseases, especially those mediated by viruses or immune dysfunction. Therapeutic trials are currently under way to evaluate whether pharmacological interruption of the neurotoxic processes involved in ADC might alleviate neurological incapacity.

SIGNIFICANCE OF AIDS DEMENTIA COMPLEX FOR OTHER
CENTRAL NERVOUS SYSTEM DISORDERS

Research on the AIDS dementia complex and CNS HIV infection has importance not only for understanding the nature and course of HIV infection, but also more generally for suggesting mechanisms involved in other infectious, immunological, and neurodegenerative diseases. The early penetration of the blood-brain barrier by HIV, the local immune response detected in the spinal fluid, and the subsequent active replication of HIV in the brain late in infection hold clues regarding the CNS ecology of HIV. How does the virus reach the brain? In lymphocytes or monocytes, or as free virus? Does it remain latent in the brain, providing a reservoir and refuge from chemotherapy? How does it later commence active replication in the brain, and what is the importance of genetic variants of the virus with enhanced capacity to replicate in the brain?

The pathogenesis of ADC involves processes that have been observed in animal models (usually of viral diseases studied as models of degenerative disorders), but that have received less attention in human diseases with a known viral cause. Unlike most other human infections, HIV infection is characterized by long latency, a seeming lack of direct nerve cell destruction in the absence of immunosuppression (which HIV first induces before then affecting the brain), and the principally indirect mechanisms of brain injury alluded to earlier. In one sense, HIV infection can be considered as an acquired genetic disease in which a tightly regulated foreign genome is transplanted into an unwelcoming host where it then causes gradual and protracted disease. The mechanisms involved in resultant neurodegeneration are likely shared by other infections, and even other degenerative and genetic conditions. Research into the mechanisms of brain injury caused by HIV infection will likely produce lessons for these other conditions, and therapies that interrupt neurotoxic processes may well be applicable to other diseases. Studies of AIDS therefore may have very real and very important spillover effects into other disease areas.

The mechanisms involved in HIV-induced brain injury and ADC are also involved in other diseases. While protracted in time and perhaps altered in its profile, cytokine activation is part of other infectious, immunological, and neurodegenerative diseases. Intermediate and final pathways of neuronal dysfunction and death are likely shared between ADC and other viral encephalitides, multiple sclerosis, postinfectious encephalomyelitis, paraneoplastic diseases, Alzheimer's disease, and even schizophrenia. Shared mechanisms may be involved whenever an abnormal gene provokes immune responses with potential to include neurotoxic responses.

CLINICAL SIGNIFICANCE OF AIDS DEMENTIA COMPLEX

The primary motivation to study ADC and HIV infection of the CNS is to treat the disability they cause. While the prevalence of ADC is still somewhat uncertain, it remains a significant complication of HIV infection, and its severe impact on the lives of patients makes it an important target of prevention and treatment. As opportunistic infections are increasingly prevented by antibiotic prophylaxis, an increase in the prevalence of ADC threatens, although such a trend has not appeared in national statistics. In evaluating antiretroviral and other therapies, the study of ADC may also prove useful, because its symptoms are a continuous variable (so small changes can be measured) and reversible. Evaluation of treatment efficacy therefore does not require monitoring of sporadic events such as opportunistic infections, as in most current AIDS clinical trials, but rather the measurement of improved performance on tests of brain function.

INTERACTIONS AMONG HIV, SUBSTANCE USE, AND MENTAL ILLNESS

The second type of interaction among HIV, the brain, and behavior relates to the unique issues associated with multiple diagnoses, that is diagnosis of any combination of HIV, drug or alcohol abuse, and mental illness. This kind of multiple diagnosis is not uncommon, and it likely affects disease progression as well as treatment strategies. It is vitally important to recognize the interactive nature of HIV infection, substance use and abuse, and mental illness in order to appropriately intervene. This, too, requires a cross-disciplinary approach.

ALCOHOL AND THE IMMUNE SYSTEM

Drinking alcohol to excess has been shown to cause damage to the immune system (Kruger and Jerrells, 1992). It therefore seems reasonable to assume that alcohol consumption in significant amounts may also render an individual more vulnerable to HIV infection and facilitate the transition from HIV infection to AIDS. However, this assumption has not been substantiated by the relatively few studies to date that have examined the relationships among alcohol, the immune system, and HIV infection. Although research suggests that alcohol generally does play a role in immune system functioning, alcohol may not advance the progression of AIDS among the HIV positive (Kaslow et al., 1989; Ostrow et al., 1990).

The effects of alcohol on the immune system and on HIV infection likely depend on a person's drinking habits. The amount, duration, and frequency of consumption, as well as the presence of liver disease may play a role. Moreover, because many of the effects of alcohol on the immune system are reversible, the relationship between the timing of alcohol consumption and the stage of HIV infection may influence alcohol's effect.

Alcohol directly alters the defensive cells, or phagocytes, that digest and degrade viruses. Alcohol also apparently suppresses the production of two important cytokines that assist phagocytes in their defensive actions. Together, these suggest that alcohol may increase the susceptibility of phagocytes to initial infection, impairing their ability to eliminate the virus in the early stages of infection, and thus increasing their potential to function as reservoirs for HIV (Kruger and Jerrells, 1992).

Alcohol also reduces the number of T-cells in the spleen, lymph nodes, thymus, and blood (Jerrells, Smith, and Eckardt, 1990; Saad and Jerrells, 1991). In addition, remaining cells may be more susceptible to initial infection upon contact. Alcohol-induced loss of cells in the immune system may accelerate the onset of clinical manifestations among HIV-infected people, but research on this issue has been inconclusive. Although it is clear that excessive alcohol consumption can impair cell-mediated immunity, this has not translated into accelerated clinical progression of HIV to AIDS in reports to date (Isaki and Gordis, 1993; Kaslow et al., 1989). The precise relationship between alcohol use and HIV/AIDS remains to be elucidated.

DRUG USE AND HIV/AIDS

The large number of drug injectors already infected with HIV pose a significant challenge to the medical care system to recognize and treat the varied clinical manifestations of HIV infection and disease in this high-risk population. Treatment of drug users who are at risk for or already infected with HIV is complicated by several factors: the fact that the clinical course of HIV infection may have special characteristics among drug injectors, the existence of complex medical and psychosocial comorbidities, and the often tenuous relationship between drug users and the health care system. Although a significant body of research has been conducted on clinical aspects of HIV disease and its management among drug users, a number of key research areas require further examination.

Natural History of HIV Infection Among Drug Users

Most studies that have described rates of progression to AIDS or clinical manifestations of HIV disease in drug users have been performed among cohorts in which the date of primary HIV infection is unknown (Des Jarlais et al., 1987; Selwyn, Alcabes, Hartel, et al., 1992). These cohorts have tended to include many with advanced HIV infection at the time of study. Although several large cohorts already exist in the United States and Europe with greater proportions of subjects with known incident HIV infection (Munoz et al., 1992; Rezza et al., 1989; Willocks et al., 1990), natural history studies of HIV disease in seroincident cohorts must continue to be conducted in the future.

Changes in the spectrum of HIV disease over time, such as the emergence or disappearance of AIDS-related illnesses among drug users as a result of medical interventions or other differences, have yet to be charted. Such changes have been noted in male homosexual populations, but these patterns must be studied over time among drug users as well (Hoover et al., 1993; Moore et al., 1992).

Clinical aspects and outcomes of certain conditions that are common in HIV-seronegative drug users (Cherubin and Sapira, 1993) but may occur more frequently in HIV-infected drug users (Mientjes et al., 1992; Selwyn, Alcabes, Hartel, et al., 1992) also demand elucidation. These include endocarditis, cellulitis or abscess, pneumonia, bacteremia, and other pyogenic bacterial infections, especially in relation to CD4 counts and degree of immunosuppression (comparing endocarditis in patients in early and late HIV infection, regarding severity, infecting organisms, and outcome, among other factors).

Preliminary data suggest that the occurrence of certain clinical conditions, such as bacterial infections and tuberculosis (TB) may hasten disease progression in HIV-infected drug users (Alcabes, Schoenbaum, and Klein, 1993; Farizo et al., 1992; Mientjes et al.,

1992; Selwyn, Alcabes, Hartel, et al., 1992; Stoneburner et al., 1988; Willocks et al., 1992). However, the prognostic importance of these conditions has yet to be fully determined. Additionally, there is a need for further epidemiologic and clinical study of tuberculosis among HIV-infected drug users, to address primary versus reactivation tuberculosis (Daley et al., 1992; Hopewell, 1992; Selwyn, Hartel, Lewis, et al., 1989), cutaneous anergy (failure to respond to TB skin tests despite infection with the TB bacterium) (Moreno et al., 1993; Selwyn, Sckell, Alcabes, et al., 1992), the observed preponderance of tuberculosis outside the lung among drug users (Braun et al.,1990), and the relationship of demographic and social variables to the observed high risk of tuberculosis among drug users (Reichman, Felton, and Edsall, 1979). The relationships among drug use (particularly drug smoking), the physical and social context of illicit drug use, and the risk of bacterial pneumonia and tuberculosis should be clarified (Caiffa et al., 1993; CDC, 1991a).

Given the relationship between HIV infection and co-infection with other organisms, the evidence of high levels of both hepatitis B and hepatitis C infection among drug users, and the key importance of liver disease in this population, it also will be important to clarify further the clinical expression and outcome of hepatitis C infection in co-infected groups (Donahue et al., 1991; Esteban et al., 1989; Haverkos and Lange, 1990; Kreek, 1983; Novick et al., 1988; Stimmel, Vernace, and Schaffner, 1975; van den Hoek et al., 1990).

Moreover, the prognostic importance of standard laboratory markers used in the assessment of HIV disease state among drug users (e.g., CD4+ T-lymphocyte subsets, Beta-2-microglobulin, neopterin, and hematologic indices) will be important to reassess, given evidence that some markers may not be as useful in drug users as in other populations. While substantial data already exist in this area, the issue can still bear further scrutiny (Alcabes et al., 1994; Chaisson et al., 1991; Davenny et al., 1990; Fernandez-Cruz et al., 1990; Munoz et al., 1992; Rezza et al., 1989; Selwyn, Alcabes, Hartel, et al., 1992).

The role of drug and alcohol use in the progression of HIV disease has received much interest in the past, but it still has not been studied definitively with respect to the hypotheses that the immunosuppressive or immunostimulatory effects of psychoactive drug use might hasten the progression of HIV infection (Kaslow et al., 1989; Rezza et al., 1989; van Griensven et al., 1990; Weber et al., 1990).

Medical Care for HIV-Infected Drug Users

As HIV infection increasingly has become a treatable condition, the focus has shifted appropriately from observational studies of disease progression toward medical interventions to alter its course. Intervention studies will have increasing relevance for drug users, regarding not only clinical management but also health services access and utilization. Here, too, however, a number of areas remain to be explored more fully.

Pharmacokinetic and other pharmacologic studies involving drugs of abuse and medications used for the treatment of HIV-related disease, as well as prescribed opioids such as methadone used to treat opiate addiction, will help determine whether interactions have potential clinical significance. Studies from the pre-AIDS era documented clinically important pharmacologic interactions between methadone and rifampin (used to treat tuberculosis), phenytoin (a treatment for epilepsy), and other medications (Kreek, 1983; Kreek et al., 1976; Tong et al., 1981). Preliminary studies with certain HIV-related medications have been performed, involving methadone and zidovudine (AZT), and more recently, rifabutin, with suggestive but inconclusive results (Sawyer et al., 1993; Schwartz et al., 1992). With the increasing number of medications continually being added to the standard therapeutic regimens of HIV-infected patients, it will be even more important in the future to assess these agents pharmacologically in relation to psychoactive drugs, both prescribed and over-the-counter drugs.

As noted above, the high background prevalence of liver disease may complicate the treatment of drug injectors, because many therapeutic agents used for the management of HIV disease (e.g., a wide range of antibiotics and antiretroviral agents) have potential liver toxicities, especially among those with preexisting liver damage. Systematic studies of drug toxicity, side effects, and the ability to tolerate standard therapeutic regimens among HIV-infected drug users will increase in importance.

Because most of the therapies used for HIV infection and related conditions (e.g., tuberculosis) require long-term medical regimens, often involving multiple medications, the levels of adherence among drug users in a variety of treatment settings must be examined. In particular, the relationship between active substance abuse and adherence to medical care is a critical question requiring further study. Preliminary data in this area are somewhat conflicting; some studies suggest that substance abuse may interfere with effective use of health services, while others have found that adherence in a medical program oriented toward drug injectors is no lower among those actively using drugs (O'Connor et al., 1992; Samet et al., 1992; Selwyn, Feingold, Iezza, et al., 1989; Selwyn et al., 1993). Interventions to promote adherence to medical care among drug users will affect both clinical research and program evaluation.

Drug injectors as a group are likely to have a high lifetime prevalence of depression, anxiety, personality disorder, and other psychiatric diagnoses (Batki, 1990a; Rounsaville et al., 1991). In addition, underlying psychopathology, especially depression, was identified as a predictive factor for persistent risk-taking behavior among drug users in one study that linked continued needle sharing to depression, and certain psychiatric disorders may be associated with lack of engagement with or follow-up with medical care for HIV infection among drug users (Batki, 1990a). The comorbidity of drug abuse and psychiatric disorders is an important area for further study, to examine both the mental health determinants of risk-taking as well as the tendency to seek or avoid health care, and to develop strategies for enhancing engagement of follow-up with care. More fundamentally, these themes highlight the importance of pursuing a research and clinical agenda that brings together mental health services, drug abuse treatment, and medical care for HIV.

Among persons with HIV infection, drug users as a group are the least likely to have sustained and consistent contacts with the health care system, especially in the areas of primary care and preventive services. They are more likely to rely on acute care services, if at all, with episodic use of emergency rooms for acute HIV-related illnesses and medical complications of injection drug use (O'Connor et al., 1992). Compared with men who have sex with men, drug injectors are less likely to receive antiretroviral therapy for HIV infection within the health care system (Moore, Hidalgo, and Sugland, 1991; Rosenberg et al., 1991; Stein et al., 1991). In spite of these findings, however, it has been clearly demonstrated that drug users can achieve high levels of adherence to HIV-related medical care, including chronic, complex outpatient regimens, when these services have been made accessible and geared specifically to their needs. Several paradigms have been developed for the provision of HIV-related medical services to drug injectors, including on-site services within methadone programs and prisons, programs linking drug treatment and primary care centers, special hospital-based services, and outreach programs such as mobile medical van services linked to needle exchange (Altice et al., 1992; Altice et al., 1993; Glaser and Greifinger, 1993; O'Connor et al., 1992; Samet et al., 1992; Selwyn, Feingold, Iezza, et al., 1989; Selwyn et al., 1993). Health planning, policy, and basic health services and evaluation research must assess more formally the effectiveness of these and other models of care for drug users with or at risk of HIV infection. These questions also hold relevance for basic policy issues concerning the integration of substance abuse treatment into mainstream medical education and practice (Lewis et al., 1987), a trend that has been stimulated in part by the AIDS epidemic (National Commission on AIDS, 1991b).

INTERVENTIONS FOR THE SERIOUSLY MENTALLY ILL

The convergence of psychiatric disorders, substance abuse, and HIV among those who are also severely mentally ill raises difficult questions about appropriate treatment, similar to issues related to treatment of injection drug users. For example, possible toxic reactions between antipsychotic and anti-HIV medications, and perhaps even antinarcotic medications, require further investigation. Moreover, little if anything is yet known about HIV disease progression among the seriously mentally ill. Given what has already been learned about the interactions of the virus and the CNS, it is possible that unique manifestations occur among people already suffering brain disorders. Yet this area remains remarkably understudied.

A larger problem is the general failure of mental health and drug abuse service providers and medical professionals to adequately address treatment issues for dual- and triple-diagnosis patients, who, because they are perceived as difficult and complicated, often are "extruded" by treatment systems (Fine, 1993). Greater sensitivity and understanding about the mental and physical health problems and needs of this population, and a willingness to address them in managed treatment, is essential both to preventing transmission of HIV among them and to treating those already infected.

THE RELATIONSHIP BETWEEN PSYCHOSOCIAL FACTORS
AND HIV INFECTION

The final type of HIV, brain, and behavior interaction addressed in this chapter is the relationship between HIV infection and certain psychiatric disorders, behavioral states, or reactions. For example, concern about HIV infection can lead to anxiety or depression. The stress of coping with the illness is not confined to the person infected, but also encompasses those who care for him or her. The management of HIV infection carries both diagnostic and therapeutic implications that may not be directly related to HIV infection *per se*. It may be difficult to distinguish depression or anxiety from the AIDS dementia complex, because many symptoms overlap. The treatment is quite different—the dementia complex may respond to drugs that inhibit HIV replication, while depression and anxiety are more likely to respond to antidepressant and antianxiety medications—and so this distinction is clinically important. Since these conditions may also coexist, and the treatments themselves may affect CNS function, clinical management of both domains overlaps.

The bidirectional relationship between psychosocial factors and HIV infection can influence disease progression and the ability to effectively treat related symptoms. These phenomena primarily have been informed by two types of research: psychoneuroimmunology and psychosocial research on coping and caregiving.

PSYCHONEUROIMMUNOLOGY

The neurobiology of AIDS involves the possible influence of the nervous system on immune function and how both respond to HIV infection. In the context of HIV/AIDS, psychoneuroimmunology is the study of how mental states might modify immune defenses and even viral replication within the immune system. Depression and other mental states may have an impact on the immune system through the hypothalamic-pituitary-adrenal axis, the autonomic nervous system, and other pathways. Stress and other nervous system perturbations may alter immune function in both animal models and humans. The complex interactions among HIV infection, immune function, and mental state have been a major theme of AIDS-related research, particularly at NIMH. Although much has been learned about the effects of HIV on psychosocial factors, less is known about the effects of psychosocial factors on HIV. The few studies undertaken so far to examine this relationship show, variously, no effects of stressors (stressful life events) on illness progression (Kessler et al., 1991) and only an indirect relationship (Blaney et al., 1990). Further investigation is needed on when and how such effects may occur (Folkman, 1993).

The direct importance of mental states on progression of HIV infection is uncertain at best, and there is no clear evidence that one or another mental disorder or state either retards or accelerates progression. Two studies published simultaneously in December 1993 reached opposite conclusions about whether depression accelerated the decline of CD4+ lymphocyte counts.

Data from the Multicenter AIDS Cohort Study in Baltimore, on the one hand, revealed no evidence that depressive symptoms independently led to worse outcomes in HIV infections. Researchers concluded that symptom reports, CD4 counts, and socioeconomic status were confounding variables. Moreover, they concluded that because depression appears to be etiologically related to AIDS-related physical symptoms, those symptoms are probably direct confounders (Lyketsos et al., 1993).

Data from the San Francisco Men's Health Study, on the other hand, found that overall depression and affective depression predicted a more rapid decline in CD4 lymphocyte counts, and that this association was not attributable to baseline physical differences. Researchers were unable to identify the actual mechanism operating, but ruled out the possibility that the association was due to perceived somatic symptoms or to differences in substance abuse. However, they, too, concluded that the association between depression and disease progression may have been confounded by the impact of both on neurological disease (Burack et al., 1993). Neither study showed a significant effect of depressive symptoms or major depression on whether an HIV-positive subject was classified as having advanced AIDS or on overall mortality. The issue of the direction of the relationship between depression and HIV disease progression—to the extent that there actually is one—remains unresolved.

It is probable that CNS modulation of immune defenses is relatively minor in relation to the overwhelming influence of the virus and other determinants on the type and potency of immune responses to HIV. The bidirectional relationship between the CNS and the immune system, including nerve cell attachments to immune organs and how those may modify immune events, is nonetheless likely to influence the dynamics of HIV infection, although measuring such effects in HIV-infected persons may be extremely difficult because of the influence of cofactors, such as substance abuse, among some such individuals.

COPING WITH HIV/AIDS

For most people, the psychological impact of AIDS begins before an HIV test has even been taken, and for those who are HIV positive, it continues to change as the disease progresses. Research in the fields of psychology, psychiatry, epidemiology, anthropology, and sociology is contributing to a knowledge and understanding of the many psychosocial aspects of HIV/AIDS and has helped to point the way toward developing appropriate interventions.

The very decision to undergo an HIV test involves a calculation of costs and benefits on the part of the individual. The most significant costs include confronting the possibility of a positive test result and fearing a breach of confidentiality (Coates, Stall, Kegeles, et al., 1988). At the same time, the benefits of testing include clarifying one's HIV status and being motivated to change one's behavior in positive ways (Siegel et al., 1989). The difficulty of making this cost-benefit calculation is evident in the fact that many people, maybe as many as 28 percent, do not obtain the result of their tests (Catania, Kegeles, and Coates, 1990; McCusker et al., 1988; Peterson et al., 1990). Among those who do learn the results of their HIV test, research has found mixed reactions. Some studies have shown a significant increase in psychiatric symptoms, including depression, among those who were notified of their serostatus, compared with those who did not receive the test results (McCusker et al., 1988; Ostrow et al., 1989). Other research, however, found no such relationship, leading the authors to hypothesize that for some people, the stress of *not* knowing one's serostatus may be as significant as that of knowing (Perry et al., 1990).

After learning that they are HIV positive, most people "manage" and "tolerate"—as opposed to "master" or "eliminate"—the psychological changes that result (Folkman, 1993). This involves employing strategies of coping and social support, which are different at different stages of the disease. Studies of asymptomatic HIV-positive people suggest that "avoidant coping"—screening out the negative implications and focusing instead on the positive— does not protect them from distress (Joseph et al., 1990; Nicholson and Long, 1990; Rabkin et al., 1990; Storosum, Van Den Boom, and Beauzekom, 1990). This finding is consistent with the general literature on coping. But it is not yet known whether HIV-related situations inherently are more stressful than others, or if avoidant coping itself is inherently maladaptive (Folkman, 1993). Cognitive coping strategies, however, such as positive reinterpretation, gaining a sense of control over events, and effecting positive changes in daily life, seem to promote psychological well-being throughout the course of the disease (Hart et al., 1990; Rabkin et al., 1991; Storosum, Van Den Boom, and Beauzekom, 1990).

Although a number of studies have focused on the psychiatric implications of HIV/AIDS, they have not been able to determine whether psychiatric disorder is an effect of HIV or existed prior to HIV. For example, among gay men psychiatric morbidity rates are high relative to the general population regardless of HIV serostatus. This may be due to the fact that these men have to deal with a host of psychological issues related to their sexual status (Atkinson et al., 1988; Tross et al., 1987; Williams et al., 1991). This finding suggests the need to understand how the context of HIV affects psychiatric symptoms among gay men, that is, what disclosure and recognition of both being gay and having HIV may mean.

There is evidence that, at least among men, strong social support—from friends or family—is related to maintaining hope and morale throughout the progression of the disease (Rabkin et al., 1991). Unlike among heterosexuals, among gay men who are HIV-positive but not yet diagnosed with AIDS, peers are more significant than family (Hays et al., 1990). But this reverses once AIDS is diagnosed. The reluctance of many gay men to turn to family may be due to larger issues of being gay, as well as to more immediate issues of being geographically distant from family and having the strong support of the gay community in close proximity.

Once a person is diagnosed with AIDS, the psychological and psychiatric implications of having HIV are presumed to gain in importance and to take precedence over other considerations (Weitz, 1989). However, research on anxiety and depression has produced essentially mixed findings. Some studies have found more depression among symptomatic and asymptomatic HIV-positive individuals than among those who are AIDS-diagnosed (Chuang et al., 1989), while others have found higher rates of depression and anxiety among diagnosed men than among untested, seronegative, seropositive-asymptomatic, or seropositive-symptomatic men (Folkman et al., 1993).

These mixed findings suggest that people adjust to living with AIDS by adopting cognitive coping strategies. Some consciously adopt strategies for minimizing stress, anxiety, and depression, while others achieve it through the actions involved in living with AIDS, such as investigating new drug therapies, educating oneself about the illness, taking control of one's legal and financial affairs, and planning the end of one's life (Folkman et al., 1993; Namir et al., 1987).

Intervention research related to ameliorating the psychosocial effects of HIV/AIDS is still underdeveloped. The few studies undertaken to date have focused on maintaining positive morale

(Fawzy, Namir, and Wolcott, 1989) and on reducing stress and depression (Folkman et al., 1993; Perry et al., 1991) among people with HIV/AIDS. Nearly all of the research on coping to date, however, has focused on gay men. Much remains to be learned about how people from various gender, racial/ethnic, and cultural groups, and with different risk factors, such as injection drug users, cope with their own and others' HIV status, including not only general psychological strategies, but also motivation or resistance to adherence to medical treatment and its implications for disease progression. Future interventions should be brief, be theory-based, be effective in teaching coping skills, include techniques for maintaining such skills, and produce manuals that enable replication of the interventions elsewhere (Folkman, 1993).

In addition to the HIV-infected person, AIDS has psychosocial implications for those around him or her. One of these is bereavement—the experience of grief and loss of a loved one. Research on bereavement suggests that it is affected by the meaning of the death involved. In the case of AIDS, death occurs at a relatively young age, it afflicts the communities in which survivors participate—raising fears about their own risks *vis-à-vis* the disease, and it afflicts numerous members of the same community (Folkman, 1993). For gay men and injection drug users, AIDS-related loss is cumulative (McKusick and Hilliard, 1991; Neugebauer et al., 1992). Some of the psychological implications of such loss include traumatic stress response, demoralization, and sleep problems (Martin, 1988). Social support, to some degree, can help people recover from grief (Lennon, Martin, and Dean, 1990; Wortman, Silver, and Kessler, in press). Current research by Folkman and colleagues at the Center for AIDS Prevention Studies in San Francisco is addressing whether social support is a factor in successful coping with bereavement over time (Folkman, 1993).

CAREGIVING FOR PEOPLE WITH HIV/AIDS

The psychosocial impact of HIV/AIDS is experienced not only by people with the disease, but also by those who care for them. A large body of literature consistently associates caregiving with psychological and physical morbidity (e.g., Cantor, 1983; Gallo, 1990; Pruchno, Kleban, and Michaels, 1990), but this literature focuses primarily on caregiving among the frail elderly, which is usually performed by a female relative. Little is known about caregiving factors among men who are likely to be the caregivers of gay men with AIDS.

At this point in time, AIDS is a chronic, episodic, debilitating, and eventually fatal disease. Increasingly, AIDS care is being provided as much (if not more so) in the patient's home and by a lover or family member as it is in hospitals by trained professionals. A broad appreciation of the AIDS caregiving issue is central to an understanding of the complexity of providing high-quality, cost-effective support to those infected. But little is yet known about either the characteristics of people giving care—formally or informally—or the psychosocial implications of their work.

Informal Caregivers

So far, there has been no systematic research on the demographic and other characteristics of people providing informal AIDS care, that is people without professional training providing physical and psychological care in a home setting. However, data from recent studies (Folkman, Chesney, and Christopher-Richards, 1994; Turner, Catania, and Gagnon, 1994) suggest that AIDS caregivers of gay men do not fit the traditional caregiver profile—an older female family member who belongs to an age cohort with more prevalent chronic illnesses and who has been socialized to be nurturing. AIDS caregivers tend to be younger, just as likely male as female, and are diverse with respect to sexual orientation and relationship to the care recipient. In major cities, for example, 26 percent of AIDS caregivers are heterosexual men, 42 percent are heterosexual women, 25 percent are gay or bisexual men, and 7 percent are lesbian or bisexual women (Turner, Catania, and Gagnon, 1994). The caregiving role is thus highly non-normative for a large proportion of AIDS caregivers.

Many caregivers are the lovers or partners of gay men with AIDS. Some are HIV-positive themselves. Usually they are young, and instead of building relationships (an appropriate developmental task at this stage of life), they are preparing for loss. The relationships between these caregivers and their ill partners are usually informal and not legally sanctioned. Moreover, since AIDS is stigmatized, caregiving is frequently hidden from the family and community (Herek, 1990; McCann and Wadsworth, 1992; Raveis and Siegel, 1991). This situation also affects older gay persons with AIDS, for whom access to family care may be especially restricted. They are more likely to be geographically separated from their families, they are generally less able to rely on parents for caregiving support, and they are more often faced with ruptured family ties because of their sexual orientation (Turner and

Pearlin, 1989). For injection drug users on the other hand, evidence from one study suggests families do play a significant role in AIDS caregiving (Schiller, Crystal, and Karus, 1990).

Recent investigations into the mental health effects of AIDS caregiving has concentrated on the population of gay men providing care to their partners (Raveis and Siegel, 1991; Turner, 1988). This likely reflects the fact that gay men constituted over 60 percent of AIDS cases reported between 1981 and 1993 (CDC, 1994) and that one-third to one-half of gay men with AIDS are cared for by gay peers (McCann and Wadsworth, 1992; Turner, Catania, and Gagnon, 1994). However, other populations of caregivers (e.g., those who care for HIV-infected drug users) also deserve attention. While some of the psychological implications for gay caregivers may be unique to their particular status *vis-à-vis* the epidemic, others probably are not.

Many caregivers are on call at all times and are intensely emotionally involved. At the same time, they may have never before given physical care to a seriously ill person and have never watched someone die. Therefore, caregivers are forced to learn a range of skills on the job, including technical tasks, such as properly administering medication and inserting and cleaning catheters, and emotional tasks, such as maintaining hope in the face of continued disease progression, providing a safe environment for the expression of fear and anger, and providing support while the care recipient is dying (Folkman, Chesney, and Christopher-Richards, 1994). It is not uncommon for caregivers to experience dysphoria—an emotional state of depression, anxiety, and restlessness (Folkman, Chesney, and Christopher-Richards, 1994). They must adjust to the partner's unpredictable illness progression, the shifting of responsibility from the person with AIDS to the caregiving partner, the stress of unexpected, temporary improvement in the partner's health, dealing with a virtually uncontrollable disease, role conflict fatigue, and concern about their own future and who will care for them if they are HIV positive.

Nevertheless, caregivers attempt to maintain positive morale all the while they are dealing with such difficult circumstances. Coping strategies include finding ways to create meaning in life, for example, by extending love through their caregiving, and savoring the ordinary, by taking pleasure in the acts of everyday life (Folkman, Chesney, and Christopher-Richards, 1994).

Parental caregivers are usually later-life families who are beyond the childrearing years and whose children have begun careers of their own. Very little is known about them and the impact on families and parents of caring for an HIV-positive child (Mellins and Ehrhardt, 1993). Family history has been noted as an important factor in family caregiving patterns during the later years. A parent's sense of affection and obligation toward a gay son with AIDS is grounded in the family's history. It is affected both by structural factors, such as parent role and birth order, and social psychological factors, such as parent/child alliances and family members' perceptions of each other's personality. These factors are important for understanding how family members relate to one another when faced with a stressful event, such as a gay son acquiring AIDS, and how they then deal with their caregiving roles and responsibilities (Frierson, Lippman, and Johnson, 1987).

The important role of families in the care of people with AIDS has not yet been adequately recognized in the health care system, which for example still focuses on individual case management plans (Goeren, Wade, and Rodriguez, 1990). In order to design a truly comprehensive plan, a family case management model might be employed that would include family treatment (medical, nursing, and psychological) and family-focused clinical trials. Expanded training of health care providers is needed in order to incorporate such a family systems approach in the care of HIV-infected individuals.

Formal Caregivers: Health Care Professionals

As with informal caregivers, not much is yet known about formal caregivers. For the most part, research has focused on how health care workers deal with the stress and burnout of providing care to AIDS patients. Some of the most significant sources of stress include working with stigmatized clients, confronting one's own sexuality, and facing dying patients who are the same age as the caregivers. The most significant predictors of the dimensions of burnout are time pressure (emotional exhaustion), vague criteria of success (reduced personal accomplishment), and stress related to client behavior (depersonalization). Research has found that people who use confrontational coping strategies are reportedly less likely to suffer burnout.

Surprisingly, stress caused by death and dying of the client is not a significant predictor of burnout among AIDS caregivers, as it has not been for caregivers in the fields of oncology and geriatrics. The confrontation with death and dying instead seems to promote the personal growth of health care personnel and the sense of meaning in their lives (Kleiber et al., 1992).

Although stress experienced by HIV caregivers is reported in professional and lay articles, research has not included systematic documentation of the incidence and prevalence of physical, psychological, occupational, or interpersonal symptoms or disorders in health care professionals who devote a substantial amount of their clinical activities to patients with HIV illness (Silverman, 1993). Surveys have revealed that fear of contagion is a significant sentiment expressed by health care professionals resistant to providing AIDS care (Silverman, 1993). Anecdotal evidence of AIDS-related nightmares, psychological numbing, aversion to patients with HIV infection, and exhaustion among professionals providing AIDS-related health care also have been reported (Friedland, 1989; Shulman and Mantell, 1988; Silverman, 1993). These symptoms, together with others related to stress and depression, suggest that some caregivers might be experiencing a form of post-traumatic stress disorder. However, according to Silverman (1993), only one published psychiatry article has addressed this possibility (Horstman and McKusick, 1986).

The psychological and physical implications of AIDS caregiving for health professionals undoubtedly is affected by their attitude toward AIDS. Surveys among nurses, physicians, dentists, social workers, psychiatrists, and health profession students are notable for revealing a consistent aversion among caregivers to the HIV/AIDS disease, to patients and their lifestyles, and to caregiving work itself (Silverman, 1993).

Future Research on Caregiving

As HIV/AIDS is shifting from a seemingly immediate, fatal disease, to a more chronic (but still apparently fatal) syndrome, the roles and responsibilities of caregivers—both informal and formal—toward people with AIDS also will change. In order to provide the best possible circumstances for both provider and recipient of AIDS care, much more research must be conducted on the psychological and social factors involved at both ends of the relationship. For example, more information is needed about which particular aspects of social support and health are associated, how this association changes over time according to the stage of the disease, and the socioeconomic and cultural characteristics of those with HIV (Green, 1993).

More information is needed about the types of individuals who typically provide informal care to persons with AIDS, including their relationship to the patient, the characteristics of both patients and caregivers that influence the acquisition and quality of informal care, the objective and subjective burden imposed by caregiving, and the impact of such burdens on the health and well-being of the caregivers (Turner, Catania, and Gagnon, 1994).

With respect to family caregivers, studying the characteristics that differentiate low-stress from high-stress families may enable professionals to develop interventions for high-stress families (Takigiku, Brubaker, and Hennon, 1993). It also will be important to include an examination of the special needs of families in which more than one member is HIV infected (Goeren, Wade, and Rodriguez, 1990).

In the particular case of parent caregivers of gay sons with AIDS, research should further develop contextual models of stress that take into account the family's ethos of affection/obligation, the unique meanings that families attach to the situations surrounding a gay son with AIDS, and how those might be influenced by gender, race/ethnicity, and the attitudes family members have toward homosexuality (Takigiku, Brubaker, and Hennon, 1993). Similar considerations should be applied to studies of caregiving among injection drug users and others.

In some instances, the parent caregiver of a person with AIDS also is HIV infected. This is frequently the situation in pediatric AIDS cases, approximately 85 percent of which result from vertical transmission (Susser et al., 1992). In these cases, caregiving is complicated by one's own illness. For example, studies have shown that HIV-positive parent caregivers are significantly more depressed and demoralized than HIV-negative parents (Susser et al., 1992). The particular needs of these parents should be identified and appropriate interventions should be developed.

With respect to formal caregiving, empirical research that can test hypotheses such as the existence of undiagnosed occupational, physical, and psychiatric morbidity related to HIV caregiving is needed. Moreover, research on stress among AIDS-related health care workers must move beyond the anecdotal and descriptive to theoretical and comparative perspectives that can locate the particular experience of AIDS caregiving within larger issues of professional stress and aversion to certain diseases and the people who suffer them. Adequate HIV/AIDS caregiving increasingly will require a deeper appreciation of the relationships between such things as social group dynamics and status and psychological and physical morbidity experienced both by people with HIV/AIDS and by their caregivers. A related issue worthy of study is the psychological and social consequences (including occupational stress) of dealing with HIV/AIDS among outreach workers and service providers (Broadhead and Fox, 1993).

CONCLUSION AND RECOMMENDATIONS

CONCLUSION

Examining the interactions among HIV infection, the central nervous system, and psychosocial factors related to disease progression and intervention makes it apparent that, although crucial insights have been gained, a number of urgent questions remain. The gaps in knowledge identified in this chapter point the way for future research at the institutes charged with focusing on the interactions of brain and behavior. Any successful approach to the prevention, treatment, and management of AIDS—especially as it becomes a more chronic disease—must combine highly focused research in many disciplines with integrative, cross-disciplinary efforts that synthesize the biological and psychosocial to address questions that range from understanding the molecular mechanisms of nerve cell dysfunction to identifying the specific health care problems of those with multiple diagnoses.

RECOMMENDATIONS FOR DISEASE PROGRESSION AND INTERVENTION

4.1 The committee recommends that NIMH continue research on the pathogenesis of HIV infection of the brain, including the factors controlling virus replication such as local immune defenses and changes in the viral genome determining neuropathogenicity.

4.2 The committee recommends that NIMH continue research on the pathobiology of nervous system injury underlying the AIDS dementia complex, including the morphological, biochemical, and molecular basis of neuronal dysfunction related to viral and cellular gene expression.

4.3 The committee recommends that NIMH support collaborative studies of the prevention and treatment of the AIDS dementia complex and other central nervous system complications of HIV infection.

4.4 The committee recommends that NIAAA, NIDA, and NIMH continue supporting research on the development of animal models for examining the basic neurochemical and behavioral changes associated with HIV/AIDS.

4.5 The committee recommends that NIAAA, NIDA, and NIMH expand research on the natural history of HIV infection among various populations, including injection drug users, other substance abusers, and the seriously mentally ill.

4.6 The committee recommends that NIAAA, NIDA, and NIMH support research on the relationship between the medical consequences of substance abuse and related behaviors and the clinical expression of HIV among the drug-using population.

4.7 The committee recommends that NIAAA, NIDA, and NIMH support research at the intersection of AIDS treatment and clinical care for substance abusers, addressing, for example, how to treat HIV/AIDS in mental health and substance abuse treatment programs.

4.8 The committee recommends that NIAAA, NIDA, and NIMH collaborate on research to investigate interactions among psychotropic (including illicit) drugs, antinarcotic and antipsychotic medications, and drugs used to treat HIV and opportunistic infections—for example, the effect of methadone on zidovudine (AZT)—including research on toxicities that might develop through such drug interactions.

4.9 The committee recommends that NIAAA, NIDA, and NIMH support more research on the neuropharmacology of anti-HIV medication.

4.10 The committee recommends that all relevant NIH institutes eliminate systemic barriers to the inclusion of injection drug users and other substance abusers in AIDS and AIDS-related clinical trials.

4.11 The committee recommends that NIAAA, NIDA, and NIMH support research on the utilization of health resources by people with AIDS, including substance abuse and mental health treatment programs. This research might include studies of the extent and manner in which the medical system acts (intentionally or not) to exclude drug users from care.

4.12 The committee recommends that NIAAA, NIDA, and NIMH support research on the relationship between adherence to HIV/AIDS medical treatment and disease progression among individuals from diverse gender, racial/ethnic, and cultural groups.

4.13 The committee recommends that NIAAA, NIDA, and NIMH support research that integrates substance abuse and mental health treatment; in particular, demonstration projects for integrated multidisciplinary treatment systems that include mental health.

4.14 The committee recommends that NIMH support research on positive as well as negative consequences of HIV, for example, how people with AIDS and their caregivers maintain positive coping strategies in the face of the disease.

4.15 The committee recommends that NIAAA, NIDA, and NIMH support research on how families (broadly defined to include persons who consider themselves to be family through mutual commitment) from diverse racial/ethnic, socioeconomic, and sexual orientation backgrounds cope with the reality of having family members who are infected with HIV or have AIDS. Special attention should be given to patterns and consequences of caregiving in such families.

PART II

Managing the AIDS Research Programs at NIAAA, NIDA, and NIMH

5

The Context of AIDS Programs at NIAAA, NIDA, and NIMH

In order to analyze the AIDS research programs of NIAAA, NIDA, and NIMH, one must understand the larger context in which they have been operating. The most significant elements of this context from the point of view of this study are the passage of the ADAMHA Reorganization Act of 1992 (PL 102-321), which separated ADAMHA's research and services entities into two different agencies (NIH and SAMHSA, respectively), and the NIH Revitalization Act of 1993 (PL 103-43), which assigned the NIH Office of AIDS Research (OAR)—housed in the office of the NIH director—new budgetary authority over the AIDS programs of all NIH institutes. These two major legislative events occurred while the committee's assessment of the ADAMHA AIDS programs was under way, and, although they were not intended to be the focus of this report, they are an important part of the overall context in which AIDS research at NIAAA, NIDA, and NIMH was conducted in the recent past and will be conducted in the future. Also, the changes will have considerable impact on the institutes' AIDS programs and their connection to AIDS services programs elsewhere in the Public Health Service (PHS). Because these changes are quite recent, much of their potential impact can only be suggested.

There are other contextual factors that also were influenced by the ADAMHA reorganization and the new authority of the NIH OAR, and that in turn affect the nature of the AIDS programs of NIAAA, NIDA, and NIMH. These are the overall and AIDS-specific budget process and the grant review process. It is important to understand the budget process because it governs the activities of all federal agencies, by circumscribing the financial constraints under which they operate from year to year. The review process is equally important to understand because it influences the scientific identity of the institutes by determining which specific research projects get funded.

THE REORGANIZATION OF ADAMHA

BACKGROUND

As outlined in Box 5.1, the organization of ADAMHA (and its predecessors) has always been problematic (IOM, 1991b). This is largely because, unlike the rest of the Public Health Service, ADAMHA included research, service, public health, and training activities all in one agency. The debate about the advantages and disadvantages of various options for administering all of these components continued (with periods of greater and lesser intensity) until Congress passed the ADAMHA Reorganization Act in 1992, which for the first time separated services and research into different agencies. On October 1, 1992, NIAAA, NIDA, and NIMH were moved organizationally to NIH, and a new agency—the Substance Abuse and Mental Health Services Administration (SAMHSA)—was created to manage the former ADAMHA service functions.

According to individuals both inside and outside of the Department of Health and Human Services (HHS), a number of complex reasons explain why the separation of research and services occurred successfully in 1992 and not earlier. First, the number of new programs and the budgets for these programs (especially those related to substance abuse) increased rapidly during the later part of the 1980s. As the agency grew, it had a more difficult time balancing the competing and sometimes conflicting missions of research and services (including the conflicting demands of constituency groups). Although internally the agency increasingly focused on research (by the late 1980s, the ADAMHA administrator and the directors of all three institutes were research scientists), the external community and HHS were more concerned about service and prevention activities. Under Bernadine Healy, NIH, which previously had fought against incorporating ADAMHA's research institutes, changed its position and actively sought the transfer of NIAAA, NIDA, and NIMH to NIH. The Office of National Drug Control Policy (ONDCP) in the White House also strongly favored the reorganization and believed that the research

Box 5.1
A Brief History of Research and Services Programs
for Mental Health and Substance Abuse

The purpose of the following chronology is to describe the chain of events that eventually led to the October 1, 1992 reorganization of ADAMHA. It is based on information from of the IOM Report—*Research and Service Programs in the PHS: Challenges in Organization* (IOM, 1991b), from a chronology prepared by the SAMHSA Legislative Office, from the Lewin and Associates (1988) study, and from the 1991 hearings on ADAMHA Reauthorization.

1929   Congress authorized a Narcotics Division within the PHS to administer two "narcotics farms."

1930   The division was renamed the Division of Mental Hygiene and its objectives were expanded to include medical and psychiatric care in federal correctional institutions.

1946   The National Mental Health Act led to the establishment of the National Institute of Mental Health (NIMH), which had three separate missions based on the premise that research, training, and services were inherently interrelated. Following considerable debate, NIMH ultimately became an institute of NIH. It was a unique institute not only because of its explicit commitment to services, but because it was the only NIH institute to strongly support behavioral and social science research.

1950s   As the service mission of NIMH grew, the NIH director began to oppose the inclusion of services within any part of the NIH program.

1960   As part of a general PHS reorganization there was an unsuccessful proposal to move the services programs of NIMH (which made up 9 percent of the budget) to other PHS bureaus. This move was defeated by the director of NIMH with congressional support.

1963   The Community Mental Health Center (CMHC) Act led to a major shift in NIMH budgetary priorities—establishing community-based psychiatric treatment and developing separate community-based treatment centers for alcohol and drug abuse.

1966   The National Center for Prevention and Control of Alcoholism (which included research, training, and services programs) and the Center for Studies of Narcotic Addiction and Drug Abuse were both established as part of NIMH. Funding for the services programs had increased to 24 percent.

continued on next page

Box 5.1 Continued

1967   A number of factors contributed to growing controversy around NIMH: the budget for the CMHC programs exceeded the NIMH budget, which caused concern within the research community that services programs had priority over research programs; NIMH targeted more of its research budget toward research into social problems, which was not viewed as an appropriate mission of NIH; NIMH was the largest NIH institute (22 percent of total NIH budget) and its leadership believed that because of its size and unique mission, it should become an independent agency.

PHS was reorganized and, despite opposition from the NIH director and the research community, NIMH became an independent agency. It was the only institute to leave NIH, and the research community believed that its research program would suffer. The intramural program remained on the NIH campus and research grants continued to be processed by the Division of Research Grants.

1968   NIMH was moved into the Health Services and Mental Health Administration, a new PHS agency established to coordinate service delivery programs.

The Comprehensive Mental Health Centers Act was amended to establish alcohol and treatment facilities and link them with mental health treatment facilities.

1970   The Comprehensive Alcohol Abuse and Alcoholism Prevention, Treatment, and Rehabilitation Act mandated the establishment of NIAAA as a separate institute within NIMH.

1972   The Drug Abuse and Treatment Act mandated the establishment of NIDA within NIMH. Although NIAAA and NIDA were part of NIMH, a 1972 internal management study concluded that all three institutes should become separate institutes working on equal terms under one administrative umbrella. NIMH was not reorganized, however, and the controversy over NIMH's mission resurfaced.

1973   As a result of the Nixon administration's efforts to limit the federal role in the provision of services, PHS was reorganized and NIMH was moved back to NIH to refocus its effort on research. At the time of the transfer, services represented 50 percent of its budget. After the reorganization Congress appropriated additional funds to treatment programs. The research community was concerned that NIMH's research programs were suffering.

Box 5.1 Continued

The Mental Health (Gordner) Task Force—established to determine how best to administer the needs for research, services, and training—presented various organizational options for restructuring NIMH activities. The task force favored integrating mental health, drug and alcohol abuse research, training, and services into the larger health care system, but also believed in a need for continued visibility and leadership (especially in the area of alcohol and drug abuse). The task force also concluded that the fields of alcohol and drug abuse should gradually be combined.

The Secretary of Health, Education, and Welfare chose that task force's option to create the Alcohol, Drug Abuse, and Mental Health Administration (ADAMHA). This option established three separate and equal institutes—NIAAA, NIDA, and NIMH. The mission of each institute continued to combine research, training, and services.

After this reorganization, a greater proportion of ADAMHA's budget was being spent on services rather than research and the research community believed that the research program was suffering because of its placement in ADAMHA.

1981 The categorical and formula grant programs at NIAAA, NIDA, and NIMH were combined into one single Alcohol, Drug Abuse, and Mental Health block grant to the states. Under this block grant system, most of the leadership responsibilities for services fell to the states. As a result, the three institutes began to focus on improving their research programs. The administration proposed eliminating social policy research.

1986 The Anti-Drug Abuse Act mandated the establishment of the Office for Substance Abuse Prevention (OSAP) to award demonstration grants to community agencies for preventing substance abuse among youth and for preventing AIDS among drug abusers. It was organizationally located in the Office of the Administrator because of fears it would not receive proper attention in the increasingly research-oriented institutes.

1987 The Homeless Assistance Act authorized additional demonstration programs and a services block grant for targeting homeless people with mental illness and substance abuse problems. The senior leadership of ADAMHA agreed that the agency should increase its research focus and explore ways of divesting itself of the service programs.

continued on next page

Box 5.1 Continued

The placement of both research and services within ADAMHA continued to be an issue, and the Senate requested a position statement from the Department of Health and Human Services (HHS). HHS commissioned Lewin and Associates to investigate the organizational options for ADAMHA, which resulted in the "Lewin Report."

1988   The Lewin Report identified five options for the reorganization of ADAMHA, yet no organizational changes occurred.

The Anti-Drug Abuse Act raised OSAP to an institute level in ADAMHA and led to the administrative creation of the Office for Treatment Improvement. Congress began to appropriate increasing amounts of money for ADAMHA prevention and treatment activities.

1991   The Institute of Medicine issued its report on the study of co-administration of services and research programs in PHS. The report indicated that the structure of the organization was less important in determining the administration of programs than the nature of the policies guiding program administration. It, therefore, recommended that agency-level organization not be used as the basis for deterring or encouraging reorganization.

In the spring of 1991, the administrator of ADAMHA sent a reorganization proposal to the assistant secretary for health to separate research and services programs into two agencies. NIH submitted a reorganization proposal to incorporate the ADAMHA research institutes into NIH as three separate institutes. In June 1991, the secretary presented his reorganization proposal which called for creating a "new ADAMHA" composed of the services programs and moving the research programs to NIH. Following the secretary's proposal, both Senate and House committees held hearings on the proposed reorganization. Although legislation authorizing the reorganization was approved by the Senate in 1991, the House could not reach agreement on all sections of the legislation and the bill had to be considered again the next year.

1992   The ADAMHA Reorganization Act authorized the separation of services and research by transferring NIAAA, NIDA, and NIMH to NIH and by establishing a new service agency—Substance Abuse and Mental Health Services Administration (SAMHSA). The proposed changes became effective October 1, 1992.

orientation of ADAMHA made it difficult to respond to immediate policy imperatives related to services—a concern also voiced by Fred Goodwin, administrator of ADAMHA, in his reorganization proposal. In addition, the budgets of the services programs grew enough to be viable as a free-standing agency within the PHS. At the same time, ADAMHA research administrators feared that if budgets were limited, the service programs would be favored at the expense of research activities. In short, a combination of factors fostered a political climate that favored reorganization.

STRUCTURAL EFFECTS OF THE ADAMHA REORGANIZATION

Overall, the reorganization appears to have had a limited effect on the research programs of the three institutes. Their organizational structure and staffing have been left largely intact, and their review process remains the same as it was at ADAMHA for the period FY 1993 through FY 1996, as mandated by the reorganization legislation. Figure 5.1 shows the structure of ADAMHA prior to the reorganization. NIAAA, NIDA, and NIMH were primarily focused on research, whereas OTI and OSAP focused on services programs. Prior to reorganization in 1992, ADAMHA had 2,186 full-time employees (FTEs). Nearly three-quarters of the ADAMHA FTEs (1,602) were related to the research programs and the remaining one-quarter (585) was related to service activities. The majority of the AIDS funding and staffing was and remains in the research institutes. (See Chapter 6.)

Figure 5.2 shows the current organization of SAMHSA. In 1992, there were 656 staff positions, which represented the 585 service positions from ADAMHA plus approximately 70 additional positions added during the reorganization, mainly in the newly created Center for Mental Health Services. The majority of these service positions came from the former OTI, OSAP, and the office of the administrator, but some were originally non-research functions in the three institutes that were subsequently transferred to SAMHSA.

Box 5.2 highlights the programs and activities that were transferred from ADAMHA to SAMHSA as a result of the reorganization. Of these 24 programs, only three are directly related to AIDS: AIDS health care worker training (moved from NIMH to CMHS); AIDS health care worker training/AIDS hotline (moved from NIDA to CSAT); and the service delivery demonstrations (also moved from NIDA to CSAT).

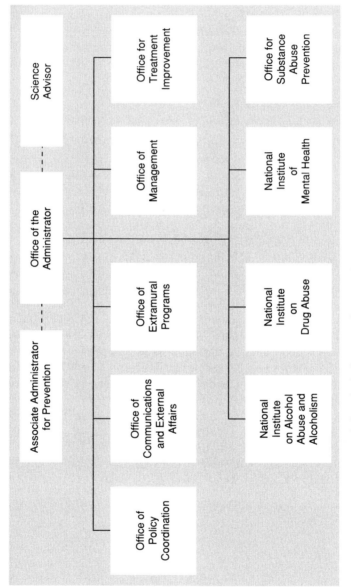

FIGURE 5.1 Organization of the Alcohol, Drug Abuse, and Mental Health Administration (ADAMHA).

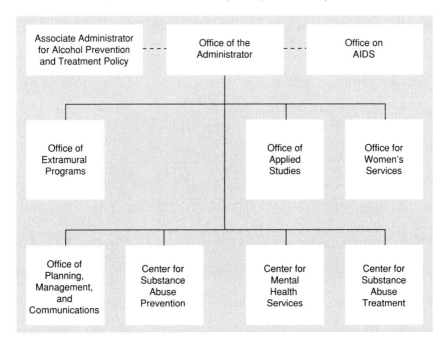

FIGURE 5.2 Organization of the Substance Abuse and Mental Health Services Administration (SAMHSA).

Figure 5.3 shows the organization of NIH after the reorganization. The reorganization added approximately 1,600 positions to NIH, all but 31 assigned directly to the three institutes. These 31 positions were research-related positions from the Office of the Administrator at ADAMHA and were assigned to the Office of the Director at NIH.

Although the reorganization appears to have had limited direct effect on the AIDS research programs of the three institutes, the Congressional Report language accompanying the Reorganization Act raised concerns about the amount of attention the three institutes devoted to AIDS. The bill required NIDA and NIMH to each create an Office on AIDS, which:

> . . . shall be responsible for the coordination of research and determining the direction of the Institute with respect to AIDS research related to: (1) Primary prevention of the spread of HIV, including transmission via drug abuse [sexual behavior in the case of NIMH]; (2) drug abuse services research [mental health services research for NIMH]; and (3) other matters determined appropriate by the Director.

The bill made no specific mention of NIAAA.

Box 5.2
ADAMHA Programs Transferred to SAMHSA as a
Result of Reorganization

Center for Mental Health Services (CMHS)	Transferred From
1. Community Support Program (CSP)	NIMH
2. Mental Health Homeless Demonstrations	NIMH
3. Alcohol Homeless Demonstrations	NIAAA
4. PATH Homeless Formula Grant	NIMH
5. Mental Health Protection and Advocacy	NIMH
6. Mental Health State Planning	NIMH
7. CMHC Construction Monitoring	NIMH
8. Mental Health Statistics Improvement Program	NIMH
9. National Reporting Program	NIMH
10. Mental Health Clinical Training	NIMH
11. AIDS Health Care Worker Training	**NIMH**
12. Refugee Mental Health	NIMH
13. Emergency Services	NIMH
14. Other Programs	NIMH
15. SEH Worker's Compensation	Office of the Administrator
16. Buildings and Facilities funds	Buildings Account
17. Mental Health Services Block Grant	OTI

Center for Substance Abuse Prevention (CSAP)	
1. Workplace Helpline	NIDA

Center for Substance Abuse Treatment (CSAT)	
1. Substance Abuse Clinical Training	OSAP
2. AIDS Health Care Worker Training/Hotline	**NIDA**
3. HRSA Service Delivery Demonstrations	**NIDA**
4. Pregnant and Post-Partum Women Program	OSAP

Office of the Administrator (OA)	
1. Quick Response Surveys and Special Projects	NIDA
2. Data Collection Programs	NIDA
3. Service System Evaluation	NIDA

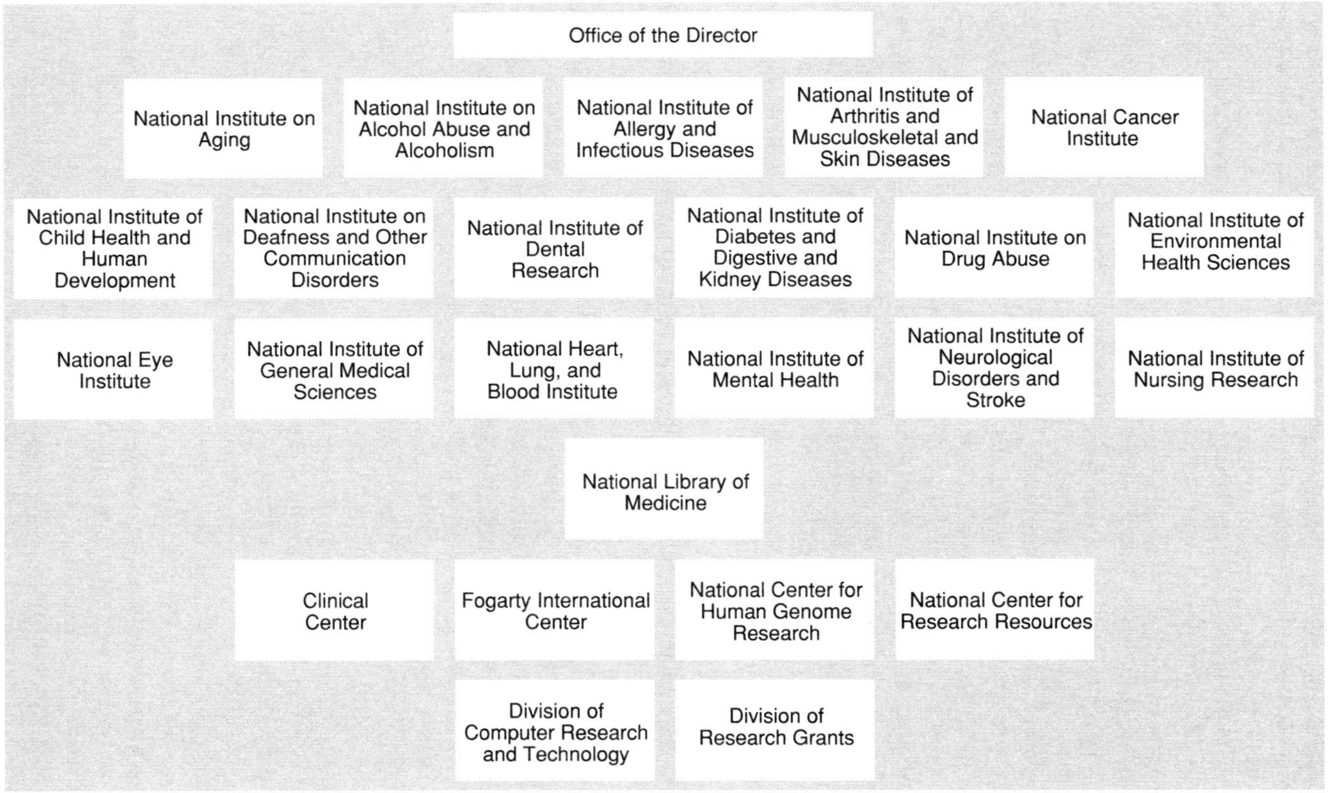

FIGURE 5.3 Organization of the National Institutes of Health.

During the 1980s, NIAAA, NIDA, and NIMH faced management demands to develop, implement, coordinate, and evaluate a rapidly growing, complex program of AIDS activities. However, ADAMHA never had an official, authorized, functioning AIDS office. Because HHS was considering reorganization, ADAMHA created an acting AIDS office rather than a permanent one. In addition, this office was headed by a part-time acting coordinator, who also directed the NIMH AIDS office. At no time during its existence did ADAMHA budget more than two or three positions for central AIDS management. Overall, the ADAMHA AIDS activity was seen as collegial and cooperative and not as directive or managerial. Consequently, each institute at ADAMHA devised its own way to manage its AIDS program, which operated quite differently from every other: NIAAA had only one or two staff acting as AIDS coordinators on a part-time basis; NIDA had an official AIDS coordinator located within one of its regular divisions; and NIMH had a formal Office on AIDS Programs with a full-time director. (Further discussion of the institute's AIDS offices appears in chapter 6.)

AIDS RESEARCH AND THE NIH REAUTHORIZATION

Simultaneous with the ADAMHA reorganization, NIH underwent changes in its leadership, and under the NIH reauthorization bill passed in 1993 developed a much more centrally managed AIDS research effort. The NIH reauthorization bill, which was signed into law June 10, 1993, contains a number of provisions concerning AIDS research supported by NIH. Some of these provisions specifically affect the planning and budgeting process for NIH. Although the law had been in effect for many months by the time this report was written, a number of provisions regarding the budget were not yet operational, given the extended time involved in the budget process. Additionally, NIH had not completed the process of implementing other legislative requests, and therefore it was not yet clear how the revamped AIDS research program would operate.

The intent of the legislation was to strengthen the central control and management of AIDS research by NIH (through the Office of AIDS Research) while maintaining research direction in the hands of individual institutes, centers, and divisions (ICDs). Despite the tensions between proponents of central control and dispersed operation, it is believed by advocates for the new OAR authority that the arrangement will create better coordination of NIH AIDS activities.

The 1993 NIH reauthorization bill builds upon previous NIH attempts to coordinate and focus its AIDS research while preserving the scientific independence of the various institutes. The Senate report accompanying the bill indicates that the legislation intends to "mandate completion of an AIDS research plan that formally states priorities and resources needs for every aspect of the nation's biomedical and behavioral research effort." The plan should ensure that overlapping expertise and information is shared and coordinated between HIV and other research endeavors by determining an overall AIDS research budget level as part of the overall budget process.

The legislation continues on a path of greater central coordination that began in 1982 with the creation of an inter-institute coordinating group to track NIH AIDS research activities and to share information among the institutes involved in AIDS research. Previous actions had included the establishment of an NIH AIDS Executive Committee in 1984, the appointment of an NIH AIDS coordinator in 1985, the administrative creation of OAR in April 1988, and the legislative authorization of OAR in November 1988. Although since its inception OAR has had an important voice in shaping the NIH AIDS program, this strength principally has resided in its incumbent director, rather than in the inherent authority of OAR. The actual statement of function for the OAR describes a classic staff office responsible for advising, supporting, coordinating, recommending, and fostering the NIH AIDS research program (IOM, 1991a).

The 1993 NIH Revitalization Act specifically provides new and greater authority to OAR with regard to the AIDS budget. The Act requires a comprehensive plan for the expenditures of appropriations, and authorizes an emergency discretionary fund for the director of OAR. According to the legislation, the plan must: provide for the conduct and support of all AIDS activities at NIH; prioritize the various AIDS activities, which are required to have objectives, measures, and a time frame; ensure that the budget is allocated according to the plan; review the plan annually and update it as needed; ensure that approval of specific projects and ongoing operation remain with the individual institute, center, and division directors; and ensure that the plan includes a range of research (including basic, applied, intramural, extramural, investigator-initiated, NIH-directed, and behavioral and social science research).

This comprehensive plan is meant to be the basis for developing the annual budget requests for AIDS research. The director of OAR (*not* the director of NIH) is required to develop a full-funding budget that provides for the ". . . amounts necessary for the agencies of the National Institutes of Health to carry out all AIDS activities determined by the Director of the Office to be appropriate, without regard to the probability that such amounts will be appropriated" for each fiscal year. This budget (called the "professional judgment budget" or "bypass budget") is to be submitted from the director of OAR directly to the president for review and submission to Congress. The NIH director, the secretary of HHS, and the AIDS Advisory Council should all have the opportunity to comment on, but not change, the budget before it is submitted. In addition, the director of OAR is required to submit another budget package as part of the normal federal budget cycle. This budget package is to include the full-funding budget, a budget based on current activities and those initiatives for which there is the most substantial need, and other budgets as appropriate. The director of NIH and the secretary of HHS are required to consider all such budget estimates when recommending their annual budgets to the president.

When AIDS funds are appropriated to NIH by Congress, they will go directly to the director of OAR. The director will allocate to the individual institutes, centers, and divisions all of the funds received in accordance with the previously approved comprehensive plan for expenditures and appropriations. Funds to support existing AIDS activities, including ". . . projects or programs for which the Agencies have made a commitment of continued support," will be allocated by the OAR director within 15 days of his or her receipt of the funds. The director will then allocate the rest of the AIDS appropriations to the institutes, centers, and divisions within 30 days, if possible. This process will be in place beginning FY 1995.

The second major change in the budgetary process created by the NIH reauthorization bill is the emergency discretionary fund from which the director of OAR, in consultation with the AIDS Advisory Council, may make expenditures to support the AIDS research activities authorized by the legislation. This fund is designed to allow the NIH to respond to rapidly changing research problems and priorities, and grew out of concerns that inflexible budget rules may prohibit important and time-sensitive research (such as research on multi-drug resistant tuberculosis). The Act provides for the appropriation of up to $100 million in each of FY

1994, 1995, and 1996, and provides limitations and safeguards on the use of the funds. In particular, the projects supported by the funds must be peer reviewed; the funds must be used for a particular set of AIDS activities that constitute either a new project or additional AIDS activities for an existing project and for which the director has determined that there is a significant need; they cannot be used for more than two years for a specific set of activities; they cannot be used for purposes that were disapproved by Congress either explicitly or implicitly; and they cannot be used for construction or renovation, nor can they be invested. The director of OAR is required to submit to Congress annually a report describing how and why the funds were used during the previous fiscal year.

THE BUDGET PROCESS

Funding of ADAMHA and NIH AIDS activities over time has taken place within the larger context of the overall federal budget process and has been directly affected by it. Appreciating the length and complexity of the budget process is critical for understanding the problems faced by rapidly changing and expanding research areas such as AIDS and by organizations that are in the process of restructuring, as were ADAMHA and NIH during the course of this study.

The overall budget process has been relatively stable over time and generally has operated similarly at ADAMHA and NIH. Although there were minor changes from time to time during the 1980s and early 1990s, and even with the reorganization of ADAMHA, the larger budget structure of PHS, HHS, the Office of Management and Budget (OMB), and Congress remained the same. In addition, PHS and HHS always had an unwritten policy of treating the research budgets of NIH and ADAMHA essentially the same.

At any one point in time, an institute (whether at ADAMHA, SAMHSA, or NIH) must consider its research program in relation to *three* separate budgets. This is illustrated in Figure 5.4, which displays the current budget calendar for an NIH institute.

At the end of calendar year 1993, the institute was in the midst of utilizing its current (FY 1994) funds (Execution), which were allocated through September 30, 1994. At the same time, the institute was involved in presenting and defending (Justification) its next year's budget (FY 1995) to reviewers ranging from OAR at NIH, HHS, OMB, and various committees within the Congress, as

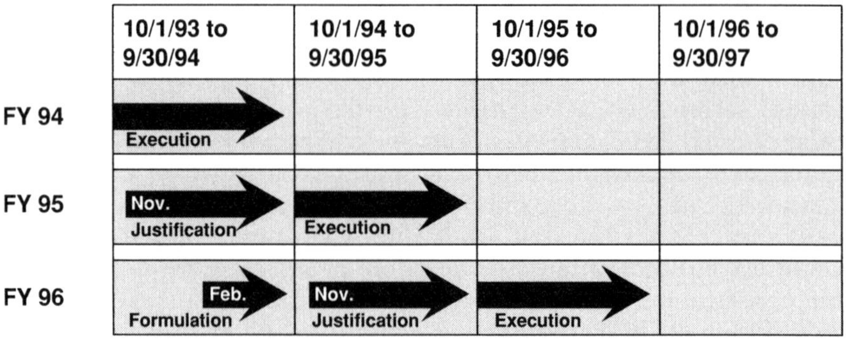

	10/1/93 to 9/30/94	10/1/94 to 9/30/95	10/1/95 to 9/30/96	10/1/96 to 9/30/97
FY 94	Execution →			
FY 95	Nov. Justification →	Execution →		
FY 96	Feb. Formulation →	Nov. Justification →	Execution →	

FIGURE 5.4 Budget Calendar.

well as to various interest groups who become more involved as the budget becomes public. Starting approximately in February 1994, the individual institutes and the NIH central budget office (and OAR) began specific plans (Formulation) for the FY 1996 budget, which will be in effect from October 1995 to September 30, 1996. In addition to dealing with issues directly related to the FY 1994 and FY 1995 budgets, the institute had to consider future budgets in relation to the "NIH Five Year Plan for HIV-Related Research" (the AIDS plan described above), the overall NIH Strategic Plan, and other cross-cutting plans that the individual institute may have had. The multi-year nature of this process is also demonstrated in Figure 5.5, which focuses on the FY 1994 budget planning cycle that began in November of 1991 and governed institute spending through September 30, 1994. (An additional complexity that is not shown in Figure 5.5 is that prior to reorganization, the White House Office on National Drug Control Policy reviewed the drug-related portions of the ADAMHA budget. In addition, the National AIDS Program Office [NAPO] assumed responsibility for reviewing the AIDS budget requests of all PHS agencies beginning in FY 1990.)

With this general overview of the budget process and its complexity in mind, one can now look at the more specific experiences of ADAMHA and NIH budgeting as they relate to AIDS funding.

ADAMHA BUDGET PROCESS, FY 1983 TO FY 1992

The budget process for ADAMHA remained relatively stable since FY 1983, when the first funds were appropriated for AIDS

1991	October	FY 1992 Begins
	November	Planning for FY 1994 Budget Begins
	December	
1992	January	Individual Institutes Formulate Budget Requests
	February	
	March	Individual Institutes Submit Budget Requests to NIH
	April	
	May	
	June	NIH Submits Budget to PHS
	July	PHS Submits Budget to HHS
	August	
	September	HHS Submits Budget to OMB
	October	FY 1993 Begins
	November	OMB Returns Budget to HHS
	December	
1993	January	
	February	President Submits Budget to Congress
	March	Appropriations Committee Deliberations Begin
	April	House Hearings
	May	Senate Hearings
	June	
	July	House Passes HHS Appropriation
	August	
	September	Senate Passes HHS Appropriation
	October	FY 1994 Begins
	November	HHS Appropriation Signed by President
	December	

FIGURE 5.5 Budget Planning Cycle, FY 1994.

research.   There were minor changes in timing and procedures over the years, but these were largely superficial.   The budget process normally began with a planning meeting in the fall between the administrator of ADAMHA and the assistant secretary for health, where overall concerns and priorities would be reviewed. Within the guidelines that may have resulted from that meeting, individual institutes and offices began their budget process in January (approximately 21 months before the fiscal year) by outlining major themes and proposing new program concepts or initiatives. This process generally took about three to four months to complete, and was informed not only by science, but also by the existing commitment base (the amount of money already committed to multi-year projects), administration policy, congressional earmarks, and the prioritization process within the specific institute. Budget decisions also were influenced by historical budget trends and the consideration of balance between mechanisms (extramural, intramural, grants, contracts, research project grants, and center grants), and the balance between AIDS and other research. Unlike other PHS organizations, the ADAMHA institutes also had to consider the balance between research and services.

The AIDS budgets from the various institutes were reviewed by the administrator of ADAMHA with the help of an analyst in the planning office. The administrator, with advice from the senior staff, would decide on an overall budget request (AIDS and non-AIDS) to submit to the Public Health Service.

The ADAMHA budget process recognized that the agency was unique in its mix of research and services programs, and the budget attempted to implement the concept of an integrated ADAMHA mission, where progress depended on linking research and services with national leadership and advocacy on substance abuse and mental health issues. This concern fundamentally differed from budgetary concerns at NIH, where there was little worry about the level of services budgets and programs in other agencies (such as Health Resources Services Administration or Centers for Disease Control and Prevention).

Historically, within ADAMHA, the three institutes approached planning and budgeting for AIDS in very different ways. NIAAA developed its overall research budget and then determined what portion was related to AIDS research. NIDA, with a large investment in AIDS research but without a formal organizational structure for AIDS programs, developed its AIDS and non-AIDS budgets jointly. NIMH, with a formal Office on AIDS Programs, developed an AIDS budget separately from its non-AIDS budget and then put the two together to develop an overall NIMH budget. The manner in which HHS treated AIDS funding, either as part of various agency budgets or as a separate entity, also affected how the institutes structured and developed their budgets.

In 1991 the budget process at NIAAA, NIDA, and NIMH became more complicated with the uncertainty about whether or not the institutes would be moved from ADAMHA to NIH. Even after the decision to reorganize was made, the institutes still were involved in implementing the FY 1992 budget as part of ADAMHA. Also, until the fall of 1992, they were developing and presenting their portions of the proposed ADAMHA budgets for FY 1993 and FY 1994. It was only in September of 1992 (the eve of FY 1993) that the three institutes began to be incorporated into the overall and AIDS-specific NIH budget processes. Obviously, the length of the budget process under normal circumstances, coupled with the type of sudden discontinuities caused by the ADAMHA reorganization, made planning difficult for all institutes and agencies involved.

WORKING WITHIN THE NIH PROCESS

Given the lead time between budget formulation and execution, most of the institute- and agency-level budget planning for FY 1993 and FY 1994—the first two years that NIAAA, NIDA, and NIMH were organizationally part of NIH—was conducted while the institutes were part of ADAMHA. The institutes first participated in the NIH budget process in September 1992, when they worked with NIH to develop materials for the HHS FY 1994 budget submission to OMB. Thus, while the three institutes had been organizationally part of NIH since October 1, 1992, the FY 1995 budget was the first NIH budget to include NIAAA, NIDA, and NIMH.

The institutes joined in the FY 1994 NIH budget process after the major internal HHS decisions about the NIH AIDS budget had been made. However, the former ADAMHA institutes were still affected by those decisions. The PHS budget request sent by the new (Clinton) administration to OMB provided $10.67 billion for NIH, including $1.3 billion for AIDS research. The allocation of the AIDS budget among the various institutes, offices, and centers was made by the director of OAR (and his staff) with the consensus of the director of NIH. The NIH director then made the final overall allocation of the NIH budget within the departmental mark, using the NIH strategic plan and her sense of where limited resources could best be utilized. While the administration proposed a 3.3 percent overall increase for NIH, including a 21 percent increase for AIDS, the allocations for the individual components ranged from negative numbers to significant double digit increases.

The FY 1994 budget review process was basically the same as it had been in recent years. Over the past few years, the major difference between the AIDS budget process and the overall process occurred before the preliminary budget was submitted by NIH. In FY 1994, these initial activities occurred before NIAAA,

NIDA, and NIMH formally became part of NIH. Also in FY 1994, the process was somewhat confused because of the change in administrations.

The major difference with the review of the AIDS budget by the NIH office of the director (OD) was the level of detail and the focus on science. Most OD-level budget review focused on mechanisms and appropriate balance, while the AIDS review was conducted on a project-by-project or, at the least, area-by-area basis. The OAR director reviewed the plan and made recommended cuts. The institutes could appeal to him to reconsider specific decisions, or the institutes also could appeal to the NIH director. After this phase, the OAR director took the proposed AIDS budget request to the NIH director and associate directors for final review. At this stage, the review broadened to include issues of program balance, mechanism balance, and magnitude of resources requested (both AIDS and non-AIDS), as well as the question of scientific opportunity. Again, unlike the rest of the NIH budget, the AIDS review did include some consideration of specific projects.

According to staff at NIAAA, NIDA, and NIMH, the FY 1994 review process was more top-down and the AIDS and non-AIDS processes were more similar than they had been in the past. NIH was given a departmental mark for AIDS and for its total budget that it then allocated to the institutes based on judgments made by the OAR director for AIDS and by the NIH director for the total budget. Apparently, the decisions in both cases were made based on judgments about where the scientific payoffs would be greatest.

In addition to considering issues of overlap and duplication, appropriate use of mechanisms, program balance, and scientific opportunities, the OD also considered the specifics of projects or project areas, the quality of the science, and the likelihood of progress when determining the NIH AIDS budget allocations. In FY 1994, as in all preceding years, once the institute received its budget allocation, the determination of which specific projects to fund was mostly a function of the grant review process, which is described next.

THE GRANT REVIEW PROCESS

The ADAMHA Reorganization Act of 1992 provided that the ADAMHA peer review systems, advisory councils, and scientific advisory committees utilized remain in effect through FY 1996 (ending September 30, 1996). The report language indicates that, while the three institutes should become full members of the NIH research community, they should also retain their independence and integrity. In addition, it recognized that the institutes' current review procedures were developed over time to meet the specific and complex needs of the alcohol, drug abuse, and mental health fields, and they provide optimal specificity for the wide array of neuroscience, behavioral, clinical, and service research responsibilities (Senate Committee Report 102-131).

In most ways, the review procedures utilized by the former ADAMHA research institutes are very similar to the procedures at NIH. Both NIH and ADAMHA have used a dual review system that separates technical and scientific assessment of projects from subsequent policy decisions concerning programmatic, scientific areas in which projects will be supported. In addition, the scientific review process is kept separate from funding to ensure that program officials are not involved in making determinations on the scientific merit of research applications. These operational procedures had evolved as part of overall development of PHS policies for extramural research grants—a joint activity of various PHS agencies.

Procedurally, the review process at NIH and ADAMHA are also very similar. All ADAMHA and NIH grant applications are mailed to the Division of Research Grants (DRG) in its role as the central receiving point for PHS research grants. In addition, DRG's major management and scientific data systems (IMPAC and CRISP, respectively) have always incorporated information about the ADAMHA research grants. The application form and basic instructions for submitting a research grant are the same for both organizations.

The major difference in processing grants is that at the former ADAMHA institutes, all grants are reviewed at institute-specific initial review groups (IRGs), while at the rest of NIH, most grants are reviewed by DRG study sections. At NIH, only the larger and more complicated grants (centers and program projects) are reviewed by institute-established special review groups (SRGs). In both cases, however, all grants receive their second-level review by the advisory council of a specific institute, and funding decisions ultimately are made by institute staff (with the director's approval).

The first level of grant review is conducted by technical experts, largely from outside the federal government, and is designed to evaluate competing applications based on scientific and technical merit. The second level of review is conducted by advisory councils to assess the quality of the first level review and to offer recommendations based on relevance of the research to the institute's mission. The recommendations of both levels of review are advisory to the federal government and the final funding decisions reside with the institute director. Funding decisions are based not only on scientific merit and policy consideration, but may also consider administration policy, funding availability, and other factors.

At the first level of review, each application is considered at a meeting of the IRG (also called a "study section") and is either given a priority score (if it contains "significant and substantial merit") or not recommended for further consideration (NRFC). Priority scores provide a number for perceived quality by the IRG and they range from outstanding (100-150) to acceptable (350-500). To help equalize the diversity of rating styles (hard and soft graders) and grade creep (the increasing proportion of applications receiving scores of 150 or better), percentile scores are calculated using the priority score for each application.

Once the first level of review is complete, the reviewers prepare a summary statement (or pink sheet) for each application. These are sent to the National Advisory Council for the second level of review. This ensures that the scientific review was appropriately conducted and generates funding recommendations to the institute. If the council disagrees with the IRG on issues related to scientific and technical merit, it may recommend that the application be referred to the same or a different IRG for further consideration. If the IRG makes the same recommendation following reconsideration, its decision is final.

The recommendation by the advisory council completes the formal ADAMHA and/or NIH review of an application. After each council meeting (they usually occur three times each year) the institute makes a funding decision and prepares a funding plan or pay plan, which is based primarily on the scientific merit of the projects (as indicated by their percentile ranking), but also on the availability of funds and balance among research areas. The funding plan is a list of projects recommended for funding by the program office or division and approved by the institute director.

Since FY 1992, NIH has used a performance standard, called the "success rate," to measure the quantity and quality of grants funded over time. The success rate is the total number of competing research project grants (RPGs) funded divided by the total number of competing RPG applications received. The success rate varies by institute and year, and it is determined not only by the number and quality of applications submitted but also by available funding.

The success of AIDS research applications has varied from institute to institute. At NIMH, AIDS grants (traditional investigator-initiated grants—R01s) have had higher success rates than non-AIDS grants; however, those success rates fell from 35.1 in 1989 to 13.5 in 1993 (Figure 5.6). At NIDA, AIDS grants (all RPGs) had higher success rates than non-AIDS grants in 1990, 1991 and 1993, but lower success rates in 1989 and 1992 (Figure 5.7). In general, NIDA RPGs consistently have had relatively high success rates (in the range of 28.4 to 41.1). Since the number of AIDS applications at NIAAA has been relatively small, the success rates may fluctuate dramatically from one year to the next (Figure 5.8). For example, in FY 1990, NIAAA received three competing AIDS applications and funded all of them. During the following year, NIAAA funded 6 of the 19 applications it received. In general, data for all institutes indicate that success rates for all research are declining, which is more likely a result of shrinking budgets and rising per-grant costs than of declining quality among grant proposals submitted.

NIH advisory committees include any committee, council, task

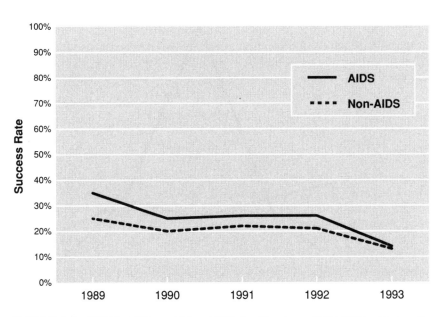

FIGURE 5.6 NIMH AIDS and Non-AIDS Applications, 1989-1993. Note: Includes R01s. Source: Office of Resource Management, NIMH.

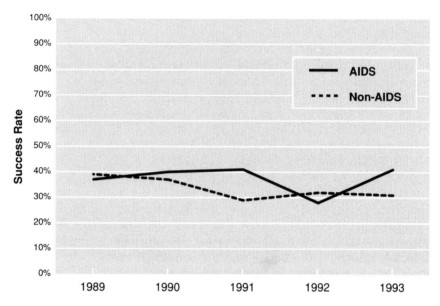

FIGURE 5.7 NIDA AIDS and Non-AIDS Applications, 1989-1993. Note: Includes R01s, P01s, R29s, R37s, R43/44s, and U01s. Source: Office of Planning and Resource Management, NIDA.

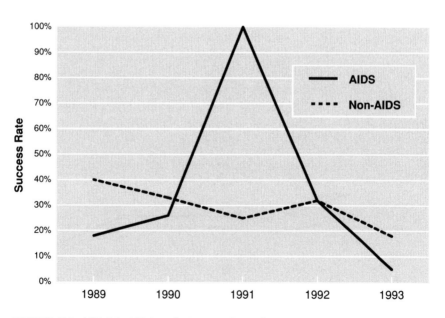

FIGURE 5.8 NIAAA AIDS and Non-AIDS Applications, 1989-1993. Note: Includes R01s and R29s. Source: Extramural Project Review Branch, NIAAA.

force, or group that is established to provide recommendations or advice on policies or other issues related to the missions of the NIH institutes. There are four distinct types of committees: scientific and technical peer review committees for research grant, cooperative agreement, and contract proposals; boards of scientific counselors to review the intramural research programs; program advisory committees to advise on specific research programs and future needs; and national advisory councils to offer advice on policies and programs and to conduct the second level of peer review. Membership on NIH advisory committees is based on demonstrated leadership and excellence in behavioral and biomedical research. Public members are chosen for an active interest in the particular mission of the committee.

NIAAA, NIDA, and NIMH each has its own National Advisory Council, Extramural Science Advisory Board, and Board of Scientific Counselors. Each institute also has several review committees (IRGs), including at least one separate review committee for AIDS research. These AIDS-specific review committees were primarily established in response to the mandatory expedited six-month review for AIDS applications (as opposed to the standard nine-month review).

NIAAA uses two scientific review committees for all applications: Alcohol Psychosocial Research Review Committee and Alcohol Biomedical Research Review Committee. All AIDS applications are reviewed by a subcommittee of the Biomedical Review Committee, called the Immunology and AIDS Subcommittee, which has twelve committee members with scientific expertise in medicine, microbiology/immunology, pathology, sociology, psychology, public health, behavioral science, cellular biology, and psychoimmunology.

NIDA has five research review committees, one of which is the Drug Abuse AIDS Research Review Committee. This committee has two subcommittees: the Biomedical and Clinical Subcommittee (DAAR-1) and the Sociobehavioral Subcommittee (DAAR-2). The twelve members of DAAR-1 represent pediatrics, pharmacology, epidemiology, anthropology, psychiatry, neurology, neuropsychology, and psychology. The thirteen members of DAAR-2 represent the fields of epidemiology, sociology, psychology, psychiatry, other social and behavioral sciences, and addiction medicine.

NIMH has more than twenty separate review committees. The Mental Health, AIDS, and Immunology Committee has two subcommittees for reviewing AIDS applications: the Behavioral, Clinical, and Psychosocial Subcommittee and the Psychobiological, Biological, and Neuroscience Subcommittee. The "psychosocial" subcommittee includes five psychologists, six psychiatrists, one epidemiologist, and representatives from the fields of public health, prevention, community research, and family studies. The "neuroscience" subcommittee includes expertise in neurology, psychology, psychiatry, physiology, pharmacology, microbiology, and immunology.

Of nearly 200 review groups of the DRG at NIH, there are seven study sections for AIDS and Related Research. All but two of them are focused on biomedical aspects of HIV/AIDS and primarily include representation from the following fields: experimental and clinical immunology, molecular biology and genetics, virology, microbiology, and clinical medicine. One study section is focused exclusively on the neuropsychologic, neuropathologic, and neurophysiologic analysis of HIV-infected individuals and includes expertise in neurology, neurobiology, psychology, pathology, and clinical medicine. Just one study section focuses on behavioral medicine and related disciplines, but it primarily includes representatives from medicine, specifically nursing, general medicine, behavioral medicine, public health, pediatrics, and psychiatry.

The second level of review at NIAAA, NIDA, and NIMH is currently conducted by the National Advisory Council of each institute. Although the ADAMHA Reorganization Act mandated that the review processes (both at the first and second levels) be maintained through 1996, it is not yet clear how AIDS research applications at the three institutes will be reviewed when this period ends. (As this report was being written, it was reported that the NIH director had requested that the former ADAMHA institutes enter into negotiations with the NIH Division of Research Grants earlier than 1996 and that the institutes agreed [Federation of Behavioral, Psychological and Cognitive Sciences, 1994].)

Given the composition of the NIH-wide AIDS study sections, some have expressed concern that applications related to the biobehavioral and social-behavioral research foci of NIAAA, NIDA, and NIMH—that is, cross-disciplinary focus—will not fare well should the three institutes be subject to the overall NIH review process. Indeed, this was a significant reason for the four-year retention of the institutes' pre-NIH review systems. While it is too soon to determine if this concern is well founded, the committee is aware that it is widespread among the institute program staff and the external research community. Furthermore, given this study's finding about the extent of cross-disciplinary research at NIAAA, NIDA, and NIMH, the committee believes that this concern deserves particular consideration.

Under current NIH procedures, described above, each member of a review panel assigns to a proposal a score from 1 (best) to 5 (worst). These ratings are averaged, giving equal weighting to each. Proposals are then ranked according to the resulting "priority score" (after multiplying by 100) and characterized by the resulting percentile. Generally speaking, proposals are funded in order, starting with the lowest percentile. In a competitive field, that might mean funding up to the 6th or 8th percentile. As a result, the only proposals likely to be funded are those receiving extremely good ratings from the great majority of panel members.

This procedure is inherently prejudicial to innovative and collaborative proposals. Unless some adjustments are made, the agencies will continue to discourage proposals involving new disciplines and multiple disciplines, or cooperation between investigators and community-based organizations. Unless instructed otherwise, responsible panel members likely would regress their scores for innovative proposals toward the mean of the scale. Because it is inherently harder to predict how such research will turn out, it is difficult to have the confidence needed to rate it as extremely good. As a result, a proposal would have to show an extraordinary degree of innovation in order to compensate for this inherent conservatism.

Review panel members also are likely to regress the scores that they give to proposals involving disciplines other than their own. They are not in a position to know what "extremely good" is in another discipline. As a result, a single-discipline proposal will be less competitive to the extent that it is judged by specialists from other disciplines. A cross-disciplinary proposal is almost guaranteed to have portions that will be unfamiliar to each reviewer.

In cases in which priority scores are compared across programs, single-discipline panels are more likely to have proposals with extremely good priority scores than are mixed-discipline panels. That could be interpreted as evidence that the single-discipline panels receive better proposals. However, it could just be that they have more unitary (or insular or ideological) evaluative standards. The more powerful a discipline is at an agency, the more likely it is to have its own review panel. Politically weaker disciplines are more likely to be combined into mixed-discipline panels. As a result, a naive interpretation of priority scores across panels is likely to create a situation where the rich get richer.

These problems arise without any deliberate attempt to create barriers to new disciplines and approaches, which might want a share of the resources allocated to a topic such as AIDS. Rather, they provide an honest way of ensuring that such prejudices are part of the evaluation system. Those interested in preserving business as usual can make candid evaluations, then let the system do the discriminating. There may be individual members of review panels who are aware of these threats, and make various efforts to overcome them. However, the extent and impact of those efforts is unknown.

These problems may be addressed either by working within the existing procedures or by changing them. Within the system, one possible solution is to weight ratings by the disciplinary competence of the raters. Although that change might reduce the (inadvertent or deliberate) censorship of other disciplines, it would not solve the problems of innovative or cross-disciplinary proposals. Another possibility is to rescale scores so that they are standardized within different categories.

More fundamental changes might include convening special review panels, affording votes to ad hoc reviewers, and dedicating funds to unconventional proposals (so that they compete amongst themselves). In implementing these proposals NIH would have to consider the appropriateness of existing review staff for creating the appropriate panels and procedures. Also, such proposals would have to be in accord with the scientific principles of evaluation (often called psychometrics).

As this report was being written, the current NIH director established a series of inter-NIH panels to examine the ways in which the peer review process could be streamlined and more innovative projects rewarded. Although this action reportedly was prompted by the "reinventing government" paradigm of the Clinton administration, it is not intended to focus solely on speeding up the process, but rather will take into account some of the issues about study section composition and scoring raised above (Federation of Behavioral, Psychological and Cognitive Sciences, 1994).

In deciding whether it is worth the effort to undertake such reforms, the primary concern in the context of this report should be the effects such reforms will have on AIDS research and the AIDS epidemic. However, an important secondary consideration should be the relationship between the agencies and the scientific community. The current evaluation system alienates scientists whose work is treated prejudicially, in particular, those who attempt to cross disciplinary boundaries. Not only will this reduce their willingness to work on AIDS-related problems, but it also will damage the reputation of existing research. Over time, that may imperil continuing public support for business as usual, if the federal research establishment is perceived to be unresponsive to the requirements of the AIDS epidemic.

CONCLUSION AND RECOMMENDATIONS

CONCLUSION

The development and management of the AIDS programs at NIAAA, NIDA, and NIMH takes place in a larger context. This context includes legislative and budgetary processes that are often in flux but still wield control over the resources available to manage the institutes' programs. In recent years, the most significant changes in this regard have been the structural reorganization of ADAMHA, which moved the institutes to NIH, and the new budgetary authority of the Office of AIDS Research at NIH, which changed the nature of how dollars will be allocated for AIDS research at the individual institutes. These changes were superimposed on the already complex budget process that governs all federal spending and together produced a climate of uncertainty for the management of the AIDS research programs at NIAAA, NIDA, and NIMH.

To maintain some stability, the institutes were allowed to retain their existing grant review procedures for four years (through FY 1996). This was seen as important for ensuring the continued support of behavioral and social research that historically had been better at ADAMHA than at NIH. The fact that this situation will be revisited in FY 1997 raises some concerns about how the cross-disciplinary research so important for advancing knowledge in HIV prevention and intervention will fare in the future.

RECOMMENDATIONS RELATED TO THE CONTEXT OF AIDS RESEARCH

5.1 The committee recommends that NIAAA, NIDA, and NIMH develop new programs and grant review procedures to encourage and facilitate innovative, collaborative, and cross-disciplinary proposals.

5.2 The committee recommends that the NIH task force charged with streamlining peer review consider alternative scoring schemes that would favor cross-disciplinary and innovative research proposals.

6

Research Funding, Programs, and Priorities at NIAAA, NIDA, and NIMH

The committee was asked to assess the adequacy of the response of NIAAA, NIDA, and NIMH to the AIDS epidemic by evaluating the scope and content of their AIDS research program activities and the balance between biomedical and behavioral research. To adequately address these two issues, the committee conducted a grant-by-grant analysis of all AIDS research projects funded by NIAAA, NIDA, and NIMH from FY 1983 (the first year of AIDS funding) through FY 1992 (the most recent year for which complete data were available). In addition, the committee reviewed a range of documents and plans produced by the institutes that describe their AIDS programs and priorities.

This approach provided the committee with comprehensive budgetary and programmatic information about the institutes' research programs that was not available in one form from any source—the institutes, ADAMHA, SAMHSA, NIH, or any other PHS office. The committee's analysis was able to link specific grants to broad institute initiatives and to actual dollars committed to these various initiatives, bringing together disparate pieces of information to guide the assessment of the institutes' AIDS programs for each fiscal year and over time.

This chapter presents an overview and analysis of the institutes' AIDS research funding, programs, and priorities, as well as the grants funded between FY 1983 and FY 1992, including a summary of the committee's main findings with respect to program activities and balance among scientific disciplines. The discussion is organized by institute, and the grant-based information is presented according to categories developed by the committee. Further information about how the grant-based analysis was conducted—including its limitations—may be found in Appendix A; the results from the research supported are included in the general discussions in Part I.

FUNDING AIDS ACTIVITIES

The committee was asked to assess the "adequacy" of funding of AIDS programs at NIAAA, NIDA, and NIMH with respect to balance in the scientific portfolios and the relationship between AIDS and non-AIDS research. "Adequacy" is a subjective term, especially since some would argue that until completely effective prevention and treatment interventions are discovered for HIV, no amount of money spent on AIDS research is adequate. The committee did not wish to engage in this discussion, nor did it wish to assess the merits of funding AIDS research relative to funding other disease-related research. Rather, the committee chose to focus on the overall situation of AIDS funding at the former ADAMHA institutes and offices, from the beginning of the epidemic to the present, and to identify areas where serious inadequacies are evident.

The historical review of AIDS funding presented here is based on the most recent *comparable* budget information provided by NIH, NIAAA, NIDA, NIMH, and SAMHSA. Therefore, expenditures are displayed and discussed using the current organizational structure of the institutes and agencies being reviewed. For example, information about SAMHSA and NIH funding reflects the current organizational splits between research and services (designated by the 1992 ADAMHA reorganization). Information about total NIH funding includes the former ADAMHA research institutes.

Despite the best efforts of various budget offices, some sets of numbers may not always be completely consistent with other sets since data were derived from a multiplicity of sources and were tabulated for a variety of purposes. In addition, other problems associated with retabulating entire budgets (to make them comparable) after the reorganization arose, such as changes in what was defined as AIDS research from year to year within an institute (i.e., coding anomalies) and differences in rounding.

CATEGORIZING AIDS RESEARCH

As mentioned earlier, the committee was charged with assessing the balance between biomedical and behavioral AIDS research at NIAAA, NIDA, and NIMH. Early in the study, however, the committee determined that these categories were too limiting for two reasons: because there were no clear definitions of "biomedical" and "behavioral," and because counterpoising these two categories masked the true level of cross-disciplinary research supported by the institutes. As the committee began to review the research portfolios grant by grant, it became apparent that labeling a project as either biomedical or behavioral was misleading, because significant portions of many projects included elements from both realms.

One option the committee faced was to find an alternative way of categorizing AIDS research, by looking at other schema employed by the Public Health Service. Since FY 1989, PHS agencies have used the following set of categories, called "Mason" categories (named after then Assistant Secretary for Health, James O. Mason): Basic Science Research, which includes biomedical research, neuroscience and neuropsychiatric research, behavioral research, therapeutic agents, vaccines, and research training and extramural construction; Risk Assessment and Prevention, which includes surveillance, population-based research, information and education/prevention services; and Clinical Health Services Research and Delivery, which includes health services grants. However, although the Mason categories are more comprehensive than the simple "biomedical-behavioral" distinction, the committee felt—as had an earlier IOM committee (IOM, 1991a)—that they were not sufficient to scientifically characterize the research programs of the institutes. In particular, it was not clear under which category(ies) psychosocial and social science research best fit. Also, prior to FY 1993, individual grants funded by the institutes could not be traced to specific Mason categories.

As a result of these problems, and in order to determine the balance of science among AIDS research grants, the committee developed its own simple matrix using four domains of science: biomedical/biobehavioral, epidemiological, psychosocial, social-structural, and two types of research: basic and applied. Figure 6.1 presents the committee's matrix.

"Biomedical/biobehavioral" research focuses on improving knowledge about basic biological mechanisms and processes, disease pathogenesis, and clinical issues related to progression and treatment of HIV/AIDS. "Epidemiological" research focuses on trans-

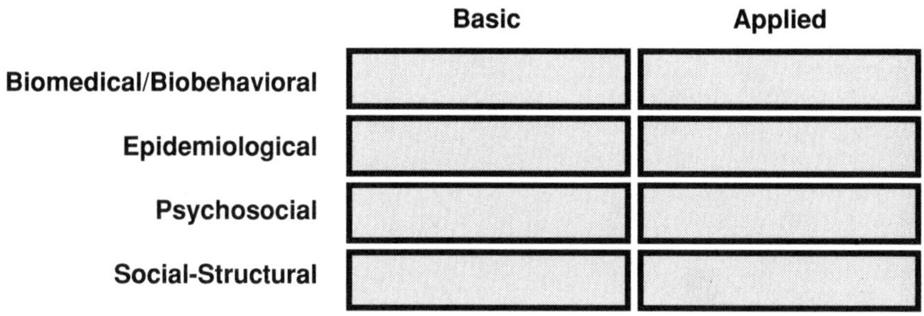

	Basic	**Applied**
Biomedical/Biobehavioral		
Epidemiological		
Psychosocial		
Social-Structural		

FIGURE 6.1 Committee Codes.

mission of HIV and the natural history of infection and disease progression. This category also includes biostatistical research to develop and refine mathematical modeling techniques for improved forecasting of HIV seroprevalence. "Psychosocial" research includes efforts to understand psychological determinants of behavior and behavior change and to develop and evaluate preventive interventions, the effect of psychosocial variables on disease progression, and the impact of HIV/AIDS on behavior and psychological functioning. "Social-structural" research examines the social context in which HIV/AIDS is transmitted and experienced, by focusing on relationships, families, communities, institutions, and cultures rather than on individuals. Social-structural research includes research on health services, evaluation, and operations. "Basic" research studies the basic mechanisms underlying biological, neurological, behavioral, and social processes and outcomes, and includes theoretical work. "Applied" research encompasses projects that test interventions.

The committee constructed an electronic database from abstracts of funded, extramural grants at NIAAA, NIDA, and NIMH from FY 1983 to FY 1992. Each AIDS grant was either single-coded with one of the four science categories or, where appropriate, multi-coded with two or more of the science categories. Generally, the committee considered the multi-coded grants to be cross-disciplinary research. In addition, each grant was coded as either basic or applied. (See Appendix A for more information about the committee's methodology.)

The committee found that a significant proportion of AIDS research at NIAAA, NIDA, and NIMH is cross-disciplinary, according to the committee's coding scheme (Figure 6.2). For example, in 1992, approximately one-third of all research project grants and research demonstrations (R18s) at NIAAA, NIDA, and NIMH were

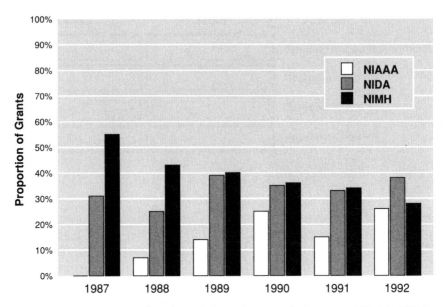

FIGURE 6.2 Proportion of Multi-coded AIDS Research Grants at NIAAA, NIDA, and NIMH, 1987-1992. Note: Includes RPGs and R18s. Source: NIH CRISP system, and IOM committee database.

multi-coded. Since 1987, the proportion of multi-coded grants at NIAAA rose significantly. At NIDA, about one-third of all grants were multi-coded from 1987 through 1992. Many of these multi-coded grants were for NIDA-sponsored drug abuse treatment research, which utilizes a wide variety of approaches for improving drug abuse treatment and reducing HIV risk behaviors (sexual and drug using), including pharmacologic and behavioral interventions as well as enhancements for improving access and retention in treatment programs. The proportion of multi-coded grants at NIMH has actually fallen from 55 percent in 1987 to 28 percent in 1992. In 1987, NIMH's AIDS portfolio was much smaller and had a high proportion of psychoneuroimmunology grants, most of which were multi-coded. Because NIMH's AIDS program grew to include research efforts targeted to the development of behavioral interventions and basic knowledge in neuro-AIDS, multi-coded grants eventually represented a smaller proportion of the total.

Using the committee's coding for basic and applied AIDS research, the analysis also discovered that most extramural AIDS research grants funded by NIAAA, NIDA, and NIMH are basic research. As demonstrated in Figure 6.3, the majority of NIAAA grants were basic research, falling from 100 percent in 1987 to 87

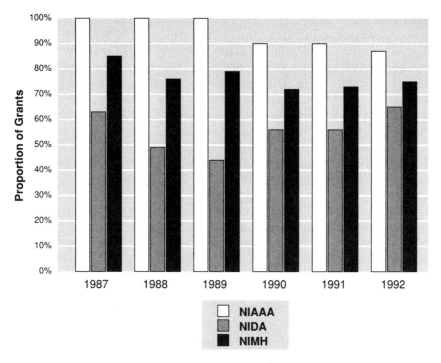

FIGURE 6.3 Proportion of Basic AIDS Research Grants at NIAAA, NIDA, and NIMH, 1987-1992. Note: Includes RPGs and R18s. Source: NIH CRISP system, and IOM committee database.

percent in 1992. Representation of basic research in NIMH's AIDS research portfolio also decreased from 85 percent in 1987 to 75 percent of the total in 1992. The proportion of basic research at NIDA has fluctuated, from as low as 44 percent in 1989 to 65 percent in 1992. This is largely due to the NADR program and the Treatment Research program, both of which were categorized as applied research.

MECHANISMS OF SUPPORT

NIAAA, NIDA, and NIMH, like all federal research institutes, employ a range of mechanisms for supporting AIDS research. The two major categories are *intramural*, which is research conducted by the institute staff itself, usually in laboratories on or near the institute, and *extramural*, which is research conducted by nonfederal scientists at universities, health centers, and other settings around the country and the world.

Extramural research mechanisms include research project grants (RPGs), centers, contracts, and other research. RPGs include: traditional investigator-initiated grants (R01s); research program projects (P01s); cooperative agreements (U01s), which support investigators at different sites working from a common research protocol with some variation in study population or mode of intervention; Small Business Innovation Research grants (SBIR-R43/44); and other research grants (including new investigator awards, first independent research support and transition [FIRST] awards, and methods to extend research in time [MERIT] awards). The vast majority of RPGs funded by NIAAA, NIDA, and NIMH are R01s. Research centers include specialized centers (P50s) and core grants (P30s), both of which support groups of researchers at a single institution working on a common theme. Other research includes research demonstrations (R18s), which typically test the efficacy of theory-driven pilot programs in an applied setting, cooperative clinical research (R10/U10), and research career program awards (K-series). There are two types of contract awards (N-series): research and development, and resource and support. Training includes individual awards (F-series) and institutional awards (T-series). Together, all of these mechanisms make up the extramural research program of an institute.

NIAAA, NIDA, and NIMH have utilized all mechanisms for supporting extramural AIDS research, but in different proportions. For example, the majority of NIAAA's extramural research grants and dollars have been committed to R01s. NIMH AIDS extramural funding has been largely committed to R01s and research centers (P50s). NIDA's extramural program has employed the widest variety of mechanisms, particularly by committing resources to research demonstration projects (R18s).

Although the committee attempted to obtain comprehensive, comparable information on all relevant funding mechanisms (i.e., extramural research project grants, contracts, intramural projects) from all three institutes, it was only able to do so for extramural grants. (Only NIMH provided complete information on its intramural program; and the contract data obtained were not comparable to the grant information.) Consequently, the analysis of grants presented below is limited to extramural research grants only. Discussions about contracts and intramural research reflect information gathered from sources other than the database. Moreover, because of the limitations of the available data (described in Appendix A)—most notably the fact that the institutes did not systematically nor consistently code grants as AIDS-related before

FY 1987—the specific analysis of the grants focuses primarily on the research portfolios beginning in FY 1987.

In the discussions of the grants in this chapter, the figures display the total proportion of research project grants, demonstration projects, and cooperative agreements (R01s, R18s, U01s, U10s, U18s) that were coded by the committee for each scientific domain. Percentages represent an institute's total level of commitment in a given scientific domain. Multi-coded grants appear in all relevant domains; for example, a grant that has both a biomedical and a psychosocial component is included in both the "biomedical/biobehavioral" and the "psychosocial" categories in the figures (as a way of illustrating how many grants include at least a component of a given scientific domain). Center grants (P50) are not included in this analysis because of their unique structure; however, they represent a significant proportion of AIDS grants (especially at NIMH) and involve cross-disciplinary research. They are, therefore, discussed elsewhere in this chapter.

Details of the differential use of mechanisms embedded in the discussions of the institutes' AIDS programs below indicate that in general, when compared to non-AIDS research, a greater proportion of AIDS research at NIAAA, NIDA, and NIMH has been directed in some way by the institutes (see Figures 6.6, 6.7, 6.11, 6.12, 6.16, and 6.17). Investigator-initiated research includes traditional R01s, whereas directed research efforts are usually funded using contracts, cooperative agreements, research demonstrations, and, to a large degree, research centers. The institutes can also help guide the field by issuing a general Program Announcement (PA) or a Request for Applications (RFA). PAs and RFAs reflect the institutes' research priorities. A program announcement is broader than an RFA, and it usually contains suggested research areas. There is no money specifically set aside to fund grants submitted in response to a PA; such grants are funded out of the institute's general funds. An RFA, on the other hand, does have specific funds set aside for grants submitted in response to its release. RFAs usually are more specific than PAs and they specify certain selection criteria. Also, RFAs have one receipt date, whereas PAs remain active for longer periods of time.

Table 6.1 lists AIDS-specific and AIDS-related PAs and RFAs issued by NIAAA, NIDA, and NIMH since the beginning of their respective AIDS programs. It does not include general program announcements for FIRST awards, small grants, and fellowships.

The level of directed research in the AIDS programs—as evidenced by PAs, RFAs, and the funding of core and center grants—

TABLE 6.1 AIDS-Specific and AIDS-Related Program Announcements (PAs) and Requests for Applications (RFAs): NIAAA, NIDA, and NIMH

Date	PA/PFA #	Title (funds available)[a]	Mechanisms	Institute(s)
1/94	PA-94-023	HIV Therapeutics in Drug Abuse	R01-R29-R03	NIDA
11/93	PA-94-010	Research on Needle Hygiene and Needle Exchange Programs	R01	NIDA
11/93	DA-94-02	Behavioral Therapies Development Program ($3 million for first year)[b]	R01-R03-R29-IRPG	NIDA
10/93	AA-94-03	Alcohol and Minorities: Biomedical and Behavioral Research ($2 million for FY 94)[c]	R01-R29	NIAAA
10/93	AA-94-01	Biomedical and Behavioral Research on Alcohol and Women[d]	R01-R29	NIAAA
10/93	AA-94-02	Biomedical and Behavioral Research on Alcohol and Youth[c]	R01-R29	NIAAA
10/93	AA-94-05	Health Services Research on Alcohol-Related Problems[c]	R01-R29-T32	NIAAA
10/93	AA-94-04	Underdeveloped Areas of Alcohol Abuse Prevention Research[c]	R01-R29	NIAAA
9/93	PA-93-111	Partner Notification to HIV-infected Drug Users	R01	NIDA
9/93	PA-93-110	Health Care Services for Persons with HIV Infection	R01	AHCPR-NIAAA-NIDA-NIMH
9/93	PA-93-106	Drug Abuse Treatment for Women of Childbearing Age and Their Children ($5 million for FY 94)[b]	R01	NIDA
8/93	PA-93-100	Research Program to Improve Drug Abuse Treatment ($10 million for FY 94)[b]	R01	NIDA
7/93	PA-93-098	Drug Abuse Aspects of AIDS (Revised)	R01-R03-R29	NIDA
6/93	AI-93-14	Center for AIDS Research/Core Support Grant (NIMH set aside $1.5 million)	P30	NIAID-NIMH
5/93	PA-93-087	National Research Service Awards (NRSA) Institutional Training Grants for AIDS	T32	NIAID-NIMH
4/93	PA-93-080	Determinants of Effective HIV Counseling	R01-R03-R29	NIDA-NIMH
2/93	PA-93-47	Preventing Alcohol-Related Problems Among Ethnic Minorities[c]	R01-R03-R29	NIAAA
1/93	PA-93-44	The Spread of Tuberculosis Among Drug Users ($3 million for FY 93)[d]	R01-R03-R29	NIDA

194

Date	PA Number	Title	Mechanisms	Institute
12/92	PA-93-28	Research to Improve Drug Abuse Treatment, Entry, Retention, Compliance, and Effectiveness[b]	R01-R03-R29	NIDA
12/92	PA-93-27	Psychotherapy, Behavior Therapy, and Counseling in Drug Treatment[b]	R01-R03-R29	NIDA
11/92	PA-93-21	Drug Abuse Treatment of Criminal Justice-Involved Populations[b]	R01	NIDA
10/92	PA-92-110	Development of Theoretically Based Psychosocial Therapies for Drug Dependence[b]	R01-R03-R29	NIDA
10/92	PA-93-009	Neural, Endocrine, Immune, and Viral Interactions, Behavior and Mental Health[d]	R01-R03-R29-P01-T32-K series-F series	NIMH-NINDS
7/92	PA-92-95	Neuro-AIDS: HIV-1 Infection and the Nervous System	R01-R29-P01	NIMH-NINDS
5/92	AA-92-03	Alcohol Research Center Grants ($1.7 million)[d]	P50	NIAAA
5/92	MH-92-11	The Role of the Family in Preventing and Adapting to HIV Infection and AIDS ($1.8 million for FY 93)	R01	NIAAA-NIDA-NIMH
3/92	PA-92-46	Research on the Prevention of Alcohol Abuse Among Youth[c]	R01-R03-R29	NIAAA
3/92	PA-92-58	Clinical Research on Human Development and Drug Abuse ($10 million for FY 93)[d]	R01-R03-R13-R29-F31-F32-T32-K20-K21	NIDA
10/91	PA-92-12	Research Grants on Alcohol and Immunology Including AIDS ($2 million for FY 92) (Revised)	R01-R03-R29	NIAAA
6/91	PA-91-75	Research on Relationships between Alcohol Use and Sexual Behaviors Associated with HIV Transmission	R01-R03-R29	NIAAA
12/90	PA-90-31	Drug Abuse Research[d] [No longer used]	R01-R03-R13-R29-R43-R44-P01-R18	NIDA
6/90	PA-90-15	Children with HIV Infection and AIDS	R01-R29	NCNR-NICHD-NIDA-NIMH-NINDS
1/90	DA-90-05	Research Demonstration Program to Enhance Drug Abuse Treatment ($10 million for FY 90)[b]	R18	NIDA
1/90	DA-90-02	A Cooperative Agreement for AIDS Community-Based Outreach/Intervention Research ($3 million for FY 90)	U01	NIDA

continued on next page

TABLE 6.1 Continued

Date	PA/PFA #	Title (funds available)[a]	Mechanisms	Institute(s)
1/90	DA-90-10	Demonstration Research on Service Delivery in Non-Traditional Settings	R18	NIDA
1/90	PA	Drug Abuse Aspects of AIDS ($15 million for FY 90) (Revised in 1/93)	R01-R03-R29-P01	NIDA
10/89	PA	National Research Service Awards for Institutional Training Grants in HIV Infection and AIDS	T series	NIAAA-NIDA-NIMH
10/89	PA	National Research Service Awards for Individual Fellows in HIV Infection and AIDS	T series	NIAAA-NIDA-NIMH
11/88	DA-89-01	Research Demonstration Program to Reduce the Spread of AIDS by Improving Treatment for Drug Abuse ($10 million for FY 89)	R18	NIDA
9/88	PA	Research Grants on Alcohol and Immunology Including AIDS (Revised in 10/91)	R01-R29-P01	NIAAA
9/88	PA	Research on Severely Mentally Ill Persons at Risk of or with HIV Infection	R01-R29	NIMH
9/88	PA	Research on Behavior Change and Prevention Strategies to Reduce Transmission of HIV	R01-R03-R29-P01-K series	CDC-NCNR-NHLBI-NIA-NIAAA-NICHD-NIDA-NIMH
9/88	PA	Measurement, Course, and Treatment of HIV-Related Mental Disorders	R01-R03-R29-P01-P50-K series	NIMH
9/88	PA	Brain, Immune System, and Behavioral and Neurological Aspects of HIV	R01-R03-R29-P01-P50-K series	NICHD-NIMH-NINCDS
9/88	PA	Central Nervous System Effects of HIV Infection: Neurobiological, Neurovirological, and Neurobehavioral Studies	R01-R03-R29-P01-P50-K series	NICHD-NIMH-NINCDS
9/88	MH-86-16	AIDS Research Centers	P50	NIDA-NIMH

Date	Number	Title		
3/88	AA-88-02	Research Grants on Alcohol Related Behavior that Increases the Risk of AIDS and/or Research on Prevention Strategies to Reduce that Risk ($1 million)	R01-R29	NIAAA
1/88	DA-88-03	AIDS Community Outreach and Counseling Demonstration Research—Phase II ($10-12 million for FY 88)	R18	NIDA
12/87	PA	Behavioral Aspects of AIDS Prevention in Children and Adolescents	not specified	NICHD-NIMH
10/87	AA-88-01	Alcohol Research Center Grants on Alcohol and Immunologic Disorders ($1.5 million)[d]	P50	NIAAA
1/87	DA-87-20	Studies of Drugs of Abuse as Potential Cofactors in the Pathogenesis of AIDS	not specified	NIDA
1/87	DA-87-14	Treatment of Intravenous Drug Abusers to Reduce the Spread of AIDS	not specified	NIDA
1/87	DA-87-13	AIDS Community Outreach: Demonstration Project ($5 million for FY 87)	R18	NIDA
1/87	DA-87-12	Studies of Heterosexual and Perinatal Transmission of AIDS Associated with Intravenous Drug Abuse	not specified	NIDA
1/87	PA-87-01	Alcohol Research Grants[a]	not specified	NIAAA
12/86	DA-87-11	Drug Abuse Aspects of AIDS (Revised in 1/90)	not specified	NIDA
11/86	DA-87-10	AIDS and the Prevention of Intravenous Drug Abuse ($1.35 million for FY 87)	not specified	NIDA
3/86	MH-86-16	AIDS Research Centers ($500,000 each for 2-3 centers for FY 86-87)	R01-R29	NIMH-NIDA
11/85	MH-86-09	Alcohol, Drug Abuse, and Mental Health Aspects of AIDS	R01-R29	NIMH-NIDA-NIAAA

[a]Funding information specified includes estimates that appeared in the PA/RFA and does not indicate what was actually spent.

[b]These PAs/RFAs call for research related to drug abuse treatment and may not include a specific reference to AIDS. However, drug abuse treatment research is one of NIDA's priority research areas for HIV/AIDS.

[c]These PAs/RFAs do not include a specific reference to AIDS, and refer only to high-risk sexual or drug-using behavior.

[d]These PAs/RFAs contain an explicit reference to HIV/AIDS, although HIV/AIDS is not the primary focus.

Source: AIDS Coordinators at NIAAA, NIDA, and NIMH.

suggests active leadership among the institute staff in encouraging investigations of specific AIDS-related topics. This kind of leadership may be more necessary in a new research field, such as AIDS, since investigators must be recruited who have been establishing careers in other, related areas of science.

NIAAA

NIAAA first began funding AIDS research in FY 1987 (Figure 6.4). AIDS was just under 3 percent of the total NIAAA budget that year, and rose to 5 percent in FY 1988. Since then, AIDS funding increased 233 percent, from $2.4 million in FY 1987 to $8 million in FY 1992 (Figure 6.5). Total NIAAA funding (AIDS and non-AIDS) grew from $83.4 million in FY 1987 to $171.5 million in FY 1992—a 106 percent increase.

NIAAA's AIDS program supports research exploring the role of alcohol as a potential biological and psychosocial factor in the transmission of HIV infection and its progression to AIDS. Specifically, NIAAA's portfolio includes studies examining the relationship between alcohol and the immune system, and studies to

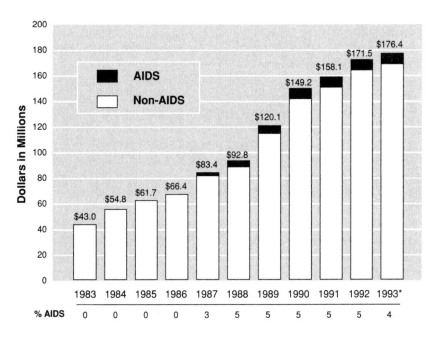

FIGURE 6.4 NIAAA Expenditures (AIDS/Non-AIDS), 1983-1993. *Estimate. Source: NIAAA Budget Office.

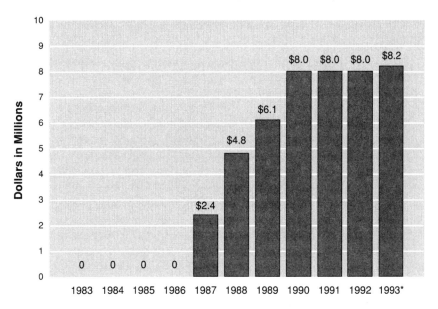

FIGURE 6.5 NIAAA AIDS Expenditures, 1983-1993. *Estimate. Source: NIAAA Budget Office.

understand the relationship between alcohol use and high-risk sexual behavior. Overall, the NIAAA AIDS program is small relative to those at NIDA and NIMH, and it has not yet included significant program initiatives on the order of those at NIDA and NIMH.

Because its AIDS program is small, NIAAA has never established an Office of AIDS and has never employed any full-time AIDS staff. Currently, NIAAA has two "part-time" coordinators—one for social and behavioral research and one for biomedical research. These coordinators perform their AIDS-related activities in addition to what amounts to full-time responsibility for other activities, and they do so without significant institutional support.

NIAAA first allocated AIDS FTEs (full-time equivalents) in FY 1987 (Table 6.2). Since that year, four extramural FTEs have been allocated to AIDS, representing a part-time commitment from program, budget, and contracting staff who support the AIDS activities of the institute. There are no individuals outside of the intramural research program who are supported full time in AIDS personnel positions. From FY 1987 through FY 1993, NIAAA's AIDS FTEs rose 114 percent, compared to a 31 percent increase in the institute's

TABLE 6.2 NIAAA AIDS Staffing (FTEs) by Administrative Area, 1987-1993

	1987	1988	1989	1990	1991	1992	1993*
Intramural research	3	3	8	9	10	7	11
RMS	4	4	4	4	4	4	4
AIDS Total	7	7	12	13	14	11	15
NIAAA Total	190	191	210	224	229	238	248

NOTE: *Estimate. RMS = Research management and support.

Source: NIAAA Budget Office.

FTEs overall. AIDS FTEs represented 6 percent of all FTEs in FY 1993.

Although the ADAMHA Reorganization Act mandated that NIDA and NIMH each establish an Office on AIDS, it was silent about NIAAA. Presumably this reflects a judgment based on the relatively small size of the NIAAA AIDS program. If so, this is a circular argument on the part of Congress: if the program is small (dollar and FTE size) then it is less significant; if it is less significant, then it will receive smaller appropriations for grants and FTEs. As a consequence, the size of the program will remain the same.

At NIAAA, the distribution of mechanisms used for AIDS research has changed from year to year (Figure 6.6), although the distribution of non-AIDS funding has remained relatively stable (Figure 6.7). The majority of AIDS funding at NIAAA includes RPGs, which increased from 45 percent of the AIDS total in FY 1987 to 73 percent in FY 1992. NIAAA's contribution to centers for AIDS research has fluctuated from as much as 30 percent of the institute's total AIDS budget in FY 1988 to as little as 1 percent in FY 1992. Use of contracts has been fairly minimal, as has NIAAA's commitment to AIDS training. As with its non-AIDS program, intramural research has constituted a significant portion of AIDS funding—accounting for 21 percent of the AIDS budget in FY 1987 and staying near 20 percent through FY 1993.

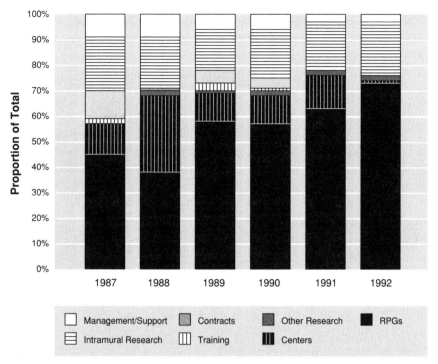

FIGURE 6.6 NIAAA AIDS Funding by Mechanism, 1987-1992. Source: NIAAA Budget Office.

PROGRAMS AND PRIORITIES

Biomedical/Biobehavioral Research

Since it first initiated its AIDS program, NIAAA has devoted much of its extramural and intramural research efforts to biomedical issues. NIAAA's broad research goal in this area is to elucidate how alcohol alters the immune system in ways that may compromise host defense against HIV. In October 1991, NIAAA issued a program announcement—*Research grants on alcohol and immunology including AIDS*—to stimulate research on effects of alcohol consumption on the biological and biochemical mechanisms involved in the etiology of immunologic dysfunction.

NIAAA's extramural research support has included research grants and supplemental funding to Alcohol Research Centers and grants for AIDS-related issues. Extramural research projects include a broad spectrum of basic and clinical immunological research, including investigations of (1) alcohol and susceptibility to infec-

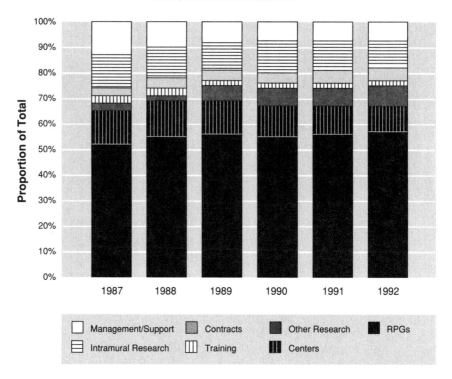

FIGURE 6.7 NIAAA Non-AIDS Funding by Mechanism, 1987-1992. Source: NIAAA Budget Office.

tion; (2) alcohol and immune system development to understand the possible role of alcohol as a cofactor of maternal transmission of HIV; (3) alcohol and cellular and humoral immunity to understand mechanisms of alcohol's effects on host resistance to HIV and related infections; (4) alcohol and neurohormonal immunomodulation to understand interactions between the nervous, endocrine, and immune systems; and (5) the murine AIDS model, which is used to understand how the virus attacks the immune system, and to test treatment modalities.

The NIAAA intramural research program primarily has focused on (1) alcohol's potential role as a cofactor in the etiology of AIDS and as a promotor of opportunistic infection in patients suffering from AIDS; (2) the effects of HIV on neuronal function; and (3) the basic mechanisms underlying lymphocyte immunosuppression. Selected research includes studies on the factors controlling T-cell maturation and proliferation, the effects of HIV proteins and related viral coat proteins on neuronal function, and the mechanisms of HIV viral coat proteins to change neuronal metabolism leading to AIDS-related dementia. Most recently, intramural researchers of the Laboratory of Clinical Studies have been investigating high-risk behaviors leading to AIDS exposure using a non-human primate model of impulsivity and habitual behavior.

Epidemiological Research

Since 1988, NIAAA has funded studies that examine the relationships between alcohol and other drug use and high-risk sexual behavior, rates of HIV seroconversion, and the development and clinical course of AIDS. These research grants include: surveys to track incidence and prevalence of high-risk behaviors among alcohol treatment inpatients; cross-sectional surveys and prospective cohort studies to examine relationships among alcohol and drug use, high-risk behavior, and HIV seropositivity among various risk groups, including alcohol-dependent adults and adolescents; a supplement to expand an ongoing prospective survey to include information on sexual practices, drug use, AIDS knowledge, and perceived risk in investigating racial/ethnic and gender differences in the relationship between alcohol consumption and AIDS-risk behaviors; and a supplement to a National Alcohol Research Center grant to develop estimates of the incidence and prevalence of sexual risk taking and drinking and an examination of beliefs, attitudes, and perceptions of AIDS risk.

Psychosocial Research

In June 1991 NIAAA issued an announcement for *Research on relationships between alcohol use and sexual behaviors associated with HIV transmission.* NIAAA has funded several grants to understand the relationship between alcohol use and high-risk sexual behavior and the development of strategies to prevent high-risk behaviors.

Most research thus far has focused on the determinants of high-risk behaviors among adolescents, women, and various racial and ethnic groups. Most recently, NIAAA has funded several projects to develop and evaluate AIDS preventive interventions. These include a culturally relevant school-based prevention program for Navajo youth and their families living on or near the Navajo Nation Reservation; an HIV risk reduction intervention for gay and bisexual males using skills-building techniques for reducing risky sexual behavior and substance use (primarily drinking); and a safer sex intervention at a substance abuse agency in San Francisco.

Social-Structural Research

None of NIAAA AIDS research grants addressed social-structural factors until 1992, when two grants investigating social influences on risk behaviors were added to the institute's portfolio. One project uses a combined qualitative-quantitative methodology to investigate how the situational context (the place and circumstances under which one drinks) interacts with the use of alcohol and sexual behavior among adolescents. Another study is collecting information on how social norms, personal beliefs, and the context of drinking influence HIV risk behaviors among African American adolescents.

GRANTS

As mentioned above, NIAAA's AIDS research program is quite small, especially relative to NIDA and NIMH. Moreover, NIAAA periodically has varied its coding scheme so that certain grants were considered AIDS-related in some years and not in others. These factors significantly impeded the committee's ability to establish the integrity of the AIDS grant data from NIAAA. Nevertheless, some general statements can be made.

From the beginning of NIAAA's AIDS efforts in 1987, the majority of NIAAA extramural research grants and dollars have been traditional investigator-initiated grants (R01s). In 1987, all AIDS-related extramural grants at NIAAA were biomedical (Figure 6.8). In most cases, these projects examined the effects of alcohol on the immune system. In 1988, NIAAA's portfolio grew to include several grants investigating alcohol use and AIDS risk behaviors. These grants were either single-coded by the committee as epidemiological or multi-coded as epidemiological and psychosocial. However, most of the research grants in 1988 continued to be biomedical. By 1990, 70 percent of NIAAA's research grants had a biomedical component, approximately one-third had a psychosocial component, and 20 percent had an epidemiological component. None of NIAAA's research grants included a social-structural perspective until 1992, as mentioned above. By 1992, the extramural AIDS research portfolio had shifted from a biomedical research focus to a more balanced portfolio including biomedical, psychosocial, and epidemiological research.

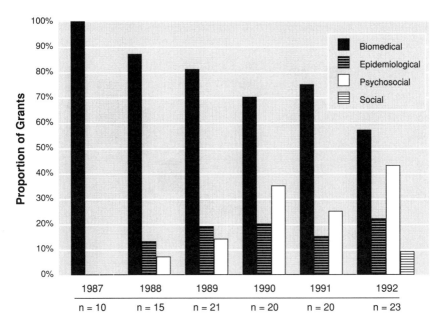

FIGURE 6.8 Proportion of NIAAA AIDS Research Grants, Coded for Each Category, 1987-1992. Note: Includes RPGs only (R01s/R29s). Multi-coded grants are included in each relevant category. Source: NIH CRISP system, and IOM committee database.

NIDA

NIDA's AIDS program began in FY 1983. Although AIDS was less than 1 percent of the total NIDA budget in FY 1983, it rose to 14.5 percent in FY 1987 and 31 percent in FY 1993 (Figure 6.9). Approximately one-third of NIDA's budget now is devoted to AIDS research. Over time, while NIDA's total budget increased by more than 500 percent, its AIDS budget rose by more than 40,000 percent—from $314,000 in FY 1983 to $125.3 million in FY 1992 (Figure 6.10).

NIDA's AIDS research portfolio includes a broad range of initiatives related to HIV/AIDS transmission and disease progression associated with drug abuse. These include studies on effective pharmacologic and/or behavioral therapies to treat drug addiction, research on prevention strategies to reduce sexual and drug-using behaviors linked to HIV/AIDS, longitudinal studies to assess seroincidence, seroprevalence, and disease progression among drug users and their sexual partners, and research to examine the relationship between drugs of abuse and the immune system.

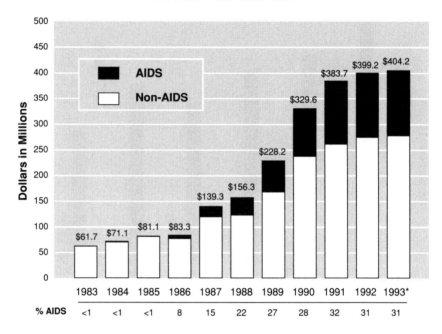

FIGURE 6.9 NIDA Expenditures (AIDS/Non-AIDS), 1983-1993. *Estimate. Source: NIDA Budget Office.

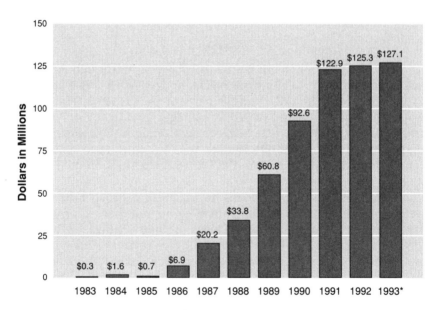

FIGURE 6.10 NIDA AIDS Expenditures, 1983-1993. *Estimate. Source: NIDA Budget Office.

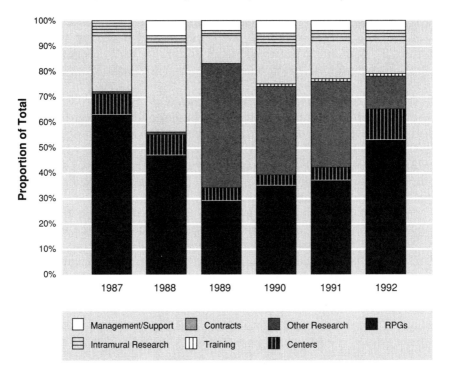

FIGURE 6.11 NIDA AIDS Funding by Mechanism, 1987-1992. Source: NIDA Budget Office.

NIDA's portfolio has included a significant proportion of re-search demonstration projects (R18s) and cooperative agreements (U01s), in addition to traditional investigator-initiated grants (R01s). The bulk of NIDA's AIDS budget, however, remains allocated to RPGs, which made up as much as 63 percent of the total AIDS budget in FY 1987, and as little as 29 percent in FY 1989 (Figure 6.11). Centers comprised 9 percent of AIDS funding in FY 1987, dropped to 4 percent in FY 1990, and then rose again to 12 percent in 1992. Treatment Research Demonstrations (shown as part of "other research") were also significant in NIDA's AIDS program. Although "other research" was less than 1 percent of the AIDS budget in FY 1987, it comprised half of the AIDS budget in FY 1989. Because the data reported here are based on comparable budget tables, they do not include the NADR program (which was transferred to OTI—now called CSAT—in 1991). Inclusion of the NADR program however, would demonstrate that R18s were one of the most significant mechanisms for the NIDA AIDS research program from FY 1987 through FY 1991. By adding the NADR funding, the "other research" category would make up approximately 34 percent of the total AIDS budget in 1987; 55 percent in 1988; 71 percent in 1989; 52 percent in 1990; and 39 percent in 1991.

Training programs were first initiated at NIDA in FY 1990, comprising one percent of the AIDS budget. Intramural research decreased slightly, from 5 percent of the NIDA AIDS budget in FY 1987 to 4 percent in FY 1992. When compared to the AIDS program, NIDA's non-AIDS program has consistently allocated a greater proportion of funding to RPGs, research management and support, and intramural research (Figure 6.12).

Although NIDA has had an AIDS coordinator since the mid-1980s, the institute only formally established an Office of AIDS in FY 1993, as required by the ADAMHA Reorganization Act. NIDA's AIDS program is designed to be decentralized, and it appears that the office has a fairly limited coordinating role. NIDA's

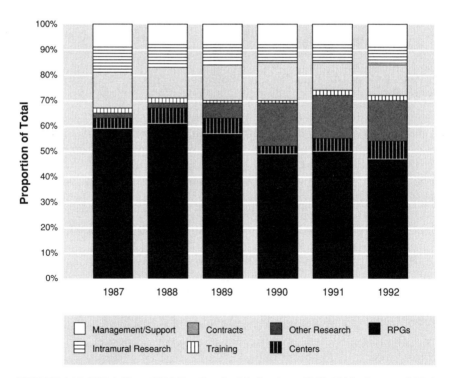

FIGURE 6.12 NIDA Non-AIDS Funding by Mechanism, 1987-1992. Source: NIDA Budget Office.

TABLE 6.3   NIDA AIDS Staffing (FTEs) by Administrative Area, 1987-1993

	1987	1988	1989	1990	1991	1992	1993*
Intramural research	1	1	1	3	15	15	15
RMS	0	13	31	50	59	59	59
AIDS Total	1	14	32	53	74	74	74
NIDA Total	205	260	282	342	356	399	395

NOTE: *Estimate. RMS = Research management and support.

Source: NIDA Budget Office.

Office of AIDS has no budgetary or oversight authority for the wide range of AIDS activities. The current director of the Office of AIDS is also the acting director of the Division of Clinical Research.

In addition, although the number of NIDA's AIDS FTEs increased from 1 to 74 between 1987 and 1991 (Table 6.3), all but two AIDS FTEs are divided among NIDA's divisions. In FY 1993, more than one-third of the AIDS staff were allocated to the Division of Clinical Research (which also received approximately one-third of the AIDS budget), and about one-fourth of the AIDS staff were allocated to the intramural research program (the Addiction Research Center). Many FTEs also were allocated to the Office of Planning and Resource Management (responsible for budgeting and grants management).

PROGRAMS AND PRIORITIES

Biomedical/Biobehavioral Research

NIDA supports biomedical research to investigate the interrelationships among HIV infection and effects of drugs of abuse on the immune, neuroendocrine, and central nervous systems. Preclinical research predominantly conducted in animal models and isolated tissues includes research on the effects of stress on the immune system and endocrine function; the effects of various drugs on stress factors; the effects of various drugs on cellular toxins, lymphokines, receptors and other cellular functions affected by HIV/AIDS; the hypothalamic and immunologic control of drug-modified HIV neurologic changes; and the physiological, biochemical, and immunological mechanisms in the pathogenesis of drug-modulated HIV encephalopathy. Clinical research, predominantly conducted with humans, is focused on the immunologic effects of opiates, marijuana, cocaine, and other drugs. Such studies specifically focus on the effects of drug-related illness and pharmacotherapeutic agents for HIV and drug abuse treatment on immune function.

Other areas of biomedical/biobehavioral AIDS research at NIDA include research related to vertical transmission of HIV (pediatric AIDS projects), development of nonreusable syringes, medications development to create new pharmacological agents for treating substance abuse and addictive disorders, and treatment research to reduce drug use and related risky behaviors.

NIDA supports pediatric AIDS projects to investigate perinatal HIV transmission and progression of pediatric HIV-related diseases related to drug abuse. Projects include research to examine the relationships between drug use patterns and health status (including HIV status) of pregnant women and their impact on perinatal HIV transmission and pregnancy outcome. The Perinatal 20 Treatment Research Demonstration Program is a related NIDA initiative focused on treating and preventing drug use among women of childbearing age. Although it is not an AIDS initiative *per se*, it contributes to the overall strategy to prevent HIV infection among women of childbearing age and their infants.

NIDA's Medication Development Division was established in 1990 to promote the identification, evaluation, and development of new medications for treating drug addiction. Opiate treatment compounds under investigation include LAAM (levo-alpha-acetylmethadol), buprenorphine, naltrexone, and ibogaine. Crack cocaine treatment compounds include a variety of dopamine agonists and antidepressants such as amantadine, desipramine, and fluoxetine. Although this research is not AIDS-specific, NIDA considers it AIDS-related because it is directed at eliminating the kinds of drug use that put people at risk for HIV infection.

Epidemiological Research

The key role of injection drug use in both current epidemiologic patterns and transmission of HIV infection makes clear the importance of basic research to understand the complex behavioral and social dimensions of drug use in relation to HIV transmission.

NIDA monitors HIV infection and risk behaviors among injection drug users through surveillance efforts that are an integral part of various program initiatives, including natural history studies, community-based outreach studies, and research on the role of the sex-for-crack phenomenon. The Seroprevalence Monitoring System is an ongoing contract that has implemented a surveillance system to monitor HIV infection among injection drug users in drug treatment programs. Initiated in 1987, this effort has allowed NIDA to systematically assess the prevalence of HIV infection among injection drug users in treatment programs in seven cities. Although data from this system suggest that levels of HIV infection among injection drug users newly admitted to methadone treatment have been fairly stable, levels of HIV risk behaviors remain high.

To better understand the dynamics of HIV/AIDS among drug users, NIDA has funded research to track HIV infection and risk behaviors among injection drug users, their sex partners, their families, and crack users. In 1984, NIDA funded its first longitudinal study to investigate risk factors for AIDS among drug users in New York City. Since the establishment of the Clinical Medicine Branch in 1987, NIDA has supported more than twenty prospective, longitudinal studies to understand the natural history of HIV transmission and disease progression among injection drug users both in and out of treatment and recruited from drug treatment programs, the criminal justice system, STD clinics, hospitals, and the street. These multidisciplinary studies incorporate biomedical, clinical, and psychosocial factors to investigate medical and behavioral risk factors for infection, clinical manifestations, immune function, and factors associated with seroconversion and disease progression.

In the face of mounting evidence that crack-smoking and sex-for-crack exchanges had the potential for spreading HIV to new populations, NIDA initiated a contract to explore the role of sex-for-crack in HIV transmission. Because the dynamics of the exchange processes were not fully understood, NIDA chose ethnography as the key research technique for studies of sex-for-crack exchanges conducted during 1990 in eight cities—Miami, Chicago, New York, San Francisco, Los Angeles, Denver, Philadelphia, and Newark. Ethnographers based in each city conducted participant observations in crack houses and other locales where crack was purchased and smoked and where sex-for-crack exchanges typically occurred. In addition, 340 crack users (233 females and 107 males) were interviewed at length regarding their drug-using and sexual behaviors.

This eight-city study indicated that crack use is closely linked with a variety of sexual behaviors that place people at risk for HIV. In addition, the study highlighted a substantial population of crack-addicted women and men living in a culture that traditional AIDS prevention initiatives may not have been reaching. An immediate response by NIDA was to extend NADR, its community-based outreach projects (see Box 6.1), initially designed for out-of-treatment injection drug users and their sexual partners, to include crack smokers.

Box 6.1
National AIDS Demonstration Research (NADR) Program

NIDA's first generation of community-based outreach programs are collectively known as the National AIDS Demonstration Research (NADR) Program, and they endured from 1987 through 1992. NADR included 41 HIV/AIDS behavior change intervention projects in 61 communities. The target populations were out-of-treatment injection drug users and their sex partners, and the overall purpose of the effort was to evaluate the efficacy of research-based interventions designed to reduce or eliminate risky behaviors for AIDS transmission, including the sharing of injection paraphernalia, abuse of multiple drugs, and unsafe sexual activities. The projects offered free HIV antibody testing as well as counseling and risk reduction in a variety of settings.

Between 1987 and 1992, the NADR initiative reached more than 150,000 people. Comparison of baseline and follow-up data brought out many significant findings: 46 percent of participants reduced or stopped injecting drugs; 37 percent reduced or stopped sharing needles; 50 percent reduced or stopped borrowing needles; 60 percent reduced or stopped sharing other injection paraphernalia; 22 percent always cleaned their needles.

In addition, 33 percent of the injection drug users contacted by the NADR effort entered treatment after the intervention, and an additional 6 percent sought treatment but were unable to access it. And most strikingly, 25 percent of the injection drug users who had never before been in drug abuse treatment entered a treatment program during the follow-up period (Brown and Beschner, 1993).

Cooperative Agreement for AIDS Community-Based Outreach/Intervention Research

The NADR program spawned a second generation of community-based outreach initiatives at NIDA, collectively known as the Cooperative Agreement for AIDS Community-Based Outreach/Intervention Research. With 22 projects at sites ranging from Anchorage to Miami and from Puerto Rico to Rio de Janeiro, this program began in 1990 and all projects are still in progress. The purposes of the projects are to: (1)

Psychosocial Research

NIDA has funded basic research on the determinants of AIDS risk behaviors, including sexual and drug-using behaviors. NIDA has also funded research grants focused specifically on AIDS prevention, and community-based AIDS prevention programs to get people into drug treatment in order to reduce their risk behaviors.

Box 6.1 Continued

prevent the further spread of HIV infection among injection drug users, crack cocaine users, and others at risk for initiating injection behavior; (2) sample and monitor the serostatus of these populations in high- and low-HIV prevalence areas; and (3) evaluate the efficacy of controlled experimental interventions designed to eliminate or reduce HIV risk behaviors.

All of the cooperative agreement projects use randomized controlled trial designs, with interventions based on theoretical models and scientific sampling strategies. Although none of these projects was completed at the time this report was written, baseline data indicate that 36 percent of the injection drug users recruited had never been in drug abuse treatment, 33 percent had not received an HIV antibody test prior to participating in the study, 43 percent were borrowing needles and/or syringes from other injectors, and 11 percent of those tested for HIV antibodies were found to be seropositive.

The cooperative agreement program also included a number of multisite studies designed to examine patterns of drug use, methods of obtaining drugs (and income and expenditures for drugs), and needle hygiene behaviors.

An important product of the NADR and cooperative agreement initiatives has been the development of a standard intervention that has had a marked effect in reducing drug-related HIV risk behaviors. Equally important, however, has been the finding that the interventions have been less effective in influencing drug users to reduce their sexual risk behaviors (NIDA Cooperative Agreement Steering Committee, 1992).

The cooperative agreement projects also included a number of contracts awarded to develop comprehensive community-based program development, intervention materials, and controlled evaluation trials for HIV risk reduction among the sex partners of injection drug users who are not themselves injectors. Data from these projects indicate that sex partners of injection drug users can be found in the community, will actively participate in risk reduction programs, and will substantially change risky behaviors, including reducing or stopping sexual practices with injection drug users and increasing condom use.

As described below, most of NIDA's treatment research projects also employ psychosocial strategies and outcome measures.

In addition to being the second largest risk group for HIV/AIDS in the United States, injection drug users represent a population that appears difficult to affect with traditional AIDS prevention messages and programs. The potential for HIV acquisition and transmission from infected paraphernalia and unsafe sex is known to virtually all drug users. Yet most are accustomed to risking death (through overdose or the violence-prone nature of the illegal drug marketplace) and disease (hepatitis and other infections) on a daily basis, and this generally fails to inhibit their drug use. For these reasons, warnings that needle sharing or unsafe sex might facilitate an infection that could cause death perhaps five or more years in the future may not be effective for many injection drug users.

Within this context, in 1987, NIDA established its AIDS community-based outreach/intervention/prevention initiative, targeting out-of-treatment drug abusers. The decision to concentrate on out-of-treatment users was based on previous work that demonstrated that this population was considerably large, the most difficult to reach, and either unwilling or unable to cease illegal drug use. At the same time, prior research by NIDA-funded investigators had demonstrated that drug injectors could be located and identified in street settings, hospital emergency rooms, and in the criminal justice system, and that they could effectively be referred to human service programs.

As described in Box 6.1, NIDA's first generation of community outreach programs—NADR—reached approximately 150,000 out-of-treatment drug users and their sex partners. NADR evaluated interventions to reduce high-risk injection drug use and sexual behaviors. The second generation of programs—the Cooperative Agreement for AIDS Community-Based Outreach/Intervention Research—uses randomized controlled trials of interventions to reduce HIV risk behaviors among drug users and their sex partners.

Investigator-initiated grants have been conducted in a variety of treatment and community settings to assess various techniques of HIV risk reduction counseling for sex and drug-related HIV risk behaviors among drug users. Most of these projects use controlled experimental designs to examine education, counseling, skills training, peer support, and other psychosocial interventions. Collectively, these studies have shown that education and counseling can influence drug users to modify their HIV risk behaviors (however, drug-related behaviors are more easily modifiable than sex-related behaviors).

Social-Structural Research

As articulated in NIDA's Five-Year Strategic Plan for AIDS research, one of the institute's primary objectives is to "explicate the transactional and dynamic aspects and the social and behavioral factors that govern high risk drug using and sexual behaviors" (NIDA, 1993). NIDA's plan also emphasizes the need for research to examine HIV risk behaviors over time and under different social circumstances using multidimensional, longitudinal studies.

Research on social factors has been integrated into existing studies, such as NIDA's treatment research initiative and community-based outreach cooperative agreement program described above. NIDA also supports research on the social networks of drug users and their role in HIV transmission. This research ranges from qualitative, ethnographic studies of the characteristics of social networks to quantitative methodological studies of advanced computer techniques for charting social networks.

In addition, NIDA's prevention agenda includes research associated with the provision of sterile drug injection equipment. Although there has been significant political pressure against it, NIDA has succeeded in funding research on needle and syringe disinfection and needle and syringe exchange evaluation (Box 6.2). Disinfection projects involve interdisciplinary basic and clinical research on the effectiveness of bleach in inactivating the HIV virus. Needle and syringe exchange research explores the effectiveness of altering an institutional dimension of injection drug use (that is, the availability of clean needles) in preventing the transmission of HIV.

Drug Abuse Treatment Research

One of NIDA's main priorities for AIDS extramural and intramural research is to develop strategies for increasing the effectiveness of drug abuse treatment. Although treatment research historically has been a priority for NIDA, the AIDS epidemic has heightened its importance (Box 6.3). Drug addiction often involves physical and psychiatric health problems in addition to environmental and social conditions that may contribute to addiction; therefore, effective treatment requires a comprehensive approach.

Box 6.2
Needle Exchange Research

Needle exchange programs in the United States date back to 1986, when activists in Boston and New Haven began trading unused or "clean" needles for used ones. The first formal program was established in Tacoma, Washington in 1988 (Lane, 1993). Although NIDA still is restricted from funding needle exchange services, even as part of clinical research, it finally was able to fund an evaluation of the New Haven needle exchange program in 1992. NIDA has also recently funded evaluations of the needle exchange programs in San Francisco and Tacoma.

The evaluation of the New Haven needle exchange program, a program legally operated by the New Haven Health Department, represents the first federally funded needle exchange research in the United States. Rather than rely on changes in self-reported risky injection behaviors, this study employed mathematical and statistical models combined with data derived from a unique syringe tracking and testing system (or STT) (Kaplan, 1991; Kaplan and O'Keefe, 1993). This system allowed for anonymity, while testing for the presence of HIV-1 proviral DNA using polymerase chain reaction (PCR) to obtain evidence of use by HIV-infected injection drug users (Heimer, Myers, Cadman, et al., 1992; Myers et al., 1993). Demographic and behavioral data were obtained from program clients at program enrollment, making it possible to relate data from the STT to individual client characteristics such as age, injection frequency, duration of drug injection and self-reported frequency of needle sharing. Researchers hypothesized that increasing the turnaround of needles would be equivalent to reducing needle circulation times, narrowing the window of time during which needle sharing can occur, and that if needles circulated for shorter durations of time, there would be fewer opportunities for needles to become infected, and the level of infection measured in needles would fall. The data derived from the STT revealed a significant drop in the portion of needles testing positive for HIV via PCR (Heimer, Kaplan, and Cadman, 1992; Heimer et al., 1993). Coincident with this trend was an increase in the portion of distributed needles returned to the program on a monthly basis, as well as a drop in observed needle circulation times (the time between needle distribution and return). The overall impact of the New Haven program was estimated to be a 33 percent reduction in new transmissions of HIV among the city's injection drug-using population (GAO, 1993; Kaplan, 1994; Kaplan and O'Keefe, 1993).

Because treatment research utilizes both pharmacologic and behavioral approaches, it is an area that cannot be easily categorized into one of the four scientific domains identified by the committee matrix. In fact, what makes these NIDA-funded research projects so unique is their emphasis on employing various combinations of pharmacologic, behavioral, and social approaches to improve the effectiveness of addiction treatment. NIDA has recognized that taking a cross-disciplinary approach in this area is the key to reducing risk of HIV transmission.

NIDA's treatment research grants are organized under three distinct categories: treatment research units (TRUs); experimental therapeutics research projects, and outcome evaluation research projects. TRUs have focused on cutting-edge treatment research, including controlled clinical trials of experimental therapeutics (psychotherapeutic and/or pharmacologic) for heroin and cocaine addiction and studies of medications development. Most TRUs also include HIV testing, counseling, and education to reduce HIV-related risk behaviors.

Experimental therapeutics research projects have also been funded to perform clinical trials of pharmacological and psychotherapy interventions for drug abuse. They include a wide variety of treatment strategies for cocaine and heroin addiction, including studies of fluoxetine, desipramine, buprenorphine, acupuncture, community reinforcement strategies, and behavioral interventions to enhance effectiveness of various medications.

Outcome evaluation research projects have focused on improving treatment effectiveness and reducing dropout rates using various psychosocial and social interventions. These include examining the impact of various treatment environments (inpatient or outpatient, varying program lengths and types) and enhancing treatment environments by adding case managers, individual counseling, or vocational training. All of these grants have used behavioral outcome measures and a few have also measured HIV seropositivity rates. Although these projects are still in progress, preliminary findings suggest that they have increased program capacity, treatment retention, and treatment effectiveness.

GRANTS

During the first decade of AIDS research funding at NIDA, a significant proportion of its AIDS grants were biomedical and psychosocial (Figure 6.13). The NADR Community Outreach Program was a significant focus of the AIDS program beginning in 1987.

Box 6.3
Treatment Research

Treatment research at NIDA has grown tremendously owing to the urgency of the AIDS epidemic. Before the first indicators of the AIDS epidemic had come to the attention of clinicians and researchers throughout the world, the drug abuse problem in the United States appeared to be under control. While heroin use had hit high rates a decade earlier, during the late 1970s the low purity of street heroin was enticing few new users, and concern over the illicit use of cocaine was limited.

In addition, treatment programs were under severe financial constraints during the 1970s as per-slot funding failed to keep pace with inflation. In the 1980s, the "New Federalism" of the Reagan administration further reduced treatment availability (Fletcher, Tims, and Inciardi, 1993). That policy sought to reduce the federal role and give states greater discretion in allocating treatment funds. The passage of the Omnibus Budget Reconciliation Act of 1981 terminated direct federal support of treatment programs and transferred funds directly to states in the form of block grants for alcohol, drug abuse, and mental health treatment. Federal treatment funding through block grants was reduced by 25 percent to reflect savings in administrative costs. Unable or unwilling to increase state allocations to replace federal administration and monitoring efforts, many states gradually reduced their own levels of treatment funding, with consequent declines in the quality and availability of public drug abuse treatment services.

At about the same time, the availability of cocaine increased, permeating all socioeconomic strata and occupational groups. And when crack cocaine became widely available on the streets of urban and rural America, cocaine use quickly became epidemic, particularly in inner-city communities. The emergence of the cocaine epidemic in the early 1980s, furthermore, was concurrent with that of the AIDS epidemic. By 1988, 28 percent of AIDS cases were among injection drug users, who with their sex partners constituted a rapidly growing risk group.

Although increased support of drug abuse treatment to combat the growing epidemics of cocaine use and AIDS was a clear need, misunderstanding and misinformation concerning the nature of drug abuse and the effectiveness of treatment were widespread. Research showed that treatment could be effective in reducing drug use and criminal behavior, but changes in patterns of drug use, in characteristics of drug users, and in the organization and structure of the treatment system created uncertainty regarding past findings on the effectiveness of treatment. Anecdotal reports suggested that typical publicly funded, community-based treatment programs developed in the 1960s and 1970s to treat heroin addiction were challenged by new patterns of drug use and were under severe strain from excessive demand, understaffing, and chronic lack of adequate re-

Box 6.3 Continued

sources and support needed to address such accompanying problems as psychiatric comorbidity and social, educational, and vocational deficits.

Although NIDA was no longer authorized to collect systematic data to monitor client flow and quality of care after 1981, surveys of the homeless, criminal justice clients, and the general household population provided evidence that the number of publicly funded treatment slots fell far short of need. It was estimated that on any given day in 1987-1988, some 5.5 million individuals needed drug treatment, while the public and private treatment capacity was estimated at only 329,000 (IOM, 1990).

Within this context there was an urgent need to expand the availability of treatment services and to improve their effectiveness—both to curb cocaine use and to slow the spread of AIDS among injection drug users. Faced with epidemics that threatened to overwhelm an already weakened treatment system, NIDA developed a program of research demonstrations to improve and expand treatment. The initiative was conceived in 1988 as part of a larger AIDS prevention effort under the premise that more effective drug abuse treatment would reduce many of the risk behaviors that were spreading HIV infection. The target populations of the effort included injection drug users as well as non-injecting drug abusers who were at risk through prostitution and sex-for-drugs exchanges.

Since 1989, approximately 30 projects have been funded through the research demonstration grant mechanism to develop, implement, and evaluate innovative treatment approaches. In addition to direct research costs, funds were provided for the support of research-related treatment costs, thereby creating new treatment capacity. The innovative projects included: special initiatives and programs targeting issues of perinatal substance abuse; enhancements to traditional treatment modalities such as methadone maintenance, residential treatment, and case management; alternative approaches for increasing retention in methadone, therapeutic community, and drug-free outpatient programs; new models for the treatment of cocaine addiction and the dually diagnosed; and such totally new initiatives as a work release therapeutic community for prisoners, and a modified day treatment therapeutic community for methadone clients.

All of these programs were funded under the R18 mechanism, but the legislation supporting this mechanism has now lapsed. There has been an attempt to stimulate new treatment research demonstrations under the R01 mechanism. However, given the high cost of treatment services associated with these projects, it is the opinion of many treatment researchers that without the R18 mechanism few new innovative projects will be funded.

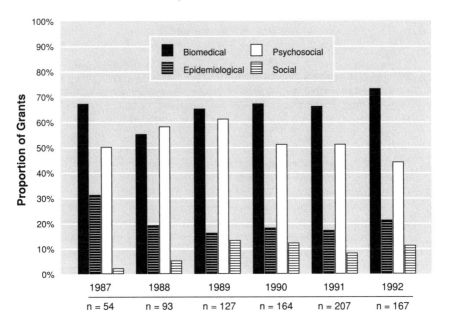

FIGURE 6.13 Proportion of NIDA AIDS Research Grants, Coded for Each Category, 1987-1992. Note: Includes RPGs (R01s, R29s, R37s, U01s, but not R43/44s); all R18s (including NADR). Multi-coded grants are included in each relevant category. Source: NIH CRISP system, and IOM committee database.

All NADR grants are categorized according to the committee's codes as applied psychosocial research. Some also include a social-structural component and are coded accordingly. The Community Outreach Cooperative Agreement Program grants—the second generation of NADR—were initially funded in 1990 and all have a psychosocial component. All of these projects are behavioral interventions aimed at reducing high-risk drug-using and sexual behaviors, and all employ the randomized controlled trial methodology, which has had the effect of eliminating the social-structural component that was present in some of the earlier, NADR projects. Approximately two-thirds of these projects also include the development of a surveillance system to monitor behaviors of out-of-treatment injection drug users (and their sex partners in some projects), and are also coded as epidemiological. Several projects also measure changes in seroprevalence rates among study participants, and are coded as biomedical.

More than 80 percent of NIDA's AIDS demonstration grants (R18s), funded between 1989 and 1992, are multi-coded. Approximately 90 percent of them have a psychosocial component, 70 percent have a biomedical component, and approximately 33 percent also include a social-structural component.

In general, NIDA's AIDS program displayed a greater commitment to social-structural research than NIAAA's or NIMH's programs did, although this was still small relative to other categories of research. Furthermore, NIDA's grant portfolio was fairly well balanced between biomedical and psychosocial research until 1990, when it shifted toward favoring biomedical research.

NIMH

NIMH has supported research on the neuroscience, neuropsychiatric, and psychosocial aspects of HIV infection and AIDS since 1983. Research has focused on the identification of determinants of high-risk behaviors and strategies to change those behaviors, as well as the mental health and neurological consequences of HIV infection.

NIMH first funded AIDS research in FY 1983, when the institute received $200,000 from supplemental funds to support several AIDS-related research project grants (R01s). While the total NIMH budget increased from $191.5 in FY 1983 to $560.5 million in FY 1992 (Figure 6.14), the AIDS budget increased from $200,000 in FY 1983 to $76.2 million in FY 1992 (Figure 6.15). AIDS accounted for less than 1 percent of the total NIMH budget from FY 1983 through FY 1985 and rose to 14 percent by FY 1990.

NIMH funding generally has been committed to R01s and P50s (research center grants). RPGs make up the bulk of the NIMH AIDS program—98 percent of AIDS funding in FY 1984, 38 percent in FY 1987, and 45 percent in FY 1992 (Figure 6.16). Centers also have been a significant mechanism for AIDS research, representing 19 percent of the AIDS budget in FY 1986 (the initial year for centers), rising to 33 percent in FY 1988, and leveling off at approximately 20 percent in FY 1991. NIMH has supported more AIDS training grants than either of the other two institutes. Training grants represent approximately 5 percent of the total NIMH AIDS budget. Contracts have constituted a small part of the AIDS program—rising from less than 1 percent in FY 1989 to 3 percent in FY 1990. Although intramural research has been an important component of the AIDS program at NIMH, it fell from 18 percent of the total AIDS budget in FY 1987 and leveled off at about 11 percent in FY 1989.

Compared to NIMH's non-AIDS funding (Figure 6.17), the dis-

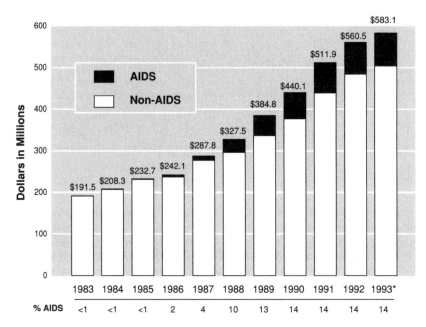

FIGURE 6.14 NIMH Expenditures (AIDS/Non-AIDS), 1983-1993. *Estimate. Source: NIMH Budget Office.

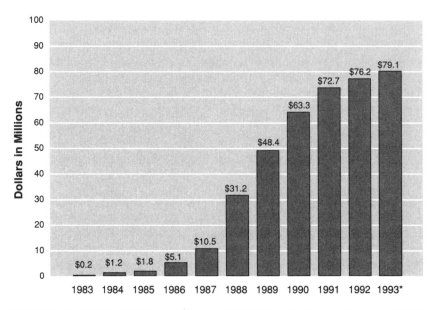

FIGURE 6.15 NIMH AIDS Expenditures, 1983-1993. *Estimate. Source: NIMH Budget Office.

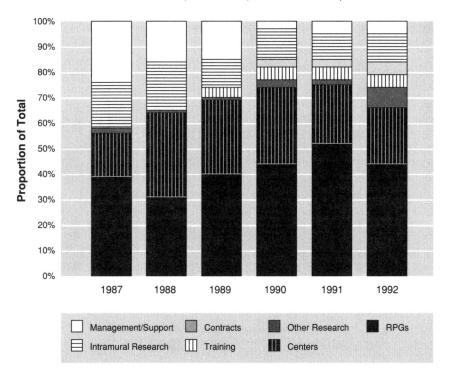

FIGURE 6.16 NIMH AIDS Funding by Mechanism, 1987-1992. Source: NIMH Budget Office.

tribution of NIMH AIDS funding by mechanism has fluctuated greatly from year to year. Unlike NIDA and NIAAA, the AIDS research program at NIMH has for some time been managed by a central AIDS office, which develops the AIDS plan (with input from outside consultants and various divisions and offices within NIMH), develops the annual AIDS budget, and directs the AIDS extramural program. While the ADAMHA Reorganization Act required the creation of a formal AIDS office at NIMH, such an office already existed administratively within the office of the director. The program continues to be centrally directed, and the majority of NIMH's extramural FTEs are located within the AIDS office, the Division of Resource Management, or the Office of Extramural Affairs (to review grants, handle grants management activities, contract, budget, and perform other administrative functions). In FY 1993, only two FTEs were allocated to other program divisions. Although NIMH AIDS FTEs rose 230 percent from FY 1986 to FY 1993, they still represent less than 5 percent of the total FTEs (Table 6.4).

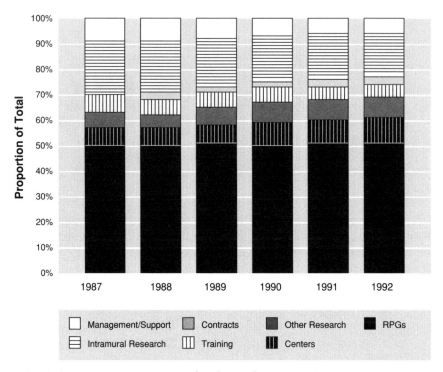

FIGURE 6.17 NIMH Non-AIDS Funding by Mechanism, 1987-1992. Source: NIMH Budget Office.

TABLE 6.4   NIMH AIDS Staffing (FTEs) by Administrative Area, 1986-1993

	1986	1987	1988	1989	1990	1991	1992	1993*
Intramural research	3	14	12	17	25	25	25	25
RMS	0	0	7	10	21	21	21	21
AIDS Total	3	14	19	27	46	46	46	46
NIMH Total	779	819	869	861	868	903	934	984

NOTE: *Estimate. RMS = Research management and support.

Source: NIMH Budget Office.

PROGRAMS AND PRIORITIES

Biomedical/Biobehavioral Research

NIMH supports intramural and extramural research on the neuroscience and neurobehavioral aspects of AIDS. When clinical researchers documented that the AIDS virus directly infected the brain, the NIMH program expanded to investigate the mechanisms of CNS HIV-1 infection.

Biomedical/biobehavioral and clinical research at NIMH is classified into several main categories, although by necessity they often overlap: the effects of HIV/AIDS on CNS function (classified as *neuroscience*); the neuropsychological, neuropsychiatric, and neurological sequelae of HIV infection on the CNS (classified as *neurobehavior*); and the biological interface relating stress and behavior to immune function (classified as *psychoneuroimmunology*).

Intramural research at NIMH has focused on the neuroscience of HIV infection and the development of animal models for more rapid exploration of the consequences of HIV infection in the brain. Intramural scientists have investigated interactions between HIV and the CNS, cognitive dysfunction and AIDS dementia, and treatment of the HIV effects on the brain. Specific intramural projects have included research on: the interaction between HIV-1 and cultured brain neurons, the role of quinolinic acid (QUIN) in CNS damage, the development of Peptide T as a potential treatment for improving neurocognitive functioning, and the impact of HIV infection on neurobehavioral functioning (visual learning, memory, and motor skills) in monkeys infected with simian immunodeficiency virus (SIV). In collaboration with investigators at the Walter Reed Army Medical Center, intramural researchers have also been studying the consequences of HIV infection on neuropsychological and neurological function in early stages of HIV infection.

To shape its extramural neuro-AIDS program, NIMH, together with the National Institute on Child Health and Human Development (NICHD) and the National Institute on Neurological Disorders and Stroke (NINDS), first issued several program announcements in September 1988 to stimulate basic neuroimmunological research on the etiology and pathology of HIV infection of the brain and to investigate the neurological and psychiatric sequelae. Research on interactions between the immune system and the brain was intended to provide important knowledge about the molecular and cellular mechanisms that affect disease susceptibility and progression. More recently, in 1992 NIMH and NINDS jointly issued a program announcement to encourage individual researchers (primarily neuroscientists) to work in partnership with researchers from the AIDS clinical trials units (ACTUs), the Multicenter AIDS Cohort Study (MACS), and the Women and Infants Transmission Study (WITS) on studies of HIV infection of the CNS. The overarching goal of AIDS-related neuroscience research is to understand the pathogenetic mechanisms involved in HIV-associated brain dysfunction. This encompasses clinical and laboratory research studies aimed at understanding the biology of HIV infection of the CNS and the mechanisms of brain dysfunction at the organismic, cellular, and molecular levels. Investigations cross many disciplines and range from clinical studies dealing with natural history, disturbed physiology, and neuroimaging, as well as clinical virology and immunology, to fundamental laboratory studies involving animal and cell culture models, as well as biochemical and molecular research.

Neurobehavioral research generally is more clinically directed and aims at defining and understanding the effects of HIV and various treatment on the neurodevelopment of infected and at-risk infants and children, and the neuropsychological, neuropsychiatric and neurological sequelae of HIV infection in infected and at-risk adults. This research involves methodological development, direct study of clinical presentation and natural history, and assessment of antiviral therapy and other interventions.

NIMH also has supported psychoneuroimmunology research in its AIDS program. This discipline focuses on the relationship between the brain (including its behavioral state) and the immune system. Its potential application to AIDS is supported by the hypothesis that behavioral states may modulate immune defenses against HIV and thereby alter the response to HIV exposure and the rate of progression to AIDS in those infected.

Epidemiological Research

Through its AIDS research centers and investigator-initiated research grants, NIMH has supported behavioral epidemiology research to identify specific populations at risk for HIV/AIDS and to understand the specific high-risk behaviors of various populations, including homosexual and bisexual men, heterosexual women and men, adolescents, injection drug users and their partners, people with severe mental illness, and the homeless. Not only is behavioral epidemiology critical for understanding risk factors associated with HIV transmission and disease progression, it is essential to the development and evaluation of preventive AIDS interventions.

Psychosocial Research

Psychosocial research investigating the determinants of risky sexual and drug-using behaviors, as well as strategies for changing these behaviors, is a major focus of the NIMH AIDS research portfolio. Beginning prior to the emergence of the epidemic and continuing into its first twelve years, political restrictions on sexual behavior and drug abuse research resulted in a relative dearth of knowledge about HIV risk behaviors. Nevertheless, NIMH was able to support a vigorous research program in this area, providing for basic psychosocial research and applied research to test the effectiveness of intervention strategies in preventing transmission of HIV infection.

Basic psychosocial research at NIMH includes theory development and testing of behavior change models, development and testing of assessments, and research on the determinants of behaviors. Basic research in this area has critically informed AIDS preventive intervention research. In the realm of applied research, NIMH has supported theory-driven preventive interventions that focus on behavior change strategies for individuals or small groups at high risk. Many of these efforts have demonstrated successful behavior change, and their generalizability is being tested in prevention strategies across multiple populations and sites in an NIMH-initiated cooperative agreement begun in 1990. This program, the Multi-Site HIV Prevention Trial, is a longitudinal five-year study targeting the chronically mentally ill, injection drug users and their partners, prisoners, young gay men, high-risk adolescents, women, and STD clinic clients.

Basic and applied psychosocial research also have been the focus of two of the five NIMH-funded centers—the Center for AIDS Prevention Studies (CAPS) at the University of California, San Francisco (UCSF), and the HIV Center for Clinical and Behavioral Studies at Columbia University/New York State Psychiatric Institute (see below for more on the centers program).

Social-Structural Research

NIMH has funded several basic research grants to explore the social context of risk behavior. These grants examine the development of social groups and crowd characteristics during early adolescence and the impact of crowd affiliation on risky behavior; the feasibility of using social network data to operationalize socioecological constructs that may influence risky behavior; the features and effects of social relationships on behavior; and the nature of structural barriers to AIDS health services and care (health services research). The NIMH agenda also emphasizes the importance of incorporating social factors into research on HIV risk behavior change and supporting research on preventive interventions at the individual, small group, institutional, and community level.

GRANTS

The most significant single domain of research at NIMH is psychosocial research, followed closely by biomedical research (Figure 6.18). Psychosocial research grants at NIMH include basic research on psychological mechanisms that underlie behavioral outcomes (including such topics as the relationship between emotion and cognition, stress and coping processes, decision-making processes, and sexual identity formation, behavioral and psychological responses to HIV testing and HIV status, and stress and coping among caregivers). Applied psychosocial research grants include

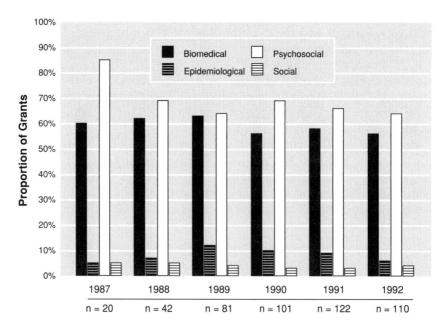

FIGURE 6.18 Proportion of NIMH AIDS Research Grants, Coded for Each Category, 1987-1992. Note: Includes RPGs only (R01s, P01s, R29s, R37s, R43/44s, and U01s). Multi-coded grants are included in each relevant category. Source: NIH CRISP system, and IOM committee database.

behavioral interventions for HIV prevention. Single-coded applied psychosocial grants use behavioral outcome measures only.

Many NIMH research grants are multi-coded for biomedical and psychosocial research components. Applied biomedical/psychosocial grants include: behavioral interventions for HIV prevention that incorporate outcome measures such as HIV seropositivity rates and/or STD rates in addition to behavioral outcome measures, and treatments and interventions for AIDS-related depression and emotional distress.

Basic biomedical/psychosocial grants include: natural history and descriptive studies examining the neuropsychological and neurobehavioral sequelae of HIV infection (studies that simultaneously gather information on biological parameters and psychosocial factors); research examining the relationship between psychosocial factors (including social stress, dominance ranking in social groups, social isolation, and social companionship) and the immune system generally with HIV disease progression specifically (in humans and non-human primates).

Most single-coded biomedical grants are basic research and include: psychoneuroimmunology and neuroimmunology research grants that focus on biological processes and mechanisms (mostly in animals, some in humans); research on neural-immune-endocrine interactions; research on neural cell functions; research on CNS pathology; and research on AIDS dementia complex. NIMH has funded several applied biomedical grants, that are therapeutic interventions.

NIMH's few grants with a social-structural component are all basic research and focus on understanding the role of social relationships and social networks in shaping an individual's behavior.

Although research centers account for a significant proportion of AIDS research funding at NIMH, they are not included in the table above. Because the centers have received funding from other institutes as well as NIMH, they are among the collaborative projects described below.

COLLABORATIVE PROJECTS

NIAAA, NIDA, and NIMH have collaborated on a number of AIDS research activities. For example, the three institutes issued joint program announcements in September 1988 for *Research on behavior change and prevention strategies to reduce transmission of HIV* (with four other NIH institutes and CDC) and for the *Role of family in preventing and adapting to HIV infection and*

AIDS. The institutes also have jointly sponsored multidisciplinary extramural AIDS research centers at institutions around the country.

AIDS RESEARCH CENTERS

AIDS research centers were first initiated in 1986 to provide support for coordinated, multidisciplinary research programs on the mental health and drug abuse aspects of HIV/AIDS. Since 1986, NIMH has supported five AIDS research centers. NIDA contributed some funding to three of these centers from 1986 through 1991.

The Center for Biopsychosocial Study of AIDS at the University of Miami was initially funded in 1986 to focus on biopsychosocial aspects of AIDS. At the intersection of biomedical and psychosocial research, the Miami center has investigated the relationship between lifestyle changes and disease progression as measured by neurocognitive and immune status.

Researchers at the UCSF Center for AIDS Prevention Studies (CAPS), also established in 1986, have conducted basic and applied research on sex and drug-related risk behaviors among a range of populations varying by sexual orientation, gender, race/ethnicity, and age. These projects include the National AIDS Behavioral Surveys (NABS), the AIDS in Multiethnic Neighborhoods (AMEN) study, studies of Latino and Latina Americans, and studies focused on improving sexual behavior research methods.

The HIV Center for Clinical and Behavioral Studies at the New York State Psychiatric Institute and Columbia University was established in 1987. This center has been committed to research on the behavioral manifestations of HIV infection and disease progression. More recently, it refined its research goals to the investigation of the determinants of sexual risk behavior for HIV and behavior change among heterosexual women and men and among the homeless mentally ill, developmental principles of sexual risk behavior during childhood and adolescence, the involvement of CNS in advanced stages of HIV disease, and improved methodological techniques.

Beginning in 1987, NIMH supported AIDS Research Centers to address key neurobiological and behavioral issues through interdisciplinary research on the CNS effects of HIV, ADC, neuropsychiatric aspects of HIV infection, brain-immune interaction, and behavior change and prevention. The HIV Neurobehavioral Research Center at the University of California, San Diego was established in 1989 to investigate neurobehavioral functioning and to identify specifically the effect of HIV on the CNS. Using neuropsychological, neuropsychiatric, and neuroimaging techniques, this center is investigating etiology, pathogenesis, and natural history of neurobehavioral disturbances associated with HIV/AIDS.

The Research Center on Molecular and Cellular Mechanisms of AIDS Dementia at the Scripps Research Institute in La Jolla, California was established in 1990 to investigate the molecular and cellular mechanisms underlying ADC. Investigators at this center have conducted multidisciplinary research to define the biological actions of persistent virus infections of the brain, the profiles of cell-to-cell signals activated by these infections, and the nature of the effects of these signals on neuron function, by conducting comparative evaluations of brain pathophysiology in AIDS patients with that found in three animal models.

Currently, NIMH is still funding four of the AIDS research centers: the Center for AIDS Prevention Studies, the HIV Center for Clinical and Behavioral Studies, the HIV Neurobehavioral Research Center, and the Research Center on Molecular and Cellular Mechanisms of AIDS Dementia. As this report was being written, NIMH announced it had funded under the "core" mechanism a new Center for AIDS Intervention Research (CAIR) at the Medical College of Wisconsin. This center will focus attention on HIV prevention and HIV mental health service intervention research.

TRAINING

Training has been an integral part of the AIDS programs at NIAAA, NIDA, and NIMH. NIAAA has funded training for AIDS-related alcohol research and has contributed to collaborative efforts to develop AIDS and substance abuse curricula for health care providers. NIDA initiated an AIDS training program in 1986 for counselors and administrators at drug abuse treatment programs. (This program was transferred to SAMHSA as a result of the ADAMHA reorganization.) NIDA also funds a number of training grants for predoctoral and postdoctoral students on research issues related to drug abuse and AIDS. NIMH training efforts are designed to prepare young scientists for careers in AIDS research. Training grants are awarded to individuals and to institutions committed to HIV-related mental health research, and the NIMH AIDS research centers provide training programs for new investigators. NIMH has trained more than 40,000 health care providers in the neuropsychiatric and psychosocial aspects of HIV/

AIDS through the NIMH AIDS Health Care Provider Training Program initiated in 1986.

THE NIH CONTEXT

Now that NIAAA, NIDA, and NIMH are located at NIH, they are part of the funding and programmatic agenda of NIH. An understanding of the overall AIDS budget and program context at NIH will provide some insight into how the former ADAMHA institutes will function in the NIH environment. Total NIH funding increased more than 100 percent between 1983 and 1993 (from $4.3 billion to $10.3 billion). While the growth in AIDS research in the same period appears to be explosive, it reflects the requirement to respond rapidly to a new disease with major public health implications (Figure 6.19). Seven NIH institutes and centers (including NIDA and NIMH) received the vast majority of AIDS funding during this period (Figure 6.20). In order of magnitude, based on FY 1992 expenditures, they are: the National Institute of Allergies and Infectious Diseases (NIAID), which received 43 percent; the National Cancer Institute (NCI), which received 16 percent; NIDA,

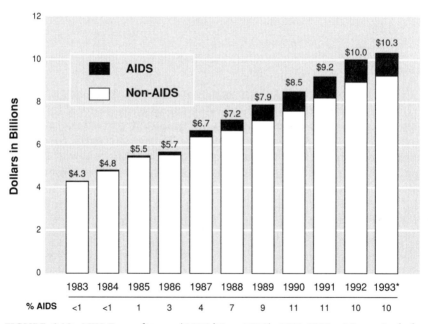

FIGURE 6.19 NIH Expenditures (AIDS/Non-AIDS), 1983-1993. Note: Includes NIAAA, NIDA, and NIMH for all years. *Estimate. Source: NIH Budget Office.

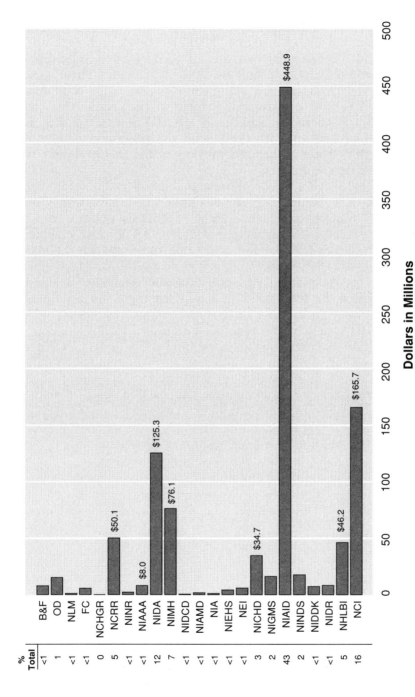

FIGURE 6.20 NIH AIDS Research Funding by Component, 1992. Source: OAR and Division of Financial Management, NIH.

which received 12 percent; NIMH, which received 7 percent; the National Center for Research Resources (NCRR) and the National Heart, Lung, and Blood Institute (NHLBI), which each received 5 percent; and the National Institute of Child Health and Human Development (NICHD), which received 3 percent. These seven institutes together received 90 percent of the total NIH AIDS budget for FY 1992 and over 90 percent of the cumulative total since 1983. With the exception of NICHD, whose funding increased suddenly in the late 1980s with the growing concern over pediatric AIDS, the number and ranking of the major players has remained fairly constant.

AIDS constituted a major portion of the budget for each of the seven institutes (Table 6.5). For example, in FY 1992 nearly half of NIAID's budget, nearly one-third of NIDA's budget, and 16 percent of NCRR's budget were devoted to AIDS. Just 2 percent of the cumulative total of the other institutes was for AIDS research.

While NIAAA, NIDA, and NIMH together represent a significant portion of the NIH AIDS budget, their funds are distributed quite differently from most of the other institutes. In FY 1992, NIAAA, NIDA, and NIMH together comprised $209.4 million or approximately 20 percent of the total NIH AIDS budget (NIAAA's portion is minor, however). According to estimates for FY 1993, the three institutes continued to account for 11 percent of the total NIH budget and 20 percent of the AIDS budget. Yet they

TABLE 6.5 AIDS Funding as Proportion of 1992 Budget, Selected NIH Institutes (Dollars in Millions)

Institute	AIDS	Total	% AIDS
NCI	165.7	1,947.6	9
NHLBI	46.2	1,190.1	4
NIAID	448.9	960.1	47
NICHD	34.7	518.6	7
NIMH	76.1	560.8	14
NIDA	125.3	399.1	31
NIAAA	8.0	171.5	5
NCRR	50.1	314.2	16
Other	94.6	3,948.4	2
TOTAL	1,049.6	10,010.4	10

Source: Division of Financial Management, NIH.

funded more than 97 percent of NIH's behavioral research (as defined by the Mason categories), 64 percent of surveillance, 54 percent of neuroscience and neuropsychiatric research, and over 30 percent of health services research and research training. On the other hand, NIAAA, NIDA, and NIMH account for less than 1 percent of the funding for therapeutic agents and 12 percent of the funding for biomedical research, two categories that together represent nearly 60 percent of the total NIH AIDS budget. It is clear that NIAAA, NIDA, and NIMH play a critical role in the overall NIH AIDS research agenda and particularly in its biobehavioral and behavioral agenda.

However, at the time this report was written, the overall NIH agenda was in the process of being reformulated, reflecting the requirements of the NIH Reauthorization Act that vested new authority for AIDS planning and budgeting within OAR. In addition to new budgetary authority, OAR also was given responsibility for developing and coordinating a five-year strategic plan for AIDS research across the NIH institutes. The general outline of that plan has been developed, and five AIDS-related research categories have been identified: natural history and epidemiology; etiology and pathogenesis; therapeutics; vaccines; and behavioral research. (Social research for the most part will likely be subsumed under the "behavioral" category.) Coordinating committees composed of NIH staff and external experts will formulate strategies regarding research priorities, goals, and objectives within these categories, across institutes. (The plan also discusses training and infrastructure and information dissemination.) Eventually, OAR will attach budget allocations to various institutes based on these strategies.

It is not clear yet how these OAR-level activities will be linked with the AIDS program activities of specific institutes. For example, although the ADAMHA Reorganization Act required that NIDA and NIMH create an Office on AIDS, it did not specify how these entities should work with the NIH OAR. Without knowing at the time this report was written how these offices plan to work together, the committee believes that all three institutes should have an AIDS coordinator for whom this job is the primary responsibility. The coordinator should be provided appropriate resources to develop and coordinate the institute's AIDS programs in cooperation with division and branch staff. The coordinator also should be linked to the OAR and the activities of its coordinating committees. It is the committee's understanding that at least in some cases, such as at NIMH, this is already occurring.

CONCLUSION AND RECOMMENDATIONS

CONCLUSION

The AIDS research programs of NIAAA, NIDA, and NIMH have developed over the past decade in response to growth and change in the HIV/AIDS epidemic itself. Increased recognition of the substance abuse and mental health aspects of AIDS is both a reflection of and encouragement for the institutes' involvement in AIDS research during this period. This is evidenced by the precipitous growth in funding of the institutes' AIDS programs, which has significantly outpaced growth in overall funding.

Characterizing and evaluating the content of the institutes' AIDS programs is a difficult task. Coding by any scheme—whether scientific domain or AIDS versus non-AIDS—is an imperfect science. Moreover, assessing the value of the research supported is hampered for applied research by a notable lack of evaluative studies, and for basic research by the recognition that the benefits of any study may not be discovered for some time after it is conducted—and that findings may end up benefitting a different area than that imagined by the investigators.

Nevertheless, the effort undertaken by the committee to assess the AIDS research programs of NIAAA, NIDA, and NIMH did reveal some important findings. Chief among these is that a significant amount of cross-disciplinary research is being supported. Much of this is directed research, which indicates a recognition on the part of the institute staff that understanding and intervening in the substance abuse, sexual behavior, and mental health aspects of AIDS requires a complex approach that takes into account the interactions of neurobiological, psychological, and social factors in the lives of individuals. The committee is encouraged by this, and would like to see the appreciation of cross-disciplinary research applied to investigator-initiated grants as well.

A related finding is that the overall balance between what could be considered "biomedical" and "behavioral" (primarily psychological) research at the institutes generally has improved over time (there is greater parity in the number and funding of grants in both domains). NIMH has most consistently balanced its portfolio; and NIAAA has moved quickly in the last couple of years to achieve greater balance. NIDA, however, moved away from its earlier balance toward favoring biomedical research, following the transfer of the NADR program out of its portfolio. In all cases, however, the "behavioral" category is primarily composed of psychosocial grants; social-structural research is notably under-supported at all three institutes.

A second important finding of the committee's analysis is that most AIDS research supported by the institutes is basic science research. This suggests that there is still a need to uncover the basic mechanisms and processes by which HIV is transmitted, experienced, and prevented in different populations. While the epidemic cries out for the quick application of basic research findings to intervention programs, this will prove ineffective in achieving its intended goal—the prevention of new HIV infections—unless basic research is solid. With respect to AIDS, although there have been significant developments in basic research on sexual behavior, drug addiction, and the effect of the HIV on the CNS, much remains to be learned.

Advances in AIDS research at NIAAA, NIDA, and NIMH—especially in the neurosciences and social sciences—will have significant implications for other areas of research at these institutes and others. These advances relate to broader phenomena, such as neurobiological drives toward addiction and sexual gratification, mental health and illness, and the role of social structure and culture in influencing individual behavior.

RECOMMENDATIONS FOR RESEARCH FUNDING, PROGRAMS, AND PRIORITIES AT NIAAA, NIDA, AND NIMH

6.1 The committee recommends that NIAAA, NIDA, and NIMH each establish a position for a full-time AIDS coordinator. The coordinator should be provided appropriate resources to develop and coordinate the institute's AIDS programs in cooperation with division and branch staff. The coordinator also should be linked to the NIH Office of AIDS Research.

6.2 The committee encourages OAR to serve as a catalyst for cross-institute and cross-PHS agency research collaborations through its funding authority and leadership role.

6.3 The committee recommends that the OAR leadership include competence in biomedical, neuroscience, behavioral, and social science perspectives.

6.4 The committee recommends that NIAAA, NIDA, and NIMH ensure the maintenance of the behavioral and social science research programs of the three institutes within the NIH context. The committee supports the recommendation

of the National Commission on AIDS (1993b) to expand research in the following behavioral and social science research perspectives: behavioral epidemiology; cognitive science; cultural and ethnographic studies; intervention research; mental health research; behavioral aspects of technological interventions; and organizational studies. The committee adds to that list cost-effectiveness research and evaluation research.

6.5 The committee notes that, of all the types of AIDS research at NIAAA, NIDA, and NIMH, social science research is the most underfunded. The committee therefore recommends that the three institutes develop new initiatives to support research on the role of social, cultural, and structural factors in HIV/AIDS transmission, prevention, and intervention.

6.6 The committee recommends that, given the prominent role of drug injection in HIV transmission and given the considerable evidence that has been assembled over the past several years regarding the efficacy of needle exchange, the U.S. government remove current restrictions barring federal funding for needle exchange programs, promote services-oriented research to help implement such programs where warranted, and evaluate these programs with an eye toward maximizing their preventive impact.

6.7 The committee recommends that drug abuse treatment research at NIDA be continued to support the design and evaluation of innovative and cross-disciplinary drug abuse treatment strategies, including collaborative efforts with SAMHSA. These strategies should include those targeted to high-risk populations, such as drug-involved offenders, prisoners, women, and crack-cocaine users. The committee urges NIDA to pay particular attention to developing treatment strategies for crack-cocaine.

6.8 The committee recommends that NIAAA, NIDA, and NIMH restore support for research demonstration projects, using a mechanism similar to the R18 that facilitates cooperation between the NIH research institute and the relevant PHS services agency or agencies.

6.9 The committee recommends that an effort be made to coordinate between institutes that have overlapping AIDS research programs (for example, HIV and CNS function at

NIMH and NINDS) by collaborating in the program development, review, and funding processes.

6.10 Given the disproportionate impact of the epidemic on men, African Americans, and Hispanics/Latinos, it is important to understand the sociocultural-specific factors—including gender, race/ethnicity, and class—that play a role in the behavioral aspects of AIDS. Therefore, the committee recommends that NIAAA, NIDA, and NIMH, with input from appropriate experts, develop a mechanism for collecting and reporting data on the gender, race/ethnicity, and socioeconomic status (class) of study populations in projects supported by the institutes. Such data collection and reporting should be guided by clear articulation of the role of these variables in the epidemic.

7

Linkages Between Research and Services

How the two worlds of researchers and service providers interact is of great concern to all those involved in AIDS activities. With respect to AIDS prevention and intervention, research findings must be disseminated to the field as quickly and effectively as possible. At the same time, service providers often are in a unique position to discover new, researchable questions. To facilitate the exchange of ideas, federal agencies charged with missions for research and services must overcome differences and develop strategies for effective coordination and communication.

This chapter examines the relationship between the AIDS research programs of NIAAA, NIDA, and NIMH and the services programs at the Substance Abuse and Mental Health Services Administration (SAMHSA) and other PHS agencies. The following discussion begins with a description of the SAMHSA AIDS programs, and then looks at how service programs in general and SAMHSA programs in particular are linked with the AIDS research programs of NIAAA, NIDA, and NIMH. Attention is also paid to the issue of collaboration and coordination beyond NIH and SAMHSA in the larger arena of PHS and HHS.

AIDS PROGRAMS AT SAMHSA

SAMHSA was officially established in FY 1992 as the new incarnation of the services activities of the former ADAMHA.

SAMHSA's major components are the Center for Mental Health Services (CMHS), the Center for Substance Abuse Prevention (CSAP)—previously the Office of Substance Abuse Prevention (OSAP)—and the Center for Substance Abuse Treatment (CSAT)—previously the Office of Treatment Improvement (OTI). The Agency's comparable total budget increased from an appropriation of $794.7 million in FY 1988 to $2.1 billion in FY 1993. During the same period, specifically identified AIDS funding decreased from $42.5 million to $28 million (falling from 5 percent of the total budget to 1 percent) (Table 7.1).

AIDS constitutes a very small part of SAMHSA funding. To some degree, this is a legacy of the ADAMHA years, during which the vast majority of AIDS funding at the agency was allocated to research activities, as Figure 7.1 shows. Research represented 100 percent of the ADAMHA AIDS budget from FY 1983 to FY 1986, declined to 62 percent in FY 1988, and rose to 89 percent of the total AIDS budget in FY 1992.

As of FY 1994, only four programs are recognized in SAMHSA's formal budget as being AIDS related. Two of these programs—which constitute the bulk of the agency's AIDS-specific funds—are located in CSAT. The first, the Demonstrations and Training Program, has three components: Linkage, Training, and Outreach. The Linkage Program, which originated at NIDA in 1989, is a joint effort with the Health Resources and Services Administration (HRSA) to support demonstration projects that link community-based primary care and substance abuse, HIV/AIDS, and mental health treatment services. The program was funded at $7.8 million in FY 1993. The Training Program, which had a $2.8 million budget in FY 1993, trains health care workers, focusing on the relationship between substance abuse, HIV/AIDS, tuberculosis, and sexually transmitted diseases in the context of treatment services. The Outreach Program is the outgrowth of the NADR program that originated at NIDA and was later transferred to OTI (see Chapters 3 and 6). The current iteration still focuses on HIV prevention outreach to out-of-treatment drug users and their sexual partners, but now includes more complete medical assessments for tuberculosis and diagnostic screening for HIV. This program supports 25 to 30 projects for up to three years and had a total budget of $10 million in FY 1993.

The second CSAT AIDS program is the Treatment Improvement Demonstration Program, also known as the Comprehensive Community Treatment Program (CCTP). This program, funded at $791,000 in FY 1993, addresses the primary care needs of sub-

TABLE 7.1 SAMHSA AIDS Program, 1986-1994 (Dollars in Millions)

	1986	1987	1988	1989	1990	1991	1992	1993[a]	1994 [b]
CMHS[c]	0	0	0	0	4.4	3.1	3.0	3.0	4.4
CSAP[d]	0	0	0	0	0	0	0	0	1.0
CSAT[e]	0	10.9	42.1	57.6	44.7	25.4	22.1	21.9	21.9
Prog. Mgt.	0.2	0.2	0.4	0.5	0.7	1.6	0.9	0.7	0.7
AIDS	0.2	11.1	42.5	58.1	49.8	30.1	26.0	25.6	28
Total	533.3	851.5	794.7	1,108.0	1,664.5	1,871.5	1,950.7	2,038.5	2,150.2
% AIDS	0	1	5	5	3	2	1	1	1

[a]Estimate.
[b]Appropriations.
[c]CMHS AIDS program includes AIDS Training and Demonstrations.
[d]CSAP AIDS program includes High Risk Youth Demonstrations.
[e]CSAT AIDS program includes Treatment Demonstrations (including NADR).

Source: SAMHSA Budget Office.

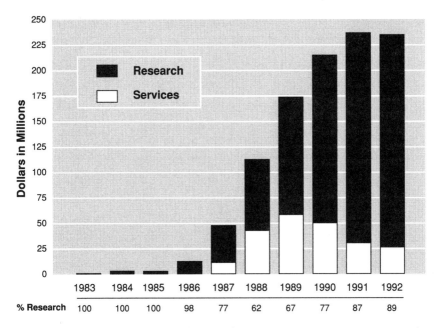

FIGURE 7.1 ADAMHA AIDS Budget Authority, 1983-1992. Note: "Research" includes former ADAMHA research activities currently with NIH (NIAAA, NIDA, NIMH, Office of Director, Buildings and Facilities); "Services" include former ADAMHA services activities currently with SAMHSA. Source: SAMHSA Budget Office.

stance abusers, including testing and prophylaxis for HIV, STDs, tuberculosis, and other illnesses, at drug treatment program entry. Overall, the CSAT AIDS program fell from $42.1 million in FY 1988 to $21.9 million in FY 1993, reflecting variations in the funding cycle of the outreach demonstration projects under the Demonstrations and Training line. The CMHS AIDS program includes Training and AIDS Training, which began at NIMH in FY 1990, and a new AIDS mental health services demonstration program, which was initiated in FY 1994. The Training Program, which was funded at $3.0 million in FY 1993, provides education and training for mental health care providers in the neuropsychiatric and psychosocial aspects of HIV infection. Eligible providers include psychiatrists, psychiatric nurses, psychiatric social workers, psychologists, and marriage and family counselors, as well as medical students, primary care residents, and nontraditional mental health care providers such as clergy, police, and alternative health care providers. The CMHS HIV/AIDS Mental Health Services Demonstration Program, developed in cooperation with HRSA and NIMH, uses the cooperative agreement mechanism to develop and evaluate effective models for delivering mental health services to people with HIV/AIDS and their loved ones and caregivers. Its FY 1994 budget of $1.2 million is intended to fund 8 to 12 new projects for up to four years (CMHS is hoping to obtain the collaboration of other agencies to ensure an even larger budget in future years). Overall, AIDS funding at CMHS decreased from $4.4 million in FY 1990 to $2.9 million in FY 1993. With the addition of the demonstrations, it rose again to $4.4 million in FY 1994.

CSAP had no AIDS program until FY 1994, when it proposed providing supplements to the Prevention Demonstrations for High Risk Youth Program to fund outreach and risk reduction activities related to HIV/AIDS, including skills building, pre-post HIV test counseling, outreach to resistant populations, and services to people who have lost friends and family members to AIDS. In FY 1994 this program was funded at $1 million, and it represents less than 1 percent of the total CSAP budget.

The goals of SAMHSA's AIDS program are fairly evident in the specific initiatives described above. First, the goal is to recognize that as AIDS becomes a chronic illness, more support will be needed from the substance abuse and mental health systems, which themselves will have to be strengthened to meet this challenge. Second, substance abuse and mental health treatment services will have to be further integrated into the primary care, general health care, and public health systems.

Indeed, the integration of substance abuse and mental health services into the general health care system is the primary goal of the SAMHSA AIDS office, which was created in 1992 by the ADAMHA reorganization bill. Currently, SAMHSA has an associate administrator for AIDS who is located in the office of the SAMHSA administrator. The associate administrator works with the three center offices on AIDS. These too were established by the ADAMHA reorganization bill, which mandated that each center have an AIDS office with an AIDS director or coordinator responsible for ensuring that HIV/AIDS issues are addressed and integrated into the overall programs of the center. The focus of the SAMHSA associate administrator for AIDS is coordination within and between the centers, SAMHSA, other federal agencies, and private organizations. An AIDS Work Group was in the planning stage at the time this report was written. This group will function under the aegis of the SAMHSA National Advisory Council and will provide a forum for discussion of planning and implementation of SAMHSA

AIDS activities. (This would be linked directly to the SAMHSA Committee for Women's Services.)

COLLABORATIONS BETWEEN RESEARCH AND SERVICES

When the ADAMHA Reorganization Act of 1992 was passed, some expressed concern that it would affect the relationship between research and services, with regard to the rapid, bidirectional transmission of information. Would research findings make their way quickly "from bench to bedside," and would observations and concerns from practitioners reach the research community in a timely manner? Those concerned about the splitting of the research and services programs of ADAMHA expressed fears that such separation could disrupt the linkages that existed within a single agency and impede the process of technology transfer. Those favoring the reorganization argued that separating the programs might well enhance relationships and thus improve linkages. This point was made in the report accompanying S-1306 the Senate bill to reorganize ADAMHA:

> It might seem logical to keep research and services under the same roof to facilitate "technology transfer," the process by which research findings are applied in the field. In practice, however, the research and services enterprises are so different that they cannot be effectively administered in one agency. Researchers and service providers share a common goal, but they speak a different language and thrive in different professional cultures. Rather than collaboration between research and services, ADAMHA has been the setting for competition between these activities, a situation compounded by overlap and confusion with respect to the duties of the institutes and the agencies. (Senate Report 102-131, p. 3)

As the Senate report notes, the problem of a lack of collaboration between the research and services communities exists beyond the federal agencies, and is based in great part on different professional cultures. The two salient features of the research culture are the drive for "knowledge for knowledge's sake" and the existence of a reward system based on number and type of publications. The pursuit of knowledge involves the employment of a scientific method that emphasizes using controlled experiments, limiting the randomness of outcomes, and producing findings that can be replicated by other scientists. It involves sophisticated mathematical and statistical methodologies and advanced verbal and written skills, and it requires objectivity and limited involvement with the subjects of the research (as much as possible) (Bailey, 1992a).

In contrast, the services world is driven by a desire to provide direct services to as many people as possible. Although the methods of service delivery are planned and evaluated, their internal integrity is often less important than the number of clients served. And while extensive reporting is often required by funding sources, this too is seen as less important to the mission of service providers than actually rendering the services—indeed, it is seen as a distraction. Furthermore, unlike researchers, service providers are trained to be subjective, to identify with and to advocate for their clients. Usually faced with funding and staffing inadequacies, and, in the case of HIV/AIDS service providers, daily experiences with severe illness and death, the services community easily can feel besieged (Bailey, 1992a).

These fundamental differences in culture and orientation between researchers and service providers result in significant barriers to collaboration. Service providers often feel that researchers are interested in their communities only for the sake of producing scientific results that will enhance the careers of individual researchers. Their experience is that, once that is accomplished, the researchers abandon the project and the client population on whom their research has been dependent. Moreover, service providers perceive researchers as coming from large, well-financed institutions that usually do not give anything back to the community they have studied once a research project is complete (Bailey, 1992a). As a result, they often feel that they and their clients are exploited by the scientific community.

At the same time, researchers often perceive service providers as unwilling to understand or appreciate the requirements of scientific research and the demand of their professional culture to get grants, teach, write, and publish. They encounter resistance to their efforts to refine or modify interventions in order to allow for rigorous scientific assessment, even though they explain to service providers the value of producing research results with scientific integrity. They often feel that service providers have unrealistic expectations about the potential applications of research findings to improved service delivery (Bailey, 1992a).

In addition to these differences in professional culture, there may be significant differences in the socioeconomic status of researchers and services providers—including their educational, racial/ethnic, and class status—that contribute to distrust and suspicion and get in the way of successful collaboration.

These kinds of conflicts are experienced at the federal level among agencies charged respectively with supporting research and services programs and are evidenced by the relatively limited collaborations between the AIDS research programs at NIAAA, NIDA, and NIMH and the AIDS services programs of SAMHSA, CDC, and HRSA, and the broader service-providing community. Even information exchange is limited. For example, each year the three research institutes sponsor many research exchange meetings, including research planning meetings, technical review meetings, workshops, and symposia. However, most of these meetings are designed to bring researchers together and very few reach beyond the research community to include service providers. Information about other linkages reported by the institutes in response to a committee request is provided below. (This is not an exhaustive review, but is meant to provide a sense of the range of existing activities.)

NIAAA

NIAAA identified only two AIDS research projects that it considers to have a direct relationship to the provision of services. The first is a longitudinal research program called The Native American Prevention Project on AIDS and Substance Abuse (NAPPASA), which developed rural school-based and community research partnerships that have produced positive outcome effects among southwestern Native American and other youth at risk. Community outreach programs were expanded to include reservation-wide, inter-reservation, statewide, regional, and national networking with Native American substance abuse and prevention groups. Workshops and conferences were cosponsored with the Navajo Tribe and with the Indian Health Service (a PHS agency). A community program coordinator representing the project has become integrated into the community and served as a member of the various prevention task forces.

The success of this continuing project is perceived to be a result of the ability of the principal investigator to form cooperative relationships between the research staff, schools, local public agencies, and the Native American Council. Staff members were hired from within the region, interventions were pretested with focus groups, and intervention materials were made available to additional school sites, which eventually requested partnerships with the research project. Both the Hopi Tribe and the Washington State Department of Indian Education have approached the principal investigator to extend his work and to form new prevention research partnerships.

The second project identified by NIAAA as linking AIDS research and services provides alcohol and drug abuse counseling to gay men in the context of AIDS prevention activities. Here, too, the success of the linkages is attributed to the ability of the principal investigator to act as a credible liaison between the research, service provider, and constituency communities. Indeed, this research project is described by NIAAA as one that was prompted by service providers in the gay community who observed an increased rate of HIV infection among heavy drinkers and identified this as an important area of research.

NIDA

NIDA has engaged in a fairly wide range of activities with other federal agencies and nongovernmental service providers related to AIDS prevention and treatment among the drug-using population. These activities include collaboration in funding and planning projects and conferences, technical assistance in research planning, service delivery, education, and information dissemination. The following is a representative sample of activities:

NIDA/HRSA Program Linking Primary Health Care and Drug Abuse Treatment

This program, which was one of those transferred to CSAT with the ADAMHA reorganization, is designed to demonstrate the feasibility of various models for linking substance abuse treatment with primary health care services for drug abusers at risk for acquiring or spreading HIV. Of the original 21 grantees, about one-third were community health centers, one-third were city or county health departments, and the remainder were other institutions such as hospitals or state agencies. Now in its second round of funding, the program already has demonstrated success in reaching historically underserved populations, including women, Hispanics/Latinos, African Americans, adolescents, and HIV-infected individuals. This project found that clients first identified through primary care were much less advanced in their drug abuse career than those identified in drug abuse treatment programs. This important finding has implications for the design of integrated HIV, drug abuse, and primary medical care models.

National AIDS Demonstration Research Program (NADR)

The National AIDS Demonstration Research Program (NADR), which began at NIDA in 1987 and was transferred to OTI/CSAT in 1991, culminated in a program of technology transfer designed to facilitate the implementation of HIV prevention outreach and intervention initiatives throughout the country. NIDA's NADR program encompassed 41 individual projects conducting studies of the efficacy of community-based interventions in nearly 50 cities. Projects were focused on reaching out-of-treatment drug users and their sexual partners, and employed the use of indigenous leaders (ex-drug users) and other community members to recruit and retain people in the intervention programs. (See Chapters 3 and 6 for further details of NADR and its successor, the Cooperative Agreement for AIDS Community-Based Outreach/Intervention Research.) As a result of these efforts, alliances and linkages were formed between university or other research groups and community-based organizations in the implementation of the intervention research program.

During 1991, NIDA, the National Association of State Alcohol and Drug Abuse Directors (NASADAD), and the NADR grantees entered into a partnership to structure, organize, and facilitate implementation of effective AIDS prevention models from the NADR projects into training workshops. NIDA published manuals that documented the implementation of those models that were found to be the most effective, that is, that had resulted in reductions of risk-taking behavior. State-level training workshops were conducted with representatives from more than 300 organizations. Moreover, perhaps as a result of the NADR program, now all states are required by law to have HIV prevention outreach programs in order to quality for block grant dollars to provide drug abuse treatment. The regulations accompanying the relevant legislation prescribe the manuals developed by NIDA for use by the states in meeting this obligation. However, as of FY 1993, the funding for the training of state representatives in the implementation of these HIV prevention programs was cut at NIDA, which may hamper the states' ability to successfully adopt the programs.

NIDA/SAMHSA HIV Prevention/Intervention Training Courses

NIDA developed a series of HIV prevention/intervention training courses that are now housed in SAMHSA (CSAT). The curricula incorporated research findings, including intervention models resulting from outreach research demonstration projects (e.g., NADR); research on the effects of drug use on immune system functioning; cofactors associated with disease progression; and relapse prevention methods used to help stabilize clients' functioning and thereby enhance their ability to practice prevention behaviors.

The contract under which the curricula were developed required dissemination to state agencies and community-based organizations. Numbers of "Training of Trainers" and "Training of Service Providers" events were specified. Participants at all training events were informally encouraged to disseminate the material to colleagues in their geographic regions. The NIDA contractor was required to maintain a list of participants who successfully completed the training in order that these individuals could serve as technical resources to governments and other public and private agencies requesting technical assistance.

Success of this program is attributed to the use of the contract mechanism, which allowed NIDA to adequately monitor performance progress and to select a contract firm with appropriate experience and expertise in HIV training and community outreach. People from that firm had numerous links with individuals and agencies at the local level, which provided a valuable resource for various activities within the program.

Outreach and Bleach Distribution

NIDA's research on the effectiveness of bleach distribution for HIV prevention among injection drug users has been directly applied in community outreach projects, beginning in San Francisco in 1986. This kind of outreach project acts as a bridge to services because it refers drug users who are not in treatment for their addiction to such treatment, as well as to primary health care services.

Bleach distribution was an important HIV preventive intervention for NIDA while the institute was precluded (by Congress) from conducting or evaluating the effectiveness of needle and syringe exchange programs in reducing HIV transmission among injection drug users (see Chapters 3 and 6). Now that prohibition has been modified, NIDA is engaging in more direct research on needle exchange programs that also bridges services through drug treatment referral.

Other Collaborations

NIDA is providing technical assistance to SAMHSA in the development of quality assurance standards in methadone maintenance programs and on AIDS-related standards for drug treatment programs. It also is collaborating with CSAT and the District of Columbia in a research demonstration project testing the comparative efficacy of model programs that link drug abuse and HIV treatment and prevention.

NIMH

AIDS Research Centers

The AIDS Research Centers (see Chapter 6) supported by NIMH (and cofunded by NIDA from 1986 to 1988) are required to include an Information Exchange Core as a built-in mechanism for communicating with service providers in their communities. The HIV Center at Columbia University, for example, set up a community-wide board to advise on all aspects of the research and services program. This arrangement is seen as responsible for the success of the center's project targeting heterosexual, gay, and lesbian adolescents considered to be at risk for HIV transmission (e.g., runaway and homeless youth). In collaboration with other researchers and community-based service providers, the principal investigator developed a training manual entitled *Adolescents Living Safely: AIDS Awareness, Attitudes, and Actions* and tested it in a research study. The Information Exchange Core of the center was instrumental in disseminating the training manual to agencies in the services arena. The manual has been translated into Russian and has been used for the past year in the St. Petersburg school system. The United Nations translated the manuals into Spanish and is currently distributing them in South America.

The Columbia University AIDS Research Center also produced video and audio tapes in collaboration with an organization called The Media Group. Three of these videos: "AIDS, Me and My Baby," "AIDS is About Secrets," and "AIDS, Not Us," have been used widely by community-based organizations, drug treatment programs, health departments, and other entities involved in HIV prevention efforts throughout the United States and in other countries. These videos have received awards from both the medical education and the media communities, both nationally and internationally.

The San Francisco AIDS Research Center was funded to develop effective prevention models and to form ongoing relationships with service organizations. An early study found that young gay men are at higher risk for HIV infection prior to confirmation with seroprevalence data. This study suggested that effective AIDS risk reduction programs should include issues concerning the meaning of life, coming out, and forming relationships. These findings were used by the San Francisco AIDS Foundation to develop a prevention campaign entitled "Life, Liberty, and the Pursuit of Happiness" targeted at young gay men.

AIDS Health Care Worker Training Program

Beginning in 1985, NIMH provided grants for training health care workers on different aspects of HIV/AIDS. Health care workers, including physicians, nurses, and social workers, were trained using the most current knowledge about AIDS, in particular HIV-related neuropsychiatric and cognitive problems. This program was one of those transferred to CMHS as part of the ADAMHA reorganization. In 1993, a book entitled *AIDS, Health and Mental Health: A Primary Sourcebook* was published as a direct outgrowth of the program and its evaluation, making possible even broader dissemination of the results.

NIMH (with CDC, HRSA, NIDA, NIAAA, and NICHD) Multisite Trial of Behavioral Strategies to Prevent the Further Spread of HIV Infection

In FY 1990, NIMH initiated a cooperative agreement to develop and test theory-driven behavior change interventions across multiple populations and sites. A major goal is to identify HIV prevention approaches that can be used readily by service providers in various communities. The cooperation of CDC and HRSA (along with NIDA, NIAAA, and NICHD) is intended to build in technology transfer and dissemination to the service provider community. This project is ongoing, and preliminary findings have not yet been released, so it is too early to measure its success in this regard.

HIV/AIDS Mental Health Services Demonstration Program

NIMH is a collaborating partner, along with HRSA, in the CMHS-sponsored demonstration program initiated in 1994 and described earlier in this chapter. NIMH will support certain aspects of the program that relate to testing and evaluating models for mental health services for people with HIV/AIDS.

Other Collaborations

Since 1990 NIMH has sponsored an annual meeting in which AIDS prevention researchers from NIAAA, NIDA, and NIMH, colleagues from other PHS agencies such as CDC and HRSA, and representatives from community-based organizations actively participate in presentations and panel discussions. One outgrowth of such meetings has been the integration of NIMH-supported researchers into the AIDS prevention activities of CDC's Division of Adolescent and School Health as advisors, reviewers, and evaluators. Another product (from the 1992 meeting) is a handbook of guidelines for HIV prevention, directed toward high-risk populations, that will be printed and distributed to state and local community-based organizations.

BARRIERS TO COLLABORATION

All but one (the CMHS demonstrations) of the examples of collaborations between research and services cited above predate the reorganization of ADAMHA. Moreover, according to institute and agency staff, these collaborations came about as a result of informal communications between individual staff. No formal mechanism existed—or yet exists—to encourage interagency cooperation. Although within ADAMHA there had been tension between the research and services entities, some fear that the organizational separation of those entities will make collaboration even more difficult. In addition to cultural differences, legal and regulatory barriers also hinder collaboration between the institutes now at NIH and the services entities at SAMHSA (as well as at HRSA and CDC). In particular, the ADAMHA reorganization legislation made it eminently clear that SAMHSA centers were not to engage in anything called "research," and that the NIH institutes were not to engage in providing anything that could qualify as "services." In the realms of substance abuse and mental health, the dichotomization of research and services is not always possible nor helpful, especially in the context of AIDS, which requires rapid information exchange between research and services. The committee does not wish to take a position on the merits or defects of the ADAMHA reorganization, but it does wish to express concern over the potential for an even greater divide between research and services. Such a divide should not be allowed to grow. Rather, the committee encourages the relaxation of cultural, legal, and regulatory barriers to collaboration between the research institutes and the service-providing agencies of the federal government.

In this regard, the committee takes heart from the new initiative sponsored by CMHS, in cooperation with NIMH and HRSA, designed to evaluate the efficacy of a range of mental health services provided to people with HIV/AIDS. The request for applications for this program was released in the spring of 1994, and applications were being submitted as this report was being written. Although it is unclear how successful this program will be, it is notable for having traversed significant organizational barriers to cooperation among the different research and services agencies, barriers made even more severe by the ADAMHA reorganization. The committee looks forward to its results.

COORDINATION OF AIDS ACTIVITIES WITHIN THE PUBLIC HEALTH SERVICE AND THE DEPARTMENT OF HEALTH AND HUMAN SERVICES

The possibility of collaborative activities between NIAAA, NIDA, and NIMH on the one hand and SAMHSA, CDC, and HRSA on the other is framed within the larger context of PHS and HHS AIDS activities. Coordination of PHS programs has resided for the past few years with the National AIDS Program Office (NAPO), and cross-agency coordination has been the function of the Federal Coordinating Committee on AIDS, chaired by PHS. In 1993, however, the Clinton administration elevated the status of federal AIDS coordination to a White House position with the appointment of a National AIDS Policy Coordinator responsible for all federal AIDS policy and programs. The activities of the newly titled Office of National AIDS Policy (ONAP) and the structures of organization and coordination within PHS and across federal agencies were still being determined at the time this report was written.

Rather than review activities of the past in this regard, the committee elected to reserve judgment about the overall coordination efforts at the PHS, HHS, and interdepartmental levels until the new organization and structures are in place. However, the committee does express its hope that mechanisms will emerge that make communication and cooperation between research and services entities more possible and collegial. Furthermore, the committee hopes that the new coordination of AIDS activities and programs seeks to eliminate duplication of efforts and ensures the appropriate use of resources throughout the responsible federal agencies.

CONCLUSION AND RECOMMENDATIONS

CONCLUSION

The reorganization of ADAMHA was intended to separate research from services activities related to mental health and substance abuse. Although the decision to do so had nothing specifically to do with AIDS, it did have implications for how the disease would be addressed. While tensions already existed between the research and services programs at ADAMHA, their formal separation made collaboration and coordination even more difficult. This is evidenced by the small number of collaborative efforts between NIAAA, NIDA, and NIMH—now at NIH—and the newly named services entities at SAMHSA.

This tension between the worlds of researchers and service providers has historical roots. Nevertheless its persistence—both inside and outside of federal government agencies—poses a barrier to effective AIDS prevention and intervention. Research institutes and service-supporting agencies must find ways to overcome the cultural and institutional barriers to collaboration if they are to see a fruitful and productive exchange of knowledge necessary for intervening in—and ultimately eradicating—AIDS.

RECOMMENDATIONS FOR LINKAGES BETWEEN RESEARCH AND SERVICES

7.1 The committee recommends that NIAAA, NIDA, and NIMH ensure adequate follow-up time and money in their AIDS intervention research grants to accelerate information dissemination activities, including technical assistance.

7.2 The committee recommends that formal mechanisms be developed within the NIH institutes and other PHS agencies to foster linkages between AIDS research and services.

7.3 The committee recommends that NIAAA, NIDA, and NIMH sponsor regular research exchange meetings with services agencies and service providers, including local, regional, and national meetings.

7.4 The committee recommends that the Assistant Secretary for Health of HHS and the Director of the Office of National AIDS Policy continue to develop a specific strategic plan for interagency cooperation and coordination among PHS AIDS activities, including an implementation plan.

Bibliography and References

Abramson, P., J. Sekler, and M. Cloud. 1989. An evaluation of an undergraduate course on AIDS. *Evaluation Review* 13:516-532.

Adam, B. 1992. Sociology and People Living with AIDS. Pp. 3-18 in J. Huber and B. Schneider, eds. *The Social Context of AIDS*. Thousand Oaks, CA: Sage Publications.

Agar, M. 1973. *Ripping and Running: A Formal Ethnography of Urban Heroin Addicts*. New York: Seminar Press.

Aggleton, P. 1993. Promoting Whose Health? Models of Health Promotion and Education About HIV Disease. Pp. 185-200 in G. Albrecht and R. Zimmerman, eds. *The Social and Behavioral Aspects of AIDS, Advances in Medical Sociology*, Vol. III. Greenwich, CT: JAI Press.

Aggleton, P., P. Davis, and G. Hart, eds. 1992. *AIDS: Responses, Policy and Care*. London: Falmer Press.

Ajzen, I. and M. Fishbein. 1977. Attitude-behavior relations: A theoretical analysis and review of empirical research. *Psychological Bulletin* 84:888-918.

Albert, E. 1986. Illness and Deviance: The Response of the Press to AIDS. Pp. 163-178 in D. Feldman and T. Johnson, eds. *The Social Dimension of AIDS: Method and Theory*. New York: Praeger.

Albrecht, G. and R. Zimmerman, eds. 1993a. *The Social and Behavioral Aspects of AIDS, Advances in Medical Sociology*, Vol. III. Greenwich, CT: JAI Press.

Albrecht, G. and R. Zimmerman. 1993b. What Does AIDS Teach Us About Social Science? Pp. 1-18 in G. Albrecht and R. Zimmerman, eds. *The Social and Behavioral Aspects of AIDS, Advances in Medical Sociology*, Vol. III. Greenwich, CT: JAI Press.

Alcabes, P., E. Schoenbaum, and R. Klein. 1993. Correlates of the rate of decline of CD4+ lymphocytes among injection drug users infected with the human immunodeficiency virus. *American Journal of Epidemiology* 137:989-1000.

Alcabes, P., P. Selwyn, K. Davenny, et al. 1994. Laboratory markers and the risk of developing HIV-1 disease among injecting drug users. *AIDS* 8:107-115.

Allen, S., A. Serufilira, J. Bogaerts, et al. 1992. Confidential HIV testing and condom promotion in Africa: Impact on HIV and gonorrhea rates. *Journal of the American Medical Association* 268:3338-3343.

Allen, S., J. Tice, P. Van de Perre, et al. 1992. Effect of serotesting with counselling on condom use and seroconversion among HIV discordant couples in Africa. *British Medical Journal* 304:1605-1609.

Altice, F., E. Fleck, P. Selwyn, et al. 1993. Provision of Health Care and HIV Counseling and Testing for Clients of the New Haven Needle Exchange Program. Paper presented: IXth Conference on AIDS. Berlin. Abstract D17-3927.

Altice, F., S. Tanguay, D. Hunt, et al. 1992. Demographics of HIV infection and utilization of medical services among IDU's in a women's prison. Paper presented: VIIIth International Conference on AIDS. Amsterdam. Abstract PoC4358.

Amaro, H. 1988. Considerations for prevention of HIV infection among Hispanic women. *Psychology of Women Quarterly* 12:429-443.

Amaro, H. 1991. Hispanic Women and AIDS: Consideration for Prevention and Research. In S. Blumenthal, A. Eichler, and G. Weissman, eds. *Women and AIDS: Promoting Healthy Behaviors*. Washington, DC: Alcohol, Drug Abuse, and Mental Health Administration.

Amaro, H. 1993. Women don't get AIDS, they just die from it. Paper presented: The American Psychological Association Convention. Toronto, Canada.

Amaro, H., L. Fried, H. Cabral, et al. 1990. Violence during pregnancy: The relationship to drug use among women and their partners. *American Journal of Public Health* 80:575-579.

Amaro, H., B. Zuckerman, and H. Cabral. 1989. Drug use among adolescent mothers: A profile of risk. *Pediatrics* 84:144-151.

American Academy of Neurology AIDS Task Force. 1991. Nomenclature and research case definitions for neurologic manifestations of human immunodeficiency virus-type 1 (HIV-1) infection. *Neurology* 41:778-785.

Anderson, R. and R. May. 1991. *Infectious Diseases of Humans: Dynamics and Control*. Oxford: Oxford University Press.

Anglin, D., Y. Hser, and W. McGlothlin. 1987. Sex differences in addict careers II: Becoming addicted. *American Journal of Drug and Alcohol Abuse* 13:59-71.

Archibald, C., M. Schechter, T. Le, et al. 1992. Evidence for a sexually transmitted cofactor for AIDS-related Kaposi's sarcoma in a cohort of homosexual men. *Epidemiology* 3:203-209.

Asamoah-Adu, A., S. Weir, M. Pappoe, et al. 1994. Evaluation of a targeted AIDS prevention intervention to increase condom use among prostitutes in Ghana. *AIDS* 8:239-246.

Atkinson, J., I. Grant, C. Kennedy, et al. 1988. Prevalence of psychiatric disorders among men infected with human immunodeficiency virus. *Archives of General Psychiatry* 45:859-864.

Auerbach, D., W. Darrow, H. Jaffe, et al. 1984. Cluster of cases of acquired immune deficiency syndrome: Patients linked by sexual contact. *American Journal of Medicine* 76:487-492.

Avins, A., W. Woods, C. Lindan, et al. 1994. HIV infection and risk behaviors among heterosexuals in alcohol treatment programs. *Journal of the American Medical Association* 271:515-518.

Baden, M. 1975. Methadone related deaths in New York City. *International Journal of the Addictions* 5:489-498.

Bailey, W. 1992a. Cultures in Conflict: Thoughts on the Conflict between AIDS Researchers and Community Based Organizations. UCLA AIDS Forum. September 18, 1992. Los Angeles, CA.

Bailey, W. 1992b. Politics, Drug Use and Sex: The HIV Primary Prevention Picture in the United States. Paper presented: VIIIth International AIDS Conference. Amsterdam.

Ball, J., W. Lange, C. Myers, et al. 1988. Reducing the risk of AIDS through methadone maintenance treatment. *Journal of Health and Social Behavior* 29:214-226.

Bandura, A. 1977. Self-efficacy: Toward a unifying theory of behavioral change. *Psychological Review* 84:191-215.

Baranowski, T. 1992/1993. Beliefs as motivational influences at stages in behavior change. *International Quarterly of Community Health Education* 13:3-29.

Barnett, T. and P. Blaikie. 1992. *AIDS in Africa: Its Present and Future Impact.* New York: Guilford Press.

Barre-Sinoussi, F., M. Nugeyre, and J. Chermann. 1985. Resistance of AIDS virus at room temperature. *Lancet* 2:721-722.

Batki, S. 1990a. Drug abuse, psychiatric disorders, and AIDS: Dual and triple diagnosis. *Western Journal of Medicine* 15:547-552.

Batki, S. 1990b. Substance Abuse and AIDS: The Need for Mental Health Services. Pp. 55-67 in S. Goldfinger, ed. *New Directions for Mental Health Services: Psychiatric Aspects of AIDS and HIV Infection.* San Francisco, CA: Jossey-Bass.

Bayer, R. 1994. AIDS Prevention and Cultural Sensitivity: Are They Compatible? Unpublished paper: Columbia University School of Public Health, HIV Center for Behavioral Studies.

Beck, E., C. Donegan, C. Cohen, et al. 1989. Risk factors for HIV-1 infection in a British population: Lessons from a London sexually transmitted disease clinic. *AIDS* 3:533-538.

Becker, M. 1974. The health belief model and sick role behavior. *Health Education Monographs* 2:409-419.

Becker, M. 1990. Theoretical models of adherence and strategies for improving adherence. In S. Shumaker, E. Schron, J. Ockene, et al., eds. *Handbook of Behavior Change.* New York: Springer.

Becker, M. and J. Joseph. 1988. AIDS and behavioral change to reduce risk: A review. *American Journal of Public Health* 78:394-410.

Benos, D., B. Hahn, J. Bubien, et al. 1994. Envelope glycoprotein gp120 of human immunodeficiency virus type 1 alters ion transport in astrocytes: Implications for AIDS dementia complex. *Proceedings of the National Academy of Sciences* 1:217-220.

Billy, J., K. Tanfer, W. Grady, et al. 1993. The sexual behavior of men in the United States. *Family Planning Perspectives* 25:52-60.

Bjorklund, A. and O. Lindvall. 1984. Pp. 55-122 in A. Bjorklund and T. Hokfelt, eds. *Handbook of Chemical Neuroanatomy.* New York: Elsevier.

Blaney, N., R. Morgan, D. Feaster, et al. 1990. Cynical hostility: A risk factor in HIV-1 infection? Unpublished paper. University of Miami School of Medicine.

Bloom, F. 1983. The endorphins: A growing family of pharmacologically pertinent peptides. *Annual Review of Pharmacology and Toxicology* 23:151-170.

Bolton, R., J. Vincke, R. Mak, et al. 1992. Alcohol and risky sex: In search of an elusive connection. *Medical Anthropology* 14:323-363.

Bortolotti, F., A. Stivanello, F. Noventa, et al. 1992. Sustained AIDS education campaigns and behavioral changes in Italian drug abusers. *European Journal of Epidemiology* 8:264-267.

Boulton, M. and R. Fitzpatrick. 1993. The Public and Personal Meanings of Bisexuality in the Context of AIDS. Pp. 77-100 in G. Albrecht and R. Zimmerman, eds. *The Social and Behavioral Context of AIDS, Advances in Medical Sociology*, Vol. III. Greenwich, CT: JAI Press.

Bounds, W. 1989. Male and female condoms. *British Journal of Family Planning* 15:14-17.

Bounds, W., J. Guillebaud, L. Stewart, et al. 1988. A female condom (Femshield): A study of its user acceptability. *British Journal of Family Planning* 14:83-87.

Bourgois, P. 1989. In search of Horatio Alger: Culture and ideology in the crack economy. *Contemporary Drug Problems* 16:619-649.

Bowser, B. 1989. Crack and AIDS: An ethnographic impression. *Journal of the National Medical Association* 81:538-540.

Boyer, C. and S. Kegeles. 1991. AIDS risk and prevention among adolescents. *Social Science and Medicine* 33:11-23.

Brady, S. and E. Carmen. 1990. AIDS Risk in the Chronically Mentally Ill: Clinical Strategies for Prevention. Pp. 83-95 in S. Goldfinger, ed. *New Directions For Mental Health Services: Psychiatric Aspects of AIDS and HIV Infection*. San Francisco, CA: Jossey-Bass.

Brandeau, M., D. Owens, C. Sox, et al. 1993. Screening women of childbearing age for human immunodeficiency virus: A model-based policy analysis. *Management Science* 39:72-92.

Braun, M., R. Byers, W. Hayward, et al. 1990. Acquired immunodeficiency syndrome and extrapulmonary tuberculosis in the United States. *Archives of Internal Medicine* 150:1913-1916.

Brenneman, D., G. Westbrook, S. Fitzgerald, et al. 1988. Neuronal cell killing by the envelope glycoprotein of HIV and its prevention by vasoactive intestinal peptide. *Nature* 335:639-642.

Brew, B., R. Bhalla, M. Paul, et al. 1989. Cerebrospinal fluid B2-microglobulin in patients with AIDS dementia complex: An expanded series including response to zidovudine treatment. *AIDS* 6:461-465.

Brew, B., R. Bhalla, M. Paul, et al. 1990. Cerebrospinal fluid neopterin in human immunodeficiency virus type 1 infection. *Annals of Neurology* 28:556-560.

Brew, B., J. Sidtis, C. Petito, et al. 1988. The Neurological Complication of AIDS and Human Immunodeficiency Virus Infection. Pp. 1-49 in F. Plum, ed. *Advances in Contemporary Neurology*. Philadelphia, PA: F. A. Davis Co.

British Journal of Family Planning. 1992. The female condom. 18:71-72.

Broadhead, R. and K. Fox. 1993. Occupational Health Risks of Harm Reduction Work: Combatting AIDS Among Injection Drug Users. Pp. 123-142 in G. Albrecht and R. Zimmerman, eds. *The Social and Behavioral Context of AIDS, Advances in Medical Sociology*, Vol. III. Greenwich, CT: JAI Press.

Brookmeyer, R. and M. Gail. 1993. *AIDS Epidemiology: A Quantitative Approach*. Oxford: Oxford University Press.

Brown, B. and G. Beschner, eds. 1993. *Handbook on Risk of AIDS: Injecting Drug Users and Sexual Partners*. Westport, CT: Greenwood Press.

Browning, F. 1993. *The Culture of Desire: Paradox and Perversity in Gay Lives Today*. New York: Crown Publishers.

Brunswick, A., A. Aidala, J. Dobkin, et al. 1993. HIV-1 seroprevalence and risk behaviors in an urban African-American community cohort. *American Journal of Public Health* 83:1390-1394.

Burack, J., D. Barrett, R. Stall, et al. 1993. Depressive Symptoms and CD4 Lymphocyte Decline Among HIV-Infected Men. *Journal of the American Medical Association* 270:2568-2573.

Burke, D. and R. Redfield. 1988. Transmission of human immunodeficiency virus (HIV). *New England Journal of Medicine* 318:1202-1203.

Caiffa, W., D. Vlahov, N. Graham, et al. 1993. Risk Factors for Bacterial Pneumonia among HIV Seropositive Intravenous Drug Users. Paper presented: IXth International Conference on AIDS. Berlin. Abstract P0-C15-2930.

Calabrese, L. and K. Gopalakrishna. 1986. Transmission of HTLV-III infection from man to woman to man. *New England Journal of Medicine* 314:987.

Calsyn, D., C. Meinecke, A. Saxon, et al. 1992. Risk reduction in sexual behavior: A condom giveaway program in a drug abuse treatment clinic. *American Journal of Public Health* 82:1536-1538.

Calsyn, D., A. Saxon, G. Freeman, et al. 1992. Ineffectiveness of AIDS education and HIV antibody testing in reducing high-risk behaviors among injection drug users. *American Journal of Public Health* 82:573-575.

Calsyn, D., A. Saxon, E. Wells, et al. 1992. Longitudinal sexual behavior changes in injecting drug users. *AIDS* 6:1207-1211.

Calzavara, L., R. Coates, J. Raboud, et al. 1993. Ongoing high-risk sexual behaviors in relation to recreational drug use in sexual encounters. *AIDS Education and Prevention* 3:272-280.

Cameron, D., F. Plummer, and J. Simonsen. 1987. Female to Male Heterosexual Transmission of HIV Infection in Nairobi. Paper presented: IIIrd International Conference on AIDS. Washington, DC.

Cantor, M. 1983. Strain among caregivers: A study of experience in the United States. *The Gerontologist* 23:597-604.

Carswell, J., G. Lloyd, and J. Howells. 1989. Prevalence of HIV-1 in East African lorry drivers. *AIDS* 3:759-761.

Castillo-Chavez, C., ed. 1989. *Mathematical and Statistical Approaches to AIDS Epidemiology*. New York: Springer-Verlag.

Castro, K., S. Lieb, H. Jaffe, et al. 1988. Transmission of HIV in Belle Glade, FL: Lessons for other communities in the United States. *Science* 239:193-197.

Catania, J., T. Coates, and R. Stall. 1991. Changes in condom use among homosexual men in San Francisco. *Health Psychology* 10:190-199.

Catania, J., T. Coates, R. Stall, et al. 1992. Prevalence of AIDS-related risk factors and condom use in the United States. *Science* 258:1101-1106.

Catania, J., D. Gibson, D. Chitwood, et al. 1990. Methodological problems in AIDS behavioral research: Influences on measurement error and participation bias in studies of sexual behavior. *Psychology Bulletin* 108:339-362.

Catania, J., S. Kegeles, and T. Coates. 1990. Psychosocial predictors of people who fail to return for their HIV test results. *AIDS* 4:262-282.

Celentano, D., D. Vlahov, S. Cohn, et al. 1991. Risk factors for shooting gallery use and cessation among intravenous drug users. *American Journal of Public Health* 81:1291-1295.

Centers for Disease Control (CDC). 1987. Antibody to human immunodeficiency virus in female prostitutes. *Morbidity and Mortality Weekly Report* 257:635-639.

Centers for Disease Control (CDC). 1990. HIV prevalence estimates and AIDS case projections for the United States: Report based upon a workshop. *Morbidity and Mortality Weekly Report* 39:1-31.

Centers for Disease Control (CDC). 1991a. Crack cocaine use among persons with tuberculosis—Contra Costa County, California, 1987-1990. *Morbidity and Mortality Weekly Report* 40:485-489.

Centers for Disease Control (CDC). 1991b. The HIV/AIDS epidemic: The first 10 years. *Morbidity and Mortality Weekly Report* 40:357-369.

Centers for Disease Control and Prevention (CDC). 1992a. The second 100,000 cases of acquired immunodeficiency syndrome—United States. *Morbidity and Mortality Weekly Report* 41:28-29.

Centers for Disease Control and Prevention (CDC). 1992b. Sexual behavior among high school students—United States, 1990. *Morbidity and Mortality Weekly Report* 40:885-888.

Centers for Disease Control and Prevention (CDC). 1992c. Youth risk behavior survey. *Morbidity and Mortality Weekly Report*.

Centers for Disease Control and Prevention (CDC). 1993a. *HIV/AIDS Surveillance Report* 5:1-18. Washington, DC: U.S. Government Printing Office.

Centers for Disease Control and Prevention (CDC). 1993b. *National Seroprevalence Surveys, 1992.* HIV/NCID/11-93/036. Washington, DC: U.S. Government Printing Office.

Centers for Disease Control and Prevention (CDC). 1993c. Use of race and ethnicity in public health surveillance, Summary of the CDC/ATSDR workshop. *Morbidity and Mortality Weekly Report*.

Centers for Disease Control and Prevention (CDC). 1994. *HIV/AIDS Surveillance Report*. Washington, DC: U.S. Government Printing Office.

Chaisson, R., E. Taylor, D. Vlahov, et al. 1991. Immune Serum Markers and CD4 Counts in HIV Infected IV Drug Users. Paper presented: VIIth International Conference on AIDS. Florence. Abstract W.B.2435.

Chen, C. 1979. Acquisition of behavioral tolerance to ethanol as a function of reinforced practice in rats. *Psychopharmacology* 63:285-288.

Cherubin, C. and J. Sapira. 1993. The medical complications of drug addiction and the medical assessment of the IV drug users: Twenty-five years later. *Annals of Internal Medicine* 119:1017-1028.

Chesney, M. and S. Folkman. 1994. Psychological impact of HIV disease and implications for intervention. *Psychiatric Clinics of North America* 17:35-55.

Chiasson, M., R. Stoneburner, D. Hildebrandt, et al. 1991. Heterosexual transmission of HIV-1 associated with the use of smokable freebase cocaine (crack). *AIDS* 5:1121-1126.

Chin, J. 1990. Current and future dimensions of the HIV/AIDS pandemic in women and children. *Lancet* 336:221-227.

Chin, J., A. Sato, and J. Mann. 1990. Projections of HIV infections and AIDS cases to the year 2000. *Bulletin of the World Health Organization* 68:1-11.

Chitwood, D., C. McCoy, and M. Comerford. 1990. Risk Behavior of Intravenous Cocaine Users: Implications for Intervention. Pp. 120-133 in C. Leukefeld, R. Battjes, and Z. Amsel, eds. *AIDS and Intravenous Drug Use, Community Intervention and Prevention.* New York: Hemisphere Publishing.

Chitwood, D., C. McCoy, J. Inciardi, et al. 1990. HIV seropositivity of needles from shooting galleries in south Florida. *American Journal of Public Health* 80:1-3.

Chitwood, D., J. Inciardi, D. McBride, et al. 1991. *A Community Approach to AIDS Intervention: Exploring the Miami Outreach Project for Injecting Drug Users and Other High Risk Groups.* Westport, CT: Greenwood Press.

Choi, K. and T. Coates. In press. Prevention of HIV infection. *AIDS*.

Chuang, J., G. Devins, J. Hunsley, et al. 1989. Psychosocial distress and well-being among gay and bisexual men with human immunodeficiency virus infection. *American Journal of Psychiatry* 146:876-880.

Cleary, P., D. Van, T. Rogers, et al. 1991. Behavior changes after notification of HIV infection. *American Journal of Public Health* 81:1586-1590.

Cleven, K., R. DeJesus, and S. Sharp. 1990. The Determination of the Knowledge

Base of Caregivers of HIV Infected Preschool Children. Paper presented: VIth International Conference on AIDS. San Francisco.

Clumeck, N., M. Robert-Guroff, P. Van de Perre, et al. 1985. Seroepidemiological studies of HTLV-III antibody prevalence among selected groups of heterosexual Africans. *Journal of the American Medical Association* 254:2599.

Coates, T. 1990. Strategies for modifying sexual behavior for primary and secondary prevention of HIV disease. *Journal of Consulting and Clinical Psychology* 58:57-69.

Coates, T. 1993. Prevention of HIV-1 infection: Accomplishments and priorities. *The Journal of NIH Research* 5:73-76.

Coates, T. and K. Haynes Sanstad. 1992. Preventing HIV disease: An agenda for behavioral science. *Psychological Science Agenda* (March/April):10-11.

Coates, T. and S. Hulley. 1992. Confidential HIV testing and condom promotion in Africa impact on HIV and gonorrhea rates. *Journal of the American Medical Association* 268:3338-3343.

Coates, T., L. McKusick, R. Kuno, et al. 1989. Stress reduction training changed number of sexual partners but not immune function in men with HIV. *American Journal of Public Health* 79:885-887.

Coates, T., R. Stall, J. Catania, et al. 1988. Behavioral factors in the spread of HIV infection. *AIDS* 2:S239-S246.

Coates, T., R. Stall, S. Kegeles, et al. 1988. AIDS antibody testing: Will it stop the epidemic? Will it help people infected with HIV? *American Psychologist* 43:859-864.

Coates, T., R. Stall, J. Mandel, et al. 1987. AIDS: A psychological research agenda. *Annals of Behavioral Medicine* 9:21-28.

Cohen, J. 1992. Sexual Transmission Associated with Commercial Sex. Paper presented: National Institute on Drug Abuse, AIDS Research Planning Meeting. January 23-24, 1992. Rockville, MD.

Cohen, J. 1993. Somber news from the AIDS front. *Science* 260:1712-1713.

Coie, J., N. Watt, S. West, et al. 1993. The science of prevention: A conceptual framework and some directions for a national research program. *American Psychologist* 48:1013-1022.

Cole, R. and S. Cooper. 1990. Lesbian exclusion in HIV/AIDS education: Ten years of low-risk identity and high-risk behavior. *SIECUS Report* (December/January).

Collier, H. 1980. Cellular site of opiate dependance. *Nature* 283:625-629.

Colon, H., R. Robles, D. Freeman, et al. 1992. Effects of an intervention program on AIDS related risk behavior among injecting drug users in Puerto Rico. Paper presented: VIIIth International Conference on AIDS. Amsterdam. Abstract PoC4279.

Colon, H., R. Robles, D. Freeman, et al. 1993. Effects of a HIV risk reduction education program among injection drug users in Puerto Rico. *Puerto Rican Health Services* 12:27-34.

Conner, R., S. Mishra, M. Lewis, et al. 1990. Theory-Based Evaluation of AIDS-Related Knowledge, Attitudes, and Behavior Changes. New Directions for Progam Evaluation. Pp. 75-85 in L. Leviton, A. Hegedus, and A. Kubrin, eds. *Evaluating AIDS Prevention: Contributions of Multiple Disciplines.* San Francisco, CA: Jossey-Bass.

Connors, M. 1992. Risk perception, risk taking and risk management among intravenous drug users: Implications for AIDS prevention. *Social Science and Medicine* 34:591-601.

Conway, G., M. Epstein, C. Hayman, et al. 1993. Trends in HIV prevalence among disadvantaged youth: Survey results from a national job training program, 1988 through 1992. *Journal of the American Medical Association* 269:2887-2889.

Cooper, M. 1992. Alcohol and increased behavioral risk for AIDS. *Alcohol Health and Research World* 16:64-72.

Corby, N., P. Barchi, and R. Wolitski. 1990. Effects of condom-skills training and HIV-testing on AIDS prevention behaviors among sex workers. Paper presented: VIth International Conference on AIDS. San Francisco. Abstract SC714.

Cournos, F., M. Empfield, E. Horwath, et al. 1991. HIV seroprevalence among patients admitted to two psychiatric hospitals. *American Journal of Psychiatry* 148:1225-1230.

Cournos, F., J. Guido, S. Coomaraswamy, et al. 1994. Sexual activity and risk of HIV infection among patients with schizophrenia. *American Journal of Psychiatry* 151:228-232.

Crystal, S. and N. Schiller. 1993. Stigma and Homecoming: Family Caregiving and the "Disaffiliated" Intravenous Drug User. Pp. 166-184 in G. Albrecht and R. Zimmerman, eds. *The Social and Behavioral Aspects of AIDS, Advances in Medical Sociology*, Vol. III. Greenwich, CT: JAI Press.

Curtis, J. and D. Patrick. 1993. Race and survival time with AIDS: A synthesis of the literature. *American Journal of Public Health* 83:1425-1428.

Daley, C., P. Small, G. Schecter, et al. 1992. An outbreak of tuberculosis with accelerated progression among persons infected with the human immunodeficiency virus. *New England Journal of Medicine* 326:231-235.

Dalton, H. 1989. AIDS in blackface: Living with AIDS part II. *Daedalus, Proceedings of the American Academy of Arts and Sciences* 118:205-225.

Darrow, W. 1991. Socioepidemiologic Responses to an Epidemic. Pp. 82-99 in R. Ulack and W. Skinner, eds. *AIDS and the Social Sciences: Common Threads.* Lexington, KY: The University Press of Kentucky.

Darrow, W. 1992. Assessing Targeted AIDS Prevention in Male and Female Prostitutes and their Clients. Pp. 215-231 in F. Paccaud, J. Vader, and F. Gutzwiller, eds. *Assessing AIDS Prevention.* Basel, Switzerland: Birkhauser Verlag.

Davenny, K., D. Buono, E. Schoenbaum, et al. 1990. Baseline Health Status of Intravenous Drug Users with and without HIV Infection. Paper presented: VIth International Conference on AIDS. San Francisco. Abstract F.B.430.

Dawson, V., T. Dawson, G. Uhl, et al. 1993. Human immunodeficiency virus type 1 coat protein neurotoxicity mediated by nitric oxide in primary cortical cultures. *Proceedings of the National Academy of Sciences* 90:3256-3259.

D'Emaro, J., M. Quadland, W. Shattls, et al. 1988. The "800 Men" project: A systematic evaluation of AIDS prevention programs demonstrating the efficacy of erotic, sexually explicit safer sex education on gay and bisexual men at risk for AIDS. Paper presented: IVth International Conference on AIDS. Stockholm. Abstract 8086.

DeMayo, M. 1991. The future of HIV/AIDS prevention programs: Learning from the experiences of gay men. *Siecus Report* 20:1-7.

Dengelegi, L., J. Weber, and S. Torquato. 1990. Drug users' AIDS-related knowledge, attitudes, and behaviors before and after AIDS education sessions. *Public Health Reports* 105:504-510.

Des Jarlais, D., A. Abdul-Quader, and H. Minkoff. 1991. Crack use and multiple AIDS risk behaviors. *Journal of Acquired Immune Deficiency Syndromes* 4:446-447.

Des Jarlais, D., C. Casriel, S. Friedman, et al. 1992. AIDS and the transition to illicit drug injection—Results of a randomized trial prevention program. *British Journal of Addiction* 87:493-498.

Des Jarlais, D. and S. Friedman. 1988. The psychology of preventing AIDS among IV drug users: A social learning conceptualization. *American Psychologist* 43:865-870.

Des Jarlais, D. and S. Friedman. 1990. The Epidemic of HIV Infection Among Injecting Drug Users in New York City: The First Decade and Possible Future Directions. Pp. 86-94 in J. Strang and G. Stimson, eds. *AIDS and Drug Misuse: The Challenge for Policy and Practice in the 1990s*. London: Routledge.

Des Jarlais, D. and S. Friedman. 1992. AIDS and legal access to sterile drug injection equipment. *Annals of the American Academy of Political and Social Science* 521:42-65.

Des Jarlais, D., S. Friedman, K. Choopanya, et al. 1992. International epidemiology of HIV and AIDS among injecting drug users. *AIDS* 6:1053-1068.

Des Jarlais, D., S. Friedman, M. Marmor, et al. 1987. HTLV-III/LAV-associated disease progression and co-factors in a cohort of IV drug users. *AIDS* 1:111-125.

Des Jarlais, D., S. Friedman, D. Novick, et al. 1989. HIV-1 infection among intravenous drug users in Manhattan, New York City, from 1977 through 1987. *Journal of the American Medical Association* 261:1008-1012.

Des Jarlais, D., S. Friedman, J. Sotheran, et al. 1994. Continuity and change within an HIV epidemic. *Journal of the American Medical Association* 271:121-127.

Des Jarlais, D., S. Friedman, and D. Strug. 1986. AIDS and Needle-Sharing Within the IV-Drug Use Subculture. Pp. 111-125 in D. Feldman and T. Johnson, eds. *The Social Dimensions of AIDS: Method and Theory*. New York: Praeger.

Des Jarlais, D., S. Friedman, and T. Ward. 1993. Harm reduction: A public health response to the AIDS epidemic among injecting drug users. *Annual Review of Public Health* 14:413-450.

Diaz, R. In press. Latino gay men and the psychocultural barriers to AIDS prevention. In M. Levine, J. Gagnon, and P. Nardi, eds. *A Plague of Our Own: The Impact of HIV on the Gay and Lesbian Communities*. Chicago, IL: University of Chicago Press.

Dickson, D., S. Lee, W. Hatch, et al. 1994. Macrophages and microglia in HIV-related CNS neuropathology. Pp. 99-118 in R. Price and S. Perry, eds. *HIV, AIDS and the Brain*. New York: Raven Press.

DiClemente, R. 1993. Preventing HIV/AIDS among adolescents—School as agents of behavior change. *Journal of the American Medical Association* 270:760-761.

DiClemente, R. and H. Houston. 1989. Health promotion strategies for prevention of human immunodeficiency virus infection among minority adolescents. *Health Education* 20:39-43.

Doll, S., F. Judson, D. Ostrow, et al. 1990. Sexual behavior before AIDS: The hepatitis b studies of homosexual and bisexual men *AIDS* 4:1067-1073.

Dommeyer, C., L. Marquard, J. Gibson, et al. 1989. The effectiveness of an AIDS education campaign on a college campus. *Journal of American College Health* 38:131-135.

Donahue, J., K. Nelson, A. Munoz, et al. 1991. Antibody to hepatitis C virus among cardiac surgery patients, homosexual men, and intravenous drug users in Baltimore, Maryland. *American Journal of Epidemiology* 134:1206-1211.

Dorfman, L., P. Derish, and J. Cohen. 1992. Hey girlfriend: An evaluation of AIDS prevention among women in the sex industry. *Health Education Quarterly* 19:25-40.

Dreyer, E., P. Kaiser, J. Offermann, et al. 1990. HIV-1 coat protein neurotoxicity prevented by calcium channel antagonists. *Science* 248:364-367.

Drucker, E. 1991. Communities at Risk: The Social Epidemiology of AIDS in New

York City. Pp. 45-63 in R. Ulack and W. Skinner, eds. *AIDS and the Social Sciences: Common Threads.* Lexington, KY: The University Press of Kentucky.

Eckholm, E. 1992. AIDS, fatally steady in the U.S., accelerates worldwide. *New York Times* (June 28):E5.

Ehrhardt, A. 1988. Preventing and treating AIDS: The expertise of the behavioral sciences. *Bulletin of the New York Academy of Medicine* 64:513-519.

Ehrhardt, A. and H. Meyer-Bahlburg. 1981. Effects of prenatal sex hormones on gender-related behavior. *Science* 211:1312-1318.

Eisen, M., G. Zellman, and A. McAlister. 1990. Evaluating the impact of a theory-based sexuality and contraceptive education program. *Family Planning Perspectives* 22:261-271.

Ekstrand, M. and T. Coates. 1990. Maintenance of safer sexual behaviors and predictors of risky sex: The San Francisco men's health study. *American Journal of Public Health* 80:973-977.

El-Bassel, N. and R. Schilling. 1992. Fifteen-month followup of women methadone patients taught skills to reduce heterosexual HIV transmission. *Public Health Reports* 107:500-504.

Epstein, L. and H. Gendelman. 1993. Human immunodeficiency virus type 1 infection of the nervous system: Pathogenetic mechanisms. *Annals of Neurology* 33:429-436.

Esteban, J., R. Esteban, L. Viladomiu, et al. 1989. Hepatitis C antibodies among risk groups in Spain. *Lancet* ii:294-297.

European Study Group. 1989. Risk factors for male to female transmission of HIV. *British Medical Journal* 298:411-415.

European Study Group. 1992. Comparison of female to male and male to female transmission of HIV in 563 stable couples. *British Medical Journal* 304:809-813.

Everall, I., P. Luthert, and P. Lantos. 1991. Neuronal loss in the frontal cortex in HIV infection. *Lancet* 337:1119-1121.

Farizo, K., J. Buehler, M. Chamberland, et al. 1992. Spectrum of disease in persons with human immunodeficiency virus infection in the United States. *Journal of the American Medical Association* 267:1798-1805.

Farmer, P. 1992. *AIDS and Accusation: Haiti and the Geography of Blame.* Berkeley, CA: University of California Press.

Fawzy, I., S. Namir, and D. Wolcott. 1989. Group intervention with newly diagnosed AIDS patients. *Psychiatric Medicine* 7:35-46.

Federation of Behavioral, Psychological and Cognitive Sciences. 1994. NIH begins to revamp the peer review process. *Federation News* (February).

Fee, E. and D. Fox, eds. 1988. *AIDS: The Burdens of History.* Berkeley, CA: University of California Press.

Fee, E. and D. Fox, eds. 1992. *AIDS: The Making of a Chronic Disease.* Berkeley, CA: University of California Press.

Fernandez, F. 1990. Psychopharmacological Interventions in HIV Infections. Pp. 43-53 in S. Goldfinger, ed. *New Directions for Mental Health Services: Psychiatric Aspects of AIDS and HIV Infection.* San Francisco, CA: Jossey-Bass.

Fernandez-Cruz, E., M. Desco, M. Montes, et al. 1990. Immunological and serological markers predictive of progression to AIDS in a cohort of HIV-infected drug users. *AIDS* 4:987-994.

Festoff, B., J. Rao, and D. Brenneman. 1990. Vasoactive intestinal polypeptide (VIP) is a secretagogue for protease nexin I (PNI) release from astrocytes. *Society for Neuroscience Abstract* 16:909.

Feucht, T., R. Stephens, and B. Gibbs. 1991. Knowledge about AIDS among intravenous drug users: An evaluation of an education program. *AIDS Education and Prevention* 3:10-20.

Fiddle, S. 1967. *Portraits From a Shooting Gallery*. New York: Harper & Row.

Fine, J. 1993. Substance use and HIV risk behavior. Paper presented: HIV/AIDS and People with Serious Mental Illness. Symposium sponsored by Columbia University and the New York Psychiatric Institute. Albany, New York.

Fischhoff, B. 1989. Making Decisions About AIDS. Pp. 168-205 in V. Mays, G. Albee, and S. Schneider, eds. *Primary Prevention of AIDS*. Thousand Oaks, CA: Sage Publications.

Fischl, M., G. Dickenson, G. Scott, et al. 1987. Evaluation of heterosexual partners, children, and household contacts of adults with AIDS. *Journal of the American Medical Association* 257:640-644.

Fishbein, M., A. Bandura, H. Triandis, et al. 1991. Factors Influencing Behavior and Behavior Change. Final report: NIMH Theorists Workshop. Washington, DC. October 3-5, 1991.

Fisher, J. 1988. Possible effects of reference group-based social influence on AIDS-risk behavior and AIDS prevention. *American Psychologist* 43:914-920.

Fisher, J. and W. Fisher. 1992. Changing AIDS-risk behavior. *Psychological Bulletin* 111:455-474.

Flaskerud, J. and A. Nyamathi. 1990. Effects of an AIDS education program on the knowledge, attitudes and practices of low income black and Latina women. *Journal of Community Health* 15:343-355.

Flaskerud, J. and G. Uman. 1993. Directions for AIDS education for Hispanic women based on analyses of survey findings. *Public Health Reports* 108:298-304.

Fletcher, B., F. Tims, and J. Inciardi. 1993. Improving Treatment: A Program for Systematic Innovation. Pp. xiii-xix in J. Inciardi, F. Tims, and B. Fletcher, eds. *Innovative Approaches in the Treatment of Drug Abuse: Program Models and Strategies*. Westport, CT: Greenwood Press.

Folkman, S. 1993. Psychosocial Effects of HIV Infection. Pp. 658-681 in L. Goldberger and S. Breznitz, eds. *Handbook of Stress: Theoretical and Clinical Aspects*. New York: The Free Press.

Folkman, S., M. Chesney, and A. Christopher-Richards. 1994. Stress and coping in partners of men with AIDS. *Psychiatric Clinics of North America* 17:163-182.

Folkman, S., M. Chesney, L. McKusick, et al. 1991. Translating coping theory into an intervention. In J. Eckenrode, ed. *The Social Context of Stress*. New York: Plenum Press.

Folkman, S., M. Chesney, L. Pollack, et al. 1993. Stress, control, coping, and depressive mood in human immunodeficiency virus-positive and -negative gay men in San Francisco. *Journal of Nervous and Mental Disease* 181:409-416.

Franzini, L., L. Sideman, K. Dexter, et al. 1990. Promoting AIDS risk reduction via behavioral training. *AIDS Education and Prevention* 2:313-321.

Friedland, G. 1989. Clinical care in the AIDS epidemic. *Daedalus* 118:59-83.

Friedland, G. and R. Klein. 1987. Transmission of human immunodeficiency virus. *New England Journal of Medicine* 317:1125-1135.

Friedman, S. 1993. AIDS as a Sociohistorical Phenomenon. Pp. 19-36 in G. Albrecht and R. Zimmerman, eds. *The Social and Behavioral Aspects of AIDS, Advances in Medical Sociology*, Vol. III. Greenwich, CT: JAI Press.

Friedman, S., D. Des Jarlais, S. Deren, et al. 1992. HIV seroconversion among street-recruited drug injectors in 14 United States cities. Paper presented: VIIIth International Conference on AIDS. Amsterdam. Abstract PoC 4251.

Friedman, S., D. Des Jarlais, and T. Ward. 1994. Social Models for Changing Health-

Relevant Behavior. Pp. 95-116 in R. DiClemente and J. Peterson, eds. *Preventing AIDS: Theories and Methods of Behavioral Interventions*. New York: Plenum Press.

Friedman, S., B. Jose, A. Neaigus, et al. 1991. Peer mobilization and widespread condom use by drug injectors. Paper presented: VIth International Conference on AIDS. Florence. Abstract W.D. 54

Friedman, S., B. Jose, A. Neaigus, et al. 1994. Consistent condom use in relationships between seropositive injecting drug users and sex partners who do not inject drugs. *AIDS* 8:357-361.

Friedman, S., M. Sufian, R. Curtis, et al. 1992. Organizing Drug Users Against AIDS. Pp. 115-130 in J. Huber and B. Schneider, eds. *The Social Context of AIDS*. Thousand Oaks, CA: Sage Publications.

Frierson, R., S. Lippman, and J. Johnson. 1987. AIDS psychological stresses on the family. *Psychosomatics* 28:65-68.

Fullilove, M. and R. Fullilove. 1989. Intersecting epidemics: Black teen crack use and sexually transmitted disease. *Journal of the American Women's Medical Association* 44:146-153.

Fullilove, R., M. Fullilove, B. Bowser, et al. 1990. Risk of sexually transmitted disease among black adolescent crack users in Oakland and San Francisco, California. *Journal of the American Medical Association* 263:851-855.

Fullilove, M., R. Fullilove, K. Haynes, et al. 1990. Black women and AIDS prevention: A view towards understanding the gender rules. *The Journal of Sex Research* 27:47-64.

Fullilove, M., M. Weinstein, R. Fullilove, et al. 1990. Race/gender issues in the sexual transmission of AIDS. *AIDS Clinical Review* 25-62.

Fullilove, M., J. Wiley, R. Fullilove, et al. 1992. Risk for AIDS in multiethnic neighborhoods of San Francisco, California—The population-based AMEN study. *West Journal of Medicine* 157:32-40.

Fullilove, M., R. Fullilove, G. Kennedy, et al. 1992. Trauma, crack and HIV risk. Paper presented: VIIIth International Conference on AIDS. Amsterdam. Abstract PoD 5477.

Gabuzda, D. and M. Hirsch. 1987. Neurologic manifestations of infection with human immunodeficiency virus. Clinical features and pathogenesis. *Annals of Internal Medicine* 107:383-391.

Gabuzda, D., D. Ho, S. de la Monte, et al. 1986. Immunohistochemical identification of HTLV-III antigen in brains of patients with AIDS. *Annals of Neurology* 20:289-295.

Gail, M., D. Preston, S. Piantadosi. 1989. Disease prevention models of voluntary confidential screening for human immunodeficiency virus (HIV). *Statistics in Medicine* 8:59-81.

Gallo, J. 1990. The effect of social support on depression in caregivers of the elderly. *Journal of Family Practice* 30:430-436.

Gardner, L., J. Brundage, D. McNeill, et al. 1989. Evidence of spread of HIV in low prevalence areas of the United States. *Journal of AIDS* 50:521-532.

Garry, R. and G. Koch. 1992. Correspondence: Tat contains a sequence related to snake neurotoxins. *AIDS* 6:1541-1542.

General Accounting Office (GAO). March 1993. *Needle Exchange Programs: Research Suggests Promise as an AIDS Prevention Strategy*. GAO/HRD-93-60. Washington, DC: General Accounting Office.

Gerrard, M. and T. Reis. 1989. Retention of contraceptive and AIDS information in the classroom. *The Journal of Sex Research* 26:315-323.

Gibson, D., J. Lovelle-Drache, M. Young, et al. 1991. Does brief counseling reduce

HIV risk in IV drug users? Final result from a randomized clinical trial. Paper presented: VIIth International Conference on AIDS. Florence. Abstract TH.D. 59.

Gibson, D., M. Young, and J. Lovelle-Drache. 1993. Randomized clinical trial to assess behavioral impact of enhanced procedures for notifying injection drug users of their antibody test results. Paper presented: IXth International Conference on AIDS. Berlin. Abstract PO-C24-3183.

Gilliam, A. and R. Seltzer. 1989. The efficacy of educational movies on AIDS knowledge and attitudes among college students. *College Health* 37:261-265.

Giulian, D., K. Vaca, and C. Noonan. 1990. Secretion of neurotoxins by mononuclear phagocytes infected with HIV-1. *Science* 250:1593-1596.

Glaser, J. and R. Greifinger. 1993. Correctional health care: A public health opportunity. *Annals of Internal Medicine* 118:139-145.

Goeders, N. and J. Smith. 1983. Cortical dopamingergic involvement in cocaine reinforcement. *Science* 221:773.

Goedert, J., M. Eyster, M. Ragni, et al. 1988. Rate of Heterosexual Transmission and Associated Risk with HIV Antigen. Paper presented: IVth International Conference on AIDS. Stockholm.

Goeren, W., K. Wade, and L. Rodriguez. 1990. Case Management of Families with HIV Infection. Paper presented: VIth International Conference on AIDS. San Francisco. Abstract SD 803.

Goldfinger, S., ed. 1990. *New Directions for Mental Health Services: Psychiatric Aspects of AIDS and HIV Infection.* San Francisco, CA: Jossey-Bass.

Goldstein, P. 1979. *Prostitution and Drugs.* Lexington, MA: Lexington Books.

Gollub, E. and Z. Stein. 1993. Commentary: The new female condom—Item I on a women's AIDS prevention agenda. *American Journal of Public Health* 83:498-500.

Gomez, C. and B. Marin. 1993. Can women demand condom use? Gender and power in safer sex. Paper presented: IXth International Conference on AIDS. Berlin.

Gonda, M., F. Wong-Staal, R. Gallo, et al. 1985. Sequence homology and morphologic similarity of HTLV-III and visna virus, a pathogenic lentivirus. *Science* 227:173-177.

Gorman, J. and R. Ketrzner. 1990. Psychoneuroimmunology at HIV infection. *Journal of Neuropsychiatry and Clinical Neurosciences* 2:241-252.

Gorski, R. 1988. Pp. 256-271 in S. Easter, K. Barald, and B. Carlson, eds. *Message to Mind.* Sunderland, MA: Sinauer Associates.

Gorski, R., J. Gordon, J. Shryne, et al. 1978. Evidence for a morphological sex difference within the medial preoptic area of the rat brain. *Brain Research* 148:333-346.

Gostin, L. 1991. The interconnected epidemics of drug dependency and AIDS. *Harvard Civil Rights-Civil Liberties Law Review* 26:114-184.

Gould, L., A. Walker, L. Crane, et al. 1974. *Connections: Notes from the Heroin World.* New Haven: Yale University Press.

Grady, W., D. Klepinger, J. Billy, et al. 1993. Condom characteristics: The perceptions and preferences of men in the United States. *Family Planning Perspectives* 25:67-73.

Grant, C. 1988. Life goes on along crack bazaar. *Miami Herald* (May 31):1B, 2B.

Gray, F., C. Geny, E. Dournon, et al. 1991. Neuropathological evidence that zidovudine reduces the incidence of HIV infection of brain. *Lancet* 337:852-853.

Green, G. 1993. Social support and HIV. *AIDS Care* 5:87-104.

Greenfield, L., G. Bigelow, and R. Brooner. 1992. HIV risk behavior in drug users:

Increased blood booting during cocaine injection. *AIDS Education and Prevention* 4:95-107.

Greve, F. 1989. Sex effect of cocaine its biggest turn-on? *Miami Herald* (October 22):1G, 6G.

Grinspoon, L. 1994. AIDS and mental health—Part II. *The Harvard Mental Health Letter* 10:1-4.

Grinspoon, L. and J. Bakalar. 1985. *Cocaine: A Drug and Its Social Evolution.* New York: Basic Books.

Grinstead, O., B. Faigeles, D. Binson, et al. 1993. Women's sexual risk for HIV: The national AIDS behavioral surveys (NABS). *Family Planning Perspectives* 25:252-256, 277.

Gross, J. 1985. A new, purified form of cocaine causes alarm as abuse increases. *New York Times* (November 29):1A.

Grossman, A. and C. Silverstein. 1993. Facilitating support groups for professionals working with people with AIDS. *Social Work* 38:144-150.

Grund, J., C. Kaplan, and N. Adriaans. 1989. Needle Exchange and Drug Sharing: A View from Rotterdam. *Newsletter of the International Working Group on AIDS and IV Drug Use.* Fourth edition.

Grund, J., C. Kaplan, N. Adriaans, et al. 1990. The limitations of the concept of needle sharing: The practice of frontloading. *AIDS* 4:819-821.

Guinan, M. 1989. Women and crack addiction. *Journal of the American Women's Medical Association* 44:129.

Guydish, J., J. Bucardo, M. Young, et al. 1993. Evaluating needle exchange: Are there negative effects? *AIDS* 7:871-876.

Guydish, J. and K. Haynes Sanstad. 1992. Behavior change among intravenous drug users: The role of community-based interventions. *Psychology of Addictive Behaviors* 6:91-99.

Hackett, G. and M. Lerner. 1987. L.A. law: Gangs and crack: The Crips and the Bloods fight for market share. *Newsweek* (April 27):35(2).

Hahn, R., I. Onorato, T. Jones, et al. 1989. Prevalence of HIV infection among intravenous drug users in the United States. *Journal of the American Medical Association* 261:2677-2684.

Hamburg, M. 1990. The epidemiology of HIV infection and AIDS in the United States. *Ear, Nose and Throat Journal* 69:394-400.

Hamburg, M. and A. Fauci. 1990. HIV Infection and AIDS: Challenges to Biomedical Research. Pp. 171-182 in L. Gostin, ed. *Hospitals, Health Care Professionals and AIDS.* New Haven: Yale University Press.

Hamer, D., S. Hu, V. Magnuson, et al. 1993. A linkage between DNA markers on the X chromosome and male sexual orientation. *Science* 261:321-326.

Hamid, A. 1990. The political economy of crack-related violence. *Contemporary Drug Problems* 17:31-78.

Hankins, C. and Handley, M. 1992. HIV disease and AIDS in women: Current knowledge and a research agenda. *Journal of Acquired Immune Deficiency Syndromes* 5:957-971.

Hanson, B., G. Beschner, J. Walters, et al. 1985. *Life with Heroin: Voices from the Inner City.* Lexington, MA: D.C. Heath.

Harris, R., K. Kavanagh, S. Hetherington, et al. 1992. Strategies for AIDS prevention—Leadership training and peer counseling for high-risk African-American women in the drug user community. *Clinical Nursing Research* 1:9-24.

Hart, C., S. Taylor, M. Kemeny, et al. 1990. Positive and negative changes in response to the threat of AIDS: Psychological adjustment as a function of severity of threat and life domain. Paper presented: VIth International Conference on AIDS. San Francisco. Abstract S.B. 371.

Hart, G., M. Boulton, R. Fitzpatrick, et al. In press. "Relapse" to Unsafe Sexual Behavior Amongst Gay Men: A Critique of Recent Behavioral HIV/AIDS Research.

Haughton, J. 1992. The Linkage: Substance Abuse Treatment and Primary Care. Secretarial Conference on Primary Care and Substance Abuse Linkage. February 26, 1992. Washington, DC.

Hausser, D., P. Lehmann, F. Dubois-Arber, et al. 1988. Evaluation of nationwide campaigns against AIDS in Switzerland. Paper presented: IVth International Conference on AIDS. Stockholm. Abstract 9553.

Hauth, A., M. Perry, J. Kelly, et al. 1993. Heavy Alcohol Use is Strongly Associated with Continued Risky Sex Among Gay Men: Risk Behavior Patterns and Alcohol-Sex Attributions. Paper presented: IXth International Conference on AIDS. Berlin.

Haverkos, H. 1990. Nitrite inhalant abuse and AIDS-related Kaposi's sarcoma. *Journal of Acquired Immune Deficiency Syndromes* 1:S47-50.

Haverkos, H. and R. Battjes. 1992. Female-to-male transmission of HIV. *Journal of the American Medical Association* 268:1855.

Haverkos, H. and W. Lange. 1990. Serious infections other than human immunodeficiency virus among intravenous drug users. *Journal of Infectious Diseases* 161:894-902.

Hays, R., J. Catania, L. McKusick, et al. 1990. Help-seeking for AIDS-related concerns: A comparison of gay men with various HIV diagnoses. *American Journal of Community Psychology* 18:743-755.

Hays, R., S. Kegeles, and T. Coates. 1993. Community mobilization promotes safer sex among young gay and bisexual men. Paper presented: IXth International Conference on AIDS. Berlin. Abstract WS-C07-1.

Healton, C. and P. Messeri. 1993. The effect of video interventions on improving knowledge and treatment compliance in the sexually transmitted disease clinic setting: Lesson for HIV health education. *Sexually Transmitted Diseases* 20:70-76.

Hearst, N. and B. Stephen. 1988. Preventing the heterosexual spread of AIDS: Are we giving our patients the best advice? *Journal of the American Medical Association* 259:2428-2432.

Heimer, R., E. Kaplan, and E. Cadman. 1992. Prevalence of HIV-infected syringes during a syringe-exchange program. *New England Journal of Medicine* 327:1883-1884.

Heimer, R., E. Kaplan, K. Khoshnood, et al. 1993. Needle exchange decreases the prevalence of HIV-1 proviral DNA in returned syringes in New Haven, Connecticut. *American Journal of Medicine* 95:214-220.

Heimer, R., S. Myers, E. Cadman, et al. 1992. Detection by polymerase chain reaction of human immunodeficiency virus type I proviral DNA sequences in needles of injecting drug users. *Journal of Infectious Diseases* 165:781-782.

Hellinger, F. 1993. The lifetime cost of treating a person with HIV. *Journal of the American Medical Association* 270:474-478.

Herek, G. 1990. Illness, Stigma, and AIDS. In P. Costa, and G. VandenBos, eds. *Psychological Aspects of Serious Illness: Chronic Conditions, Fatal Diseases, and Clinical Care.* Washington, DC: American Psychological Association.

Herek, G. and J. Capitanio. 1993. Public reactions to AIDS in the United States: A second decade of stigma. *American Journal of Public Health* 83:574-577.

Hernandez-Avila, M. 1992. Report to Wisconsin Pharmacal Company: Acceptability of Female Condoms Among Female Prostitutes in Mexico City—Preliminary Findings. Letter to Dr. Mary Ann Leeper, Center for Public Health Research, National Institute of Public Health, Mexico.

Heyes, M., B. Brew, A. Martin, et al. 1991. Quinolinic acid in cerebrospinal fluid and serum in HIV-1 infection: Relationship to clinical and neurological status. *Annals of Neurology* 29:202-209.

Heyes, M., B. Brew, K. Saito, et al. 1992. Inter-relationships between neuroactive kynurenines, neopterin and B2 microglobulin in cerebrospinal fluid and serum of HIV-1-infected patients. *Journal of Neuroimmunology* 40:71-80.

Heyes, M., K. Saito, S. Crowley, et al. 1992. Quinolinic acid and kynurenine pathway metabolism in inflammatory and non-inflammatory neurological disease. *Brain* 115:1249-1274.

Hill, J. and D. Brenneman. 1990. GP 120-induced retardation of behavioral development in neonatal rats: Prevention by peptide T. *Society for Neuroscience Abstracts* 16:615.

Himmelsbach, C. 1943. With reference to physical dependence. Symposium: Can the Euphoric, Analgetic, and Physical Dependence Affects of Drugs be Separated. *Federation Proceedings* 2:201.

Hinkle, Y., E. Johnson, D. Gilbert, et al. In press. Black males who always use condoms: Their attitudes, knowledge about AIDS and sexual behavior. *Journal of the National Medical Association.*

Ho, D., D. Bredesen, H. Vinters, et al. 1989. The acquired immunodeficiency syndrome (AIDS) dementia complex [clinical conference]. *Annals of Internal Medicine* 111:400-410.

Hobfoll, S., A. Jackson, J. Lavin, et al. 1993. Safer sex knowledge, behavior, and attitudes of inner-city women. *Health Psychology* 12:481-488.

Holmberg, S., C. Horsburg, J. Ward, et al. 1989. Biological factors in the heterosexual transmission of human immunodeficiency virus. *Journal of Infectious Diseases* 160:116-125.

Holtgrave, D., R. Valdiserri, and A. Gerber. 1993. HIV counseling, testing, referral, and partner notification services: A cost-benefit analysis. *Archives of Internal Medicine* 153:1225-1230.

Hoover, D., A. Saah, H. Bacella, et al. 1993. Clinical manifestations of AIDS in the era of pneumocystis prophylaxis. *New England Journal of Medicine* 329:1922-1926.

Hopewell, P. 1992. Impact of human immunodeficiency virus infection on the epidemiology, clinical features, management, and control of tuberculosis. *Clinical Infectious Diseases* 15:540-547.

Horstman, W. and L. McKusick. 1986. The Impact of AIDS on the Physician. In L. McKusick, ed. *What To Do About AIDS.* Berkeley, CA: University of California Press.

Howard, M. and J. McCabe. 1990. Helping teenagers postpone sexual involvement. *Family Planning Perspectives* 22:21-26.

Hser, Y., D. Anglin, and W. McGlothlin. 1987. Sex differences in addict career, I: Initiation of use. *American Journal of Drug and Alcohol Abuse* 11:1-16.

Hunter, J., M. Rotheram-Borus, M. Reid, et al. 1992. Sexual and Substance Abuse Acts that Place Lesbians at Risk for HIV. Poster presented: VIIIth International Conference on AIDS. Amsterdam.

Icard, L., R. Schilling, N. El-Bassel, et al. 1992. Preventing AIDS among black gay men and black gay and heterosexual male intravenous drug users. *Social Work* 37:440-445.

Icovics, J. and R. Rodin. 1992. Women and AIDS in the United States: Epidemiology, natural history, and mediation mechanisms. *Health Psychology* 11:1-16.

Inciardi, J. 1987. Beyond cocaine: Basuco, crack, and other coca products. *Contemporary Drug Problems* 14:461-492.

Inciardi, J. 1989. Trading sex for crack among juvenile drug users: A research note. *Contemporary Drug Problems* 16:689-700.

Inciardi, J. 1990a. AIDS—a strange disease of uncertain origins. *American Behavioral Scientist* 33:397-407.

Inciardi, J. 1990b. Federal efforts to control the spread of HIV and AIDS among IV drug users. *American Behavioral Scientist* 20:267-280.

Inciardi, J. 1992. *The War on Drugs II: The Continuing Epic of Heroin, Cocaine, Crack, Crime, AIDS, and Public Policy.* Mountain View, CA: Mayfield.

Inciardi, J. 1993. Kingrats, Chicken Heads, Slow Necks, Freaks, and Blood Suckers: A Glimpse at the Miami Sex-for-Crack Market. Pp. 37-67 in M. Ratner, ed. *Crack Pipe As Pimp: An Ethnographic Investigation of Sex-for-Crack Exchanges.* New York: Lexington Books.

Inciardi, J., D. Chitwood, and C. McCoy. 1992. Special risks for the acquisition and transmission of HIV infection during sex in crack houses. *Journal of Acquired Immune Deficiency Syndromes* 5:951-952.

Inciardi, J., D. Lockwood, and A. Pottieger. 1993. *Women and Crack-Cocaine.* New York: Macmillan.

Inciardi, J. and J. Page. 1991. Drug sharing among intravenous drug users. *AIDS* 5:772-774.

Inciardi, J., F. Tims, and B. Fletcher, eds. 1993. *Innovative Approaches in the Treatment of Drug Abuse: Program Models and Strategies.* Westport, CT: Greenwood Press.

Institute of Medicine (IOM). 1986. *Confronting AIDS: Directions for Public Health, Health Care, and Research.* Washington, DC: National Academy Press.

Institute of Medicine (IOM). 1988. *Confronting AIDS: Update 1988.* Washington, DC: National Academy Press.

Institute of Medicine (IOM). 1990. Gerstein, D., and H. Harwood, eds. *Treating Drug Problems: A Study of the Evolution, Effectiveness, and Financing of Public and Private Drug Treatment Systems.* Washington, DC: National Academy Press.

Institute of Medicine (IOM). 1991a. *The AIDS Research Program of the National Institutes of Health.* Washington, DC: National Academy Press.

Institute of Medicine (IOM). 1991b. *Research and Service Programs in the PHS: Challenges in Organization.* Washington, DC: National Academy Press.

Institute of Medicine (IOM). 1994. *Development of Anti-addiction Medications: Issues for the Government and Private Sector.* Washington, DC: National Academy Press.

Isaki, L. and E. Gordis. 1993. Alcohol and immunology—Progress and questions. *Alcoholism, Clinical and Experimental Research* 17:725-726.

Izazola, J., J. Valdespino, and J. Sepulveda. 1988. Indicators of behavior modification due to the campaign for the prevention of AIDS in Mexico. Paper presented: IVth International Conference on AIDS. Stockholm. Abstract 9551.

Jaffe, J. and S. Sharpless. 1968. Pharmacological denervation supersensitivity in the cenrtal nervous system: A theory of physical dependence. *Research Publications—Association for Research in Nervous and Mental Disease* 46:226-246.

Jager, J. and E. Ruitenberg, eds. 1992. *AIDS Impact Assessment: Modelling and Scenario Analysis.* New York: Elsevier.

Jemmott, J., L. Jemmott, and G. Fong. 1992. Reductions in HIV risk-associated sexual behaviors among black male adolescents: Effects of an AIDS prevention intervention. *American Journal of Public Health* 82:372-377.

Jemmott, L. and J. Jemmott III. 1992. Increasing condom-use intentions among sexually active black adolescent women. *Nursing Research* 41:273-279.

Jerrells, T., W. Smith, and M. Eckardt. 1990. Murine model of ethanol-induced immunosuppression. *Alcoholism: Clinical and Experimental Research* 14:546-550.

Johnson, A. 1988. Heterosexual transmission of human immunodeficiency virus. *British Medical Journal* 296:1017-1020.

Johnson, A., H. Coirini, G. Ball, et al. 1989. Anatomical localization of the effects of 17 beta-estradiol on oxytocin receptor binding in the ventromedial hypothalamic nucleus. *Endocrinology* 124:207-211.

Johnson, A., H. Coirini, B. McEwen, et al. 1989. Testosterone modulates oxytocin binding in the hypothalamus of castrated male rats. *Neuroendocrinology* 50:199-203.

Johnson, A. and M. Laga. 1988. Heterosexual transmission of HIV. *AIDS* 2:S49-S56.

Johnson, A., A. Petherick, S. Davidson, et al. 1989. Transmission of HIV to heterosexual partners of infected men and women. *AIDS* 3:367-372.

Johnson, B., P. Goldstein, E. Preble, et al. 1985. *Taking Care of Business: The Economics of Crime by Heroin Users.* Lexington, MA: D.C. Heath.

Johnson, R. 1994. Questions and Prospects Related to HIV-1 and the Brain. In R. Price and S. Perry, eds. *HIV, AIDS and the Brain.* New York: Raven Press.

Jose, B., S. Friedman, A. Neaigus, et al. 1993. Syringe-mediated drug-sharing (backloading): A new risk factor for HIV among injecting drug users. *AIDS* 7:1653-1660.

Joseph, J., S. Caumartin, M. Tal, et al. 1990. Psychological functioning in a cohort of gay men at risk for AIDS: A three-year descriptive study. *Journal of Nervous and Mental Disease* 178:607-615.

Joseph, S. and D. Des Jarlais. 1989. Needle and syringe exchange as a method of AIDS epidemic control. *AIDS Updates* 2:1-8.

Kahn, J. 1993. Are NEP's Cost-Effective in Preventing HIV Infection? Pp. 475-509 in P. Lurie and A. Reingold, eds. *The Public Health Impact of Needle Exchange Programs in the United States and Abroad.* San Francisco, CA: Institute for Health Policy Studies, University of California, San Francisco.

Kaiser, P., J. Offerman, and S. Lipton. 1990. Neuronal injury due to HIV-1 envelope protein is blocked by anti-gp-120 antibodies but not by anti-CD4 antibodies. *Neurology* 40:1757-1761.

Kalichman, S., J. Kelly, T. Hunter, et al. 1993. Culturally tailored HIV-AIDS risk-reduction messages targeted to African-American urban women: Impact on risk sensitization and risk reduction. *Journal of Consulting and Clinical Psychology* 61:291-295.

Kalichman, S., J. Kelly, J. Johnson, et al. 1994. Factors associated with risk for HIV infection among chronic mentally ill adults. *American Journal of Psychiatry* 151:221-227.

Kamenga, M., R. Ryder, M. Jingu, et al. 1991. Evidence of marked sexual behavior change associated with low HIV-1 seroconversion in 149 married couples with discordant HIV-1 serostatus: experience at an HIV counseling center in Zaire. *AIDS* 5:61-67.

Kaplan, E. 1991. Evaluating needle exchange programs via syringe tracking and testing (STT). *AIDS and Public Policy Journal* 6:109-115.

Kaplan, E. 1994. Operational modeling of needle exchange programs, in Needle Exchange and Bleach Distribution Programs. Paper presented: National Research

Council Panel on Needle Exchange and Bleach Distribution Programs, Committee on AIDS Research in the Behavioral, Social and Statistical Sciences. Washington, DC. National Academy Press.

Kaplan, E. and M. Brandeau, eds. 1994. *Modeling the AIDS Epidemic: Planning, Policy and Prediction.* New York: Raven Press.

Kaplan, E. and R. Heimer. 1994. HIV incidence among needle exchange participants: Estimates from syringe tracking and testing data. *Journal of Acquired Immune Deficiency Syndromes* 7:182-189.

Kaplan, E. and A. Novick. 1990. Self-deferral, HIV infection and the blood supply: Evaluating an AIDS intervention. *Evaluation Review* 14:686-700.

Kaplan, E. and E. O'Keefe. 1993. Let the needles do the talking! Evaluating the New Haven needle exchange. *Interfaces* 23:7-26.

Kaplan, E. and R. Heimer. 1994. A circulation theory of needle exchange. *AIDS* 8:567-574.

Kaplan, J. 1983. *The Hardest Drug: Heroin and Public Policy.* Chicago: University of Chicago Press.

Kaslow, R. and D. Francis, eds. 1989. *The Epidemiology of AIDS: Expression, Occurrence, and Control of Human Immunodeficiency Virus Type 1 Infection.* New York: Oxford University Press.

Kaslow, R., W. Blackwelder, D. Ostrow, et al. 1989. No evidence for a role of alcohol or other psychoactive drugs in accelerating immunodeficiency in HIV-1-positive individuals, a report from the multicenter AIDS cohort study. *Journal of the American Medical Association* 261:3424-3429.

Kayal, P. 1993. The Sociological Imagination in AIDS Prevention Education Among Gay Men. Pp. 201-221 in G. Albrecht and R. Zimmerman, eds. *The Social and Behavioral Aspects of AIDS. Advances in Medical Sociology,* Vol. III. Greenwich, CT: JAI Press.

Kegeles, S., R. Hays, and T. Coates. 1993. A community-level risk reduction intervention for young gay and bisexual men. Paper presented: IXth International Conference on AIDS. Berlin. Abstract WSC071.

Kelly, J., D. Murphy, R. Bahr, et al. 1992. AIDS/HIV risk behavior among the chronically mentally ill. *American Journal of Psychiatry* 149:886-889.

Kelly, J., D. Murphy, and R. Roffman, et al. 1992. Acquired immunodeficiency syndrome/human immunodeficiency virus risk behavior among gay men in small cities: Findings of a 16-city national sample. *Archives of Internal Medicine* 152:2293-2297.

Kelly, J., D. Murphy, K. Sikkema, et al. 1993. Psychological interventions to prevent HIV infection are urgently needed: New priorities for behavioral research in the second decade of AIDS. *American Psychologist* 48:1023-1034.

Kelly, J., D. Murphy, C. Washington, et al. In press. Effects of HIV/AIDS prevention groups for high-risk women in urban primary health care clinics. *American Journal of Public Health.*

Kelly, J. and J. St. Lawrence. 1988. *The AIDS Health Crisis—Psychological and Social Interventions.* New York: Plenum Press.

Kelly, J., J. St. Lawrence, R. Betts, et al. 1990. A skills-training group intervention model to assist persons in reducing risk behaviors for HIV infection. *AIDS Education and Prevention* 2:24-35.

Kelly, J., J. St. Lawrence, and T. Brasfield. 1991. Predictors of vulnerability to AIDS risk behavior relapse. *Journal of Consulting and Clinical Psychology* 59:163-166.

Kelly, J., J. St. Lawrence, Y. Diaz, et al. 1991. HIV risk behavior reduction following intervention with key opinion leaders of population: An experimental analysis. *American Journal of Public Health* 81:168-171.

Kelly, J., J. St. Lawrence, H. Hood, et al. 1989. Behavioral intervention to reduce AIDS risk activities. *Journal of Consulting and Clinical Psychology* 57:60-67.

Kelly, J., J. St. Lawrence, Y. Stevenson, et al. 1992. Community AIDS/HIV risk reduction: The effects of endorsements by popular people in three cities. *American Journal of Public Health* 82:1483-1489.

Kelly, J., R. Winett, R. Roffman, et al. 1993. Social Diffusion Models Can Produce Population-Level HIV Risk Behavior Reduction: Field Trial Results and Mechanisms Underlying Change. Paper presented: IXth International Conference on AIDS. Berlin. Abstract POC233167.

Kerr, P. 1986a. Crack users' babies crowding hospital nurseries (in New York). *New York Times* (August 25):15,B1.

Kerr, P. 1986b. New York crack cases strain its justice system. *New York Times* (November 24):13,A1.

Kerr, P. 1988. Addiction's hidden toll: Poor families in turmoil. *New York Times* (June 23):1,A1.

Kerr, P. 1989. Crack and resurgence of syphilis spreading AIDS among the poor. *New York Times* (November):1.

Kessler, R., C. Foster, J. Joseph, et al. 1991. Stressful life events as predictors of symptoms onset in HIV infection. *American Journal of Psychiatry* 145:733-738.

Khachaturian, H., M. Lewis, K. Tsou, et al. 1985. Pp. 216-272 in A. Bjorklund and T. Hokfelt, eds. *Handbook of Chemical Neuroanatomy*. New York: Elsevier.

Kingsley, L., R. Detels, R. Kaslow, et al. 1987. Risk factors for seroconversion to human immundeficiency virus among male homosexuals: Results from the Multicenter AIDS Cohort Study. *Lancet* 1:345-349.

Kingsley, L., S. Zhou, H. Bacellar, et al. 1991. Temporal trends in human immuodeficiency virus type 1 seroconversion 1984-1989. *American Journal of Epidemiology* 134:331-339.

Kippax, S., G. Dowsett, M. Davis, et al. 1991. Social Aspects of the Prevention of AIDS. Technical Report: Australian Federation of AIDS Organizations and the AIDS Council of New South Wales. Sustaining Safe Sex Survey. Sydney, Australia: Macquarie University, AIDS Research Unit.

Kirby, D., R. Barth, N. Leland, et al. 1991. Reducing the risk: Impact of a new curriculum on sexual risk-taking. *Family Planning Perspectives* 23:253-263.

Kleiber, D., B. Gusy, D. Enzmann, et al. 1992. Causes and Prevalence of Stress and Burnout among Healthcare Personnel in the Field of AIDS. Paper presented: VIIIth International Conference on AIDS. Amsterdam. Abstract POB3433.

Klepinger, D., J. Billy, K. Tanfer, et al. 1993. Perceptions of AIDS risk and severity and their association with risk-related behavior among U.S. men. *Family Planning Perspectives* 25:74-82.

Kline, A., E. Kline, and E. Oken. 1992. Minority women and sexual choice in the age of AIDS. *Social Science and Medicine* 34:447-457.

Kline, A. and J. Strickler. 1993. Perceptions of risk for AIDS among women in drug treatment. *Health Psychology* 12:313-323.

Klovdahl, A. 1985. Social networks and the spread of infectious diseases: The AIDS example. *Social Science and Medicine* 21:1203-1216.

Klovdahl, A., J. Potterat, D. Woodhouse, et al. 1994. Social networks and infectious disease: The Colorado Springs study. *Social Science and Medicine* 38:79-88.

Knopf, A. 1989a. Syphilis and crack linked in Connecticut. *Substance Abuse Report* (August 1):1-2.

Knopf, A. 1989b. Syphilis and gonorrhea on the rise among inner-city drug addicts. *Substance Abuse Report* (June 1):1-2.

Koenig, S., H. Gendelman, J. Orenstein, et al. 1986. Detection of AID virus in macrophages in brain tissue from AIDS patients with encephalopathy. *Science* 233:1089-1093.

Koob, G. and F. Bloom. 1988. Cellular and molecular mechanisms of drug dependence. *Science* 242:715-723.

Koob, G., H. Le, and I. Creese. 1987. The D1 dopamine receptor antagonist SCH 23390 increases cocaine self-administration in the rat. *Neuroscience Letters* 79:315-320.

Koppel, B. 1992. Neurological complications of AIDS and HIV infection. Pp. 315-348 in G. Wormser, ed. *AIDS and Other Manifestations of HIV Infection*. New York: Raven Press.

Kreek, M. 1983. Health Consequences Associated with the Use of Methadone. Pp. 456-482 in J. Cooper, F. Altman, F. Brown, et al., eds. *Research on the Treatment of Narcotic Addiction*. Rockville, MD: National Institute on Drug Abuse.

Kreek, M., T. Garfield, C. Gutjahr, et al. 1976. Rifampin-induced methadone withdrawal. *New England Journal of Medicine* 294:1104-1106.

Kreiss, J., D. Koech, and F. Plummer. 1986. AIDS virus infection in Nairobi prostitutes: Spread of the epidemic in East Africa. *New England Journal of Medicine* 314:414-418.

Kruger, T. and T. Jerrells. 1992. Potential role of alcohol in human immunodeficiency virus infection. *Alcohol Health and Research World* 16:57-63.

Kyes, K. 1990. The effect of a "safer sex" film as mediated by erotophobia and gender on attitudes towards condoms. *The Journal of Sex Research* 27:297-303.

L'Age-Stehr, J., A. Schwarz, and G. Offermann. 1985. HTLV-III infection in kidney transplant recipients. *Lancet* 2:1361-1362.

Laga, M., H. Taelman, L. Bonneux, et al. 1988. Risk Factors for Heterosexual Partners of HIV-Infected Africans and Europeans. Paper presented: IVth International Conference on AIDS. Stockholm.

Laga, M., H. Taelman, P. Van der Stuyft, et al. 1989. Advanced immunodeficiency as a risk factor for heterosexual transmission of HIV. *AIDS* 3:361-366.

Lamar, J. 1986. Crack. *Time* (June 2):16-18.

Lamptey, P. 1991. An Overview of AIDS Interventions in High-Risk Groups: Commercial Sex Workers and Their Clients. In *AIDS and Women's Reproductive Health*. New York: Plenum Press.

Lane, S. 1993. How and Why Did NEPs Develop? Pp. 139-169 in P. Lurie and A. Reingold, eds. *The Public Health Impact of Needle Exchange Programs in the United States and Abroad*. San Francisco, CA: Institute for Health Policy Studies, University of California, San Francisco.

Larson, A. 1989. Social context of human immunodeficiency virus transmission in Africa: Historical and cultural bases of east and central African sexual relations. *Reviews of Infectious Diseases* 11:716-731.

Latkin, C., W. Mandell, M. Oziemkowska, et al. 1993. The Relationship Between Sexual Behavior, Alcohol, Cocaine, Heroin Use, and Social Network Characteristics in Injecting Drug Users in the SAFE Study. NIAAA workshop on AIDS and Alcohol. Bethesda, MD.

Laumann, E., J. Gagnon, S. Michaels, et al. 1993. Monitoring AIDS and other rare population events: A network approach. *Journal of Health and Social Behavior* 34:7-22.

Lawlor, J. 1986. USA Battles Souped-Up Cocaine. *USA Today* (June 16):1A-2A.

Lawrance, L., S. Levy, and L. Rubinson. 1990. Self-efficacy and AIDS prevention for pregnant teens. *Journal of School Health* 60:19-24.

Lazzarin, A., A. Saracco, M. Musicco, et al. 1991. Man-to-woman sexual transmission of the human immunodeficiency virus: Risk factors related to sexual behavior, man's infectiousness, and woman's susceptibility. *Annals of Internal Medicine* 151:2411-2416.

LeBlanc, A., R. Gibbins, and H. Kalant. 1973. Behavioral augmentation of tolerance to ethanol in the rat. *Psychopharmacologia* 30:117-122.

Lee, F. 1988. Neighbors frustrated by invasion of crack. *Miami Herald* (April 24):1A.

Lee, P. and A. Moss. 1987. AIDS prevention: Is cost-benefit analysis appropriate? *Health Policy* 8:193-196.

Leeper, M. 1990. Preliminary evaluation of REALITY: A condom for women to wear. *AIDS Care* 2:287-290.

Leeper, M. and M. Conrardy. 1989. Preliminary evaluation of REALITY: A condom for women to wear. *Advances in Contraception* 5:229-235.

Lefrere, J., D. Vittecoq, M. North, et al. 1988. Risk of female to male transmission of HIV from women infected by transfusion. *AIDS* 2:137-138.

Lehmann, P., D. Hausser, B. Somaini, et al. 1987. Campaign against AIDS in Switzerland: evaluation of a nationwide educational programme. *British Medical Journal* 295:1118-1120.

Leigh, B. and R. Stall. 1993. Substance use and risky sexual behavior for exposure to HIV: Issues in methodology, interpretation, and prevention. *American Psychologist* (October):1035-1045.

Leigh, B., M. Temple, and K. Trocki. 1993. The sexual behavior of U.S. adults: Results from a national survey. *American Journal of Public Health* 83:1400-1408.

Lennon, M., J. Martin, and L. Dean. 1990. The influence of social support on AIDS-related grief reaction among gay men. *Social Science and Medicine* 31:477-484.

LeVay, S. 1991. A difference in hypothalamic structure between heterosexual and homosexual men. *Science* 253:1034-1037.

Levy, J. and G. Albrecht. 1989. Methodological Considerations in Research on Sexual Behavior and AIDS Among Older People. Pp. 96-123 in M. Riley, M. Ory, and D. Zablotsky, eds. *AIDS in an Aging Society*. New York: Springer.

Lewin and Associates. 1988. *Examination of the Advisability and Feasibility of Restructuring Federal Alcohol, Drug Abuse, and Mental Health Activities.* Washington, DC: Lewin and Associates.

Lewis, D., R. Niven, D. Czechowicz, et al. 1987. A review of medical education in alcohol and other drug abuse. *Journal of the American Medical Association* 257:2945-2948.

Linville, P., Fischer, G., and B. Fischhoff. In press. Perceived Risk and Decision Making Involving AIDS. In J. Pryor and G. Reeder, eds. *The Social Psychology of HIV Infection*. Hillsdale, NJ: Erlbaum.

Lipton, S. 1991. Requirement for macrophages in neuronal injury induced by HIV envelope protein gp 120. *Neurological Report* 3:913-915.

Lipton, S. 1992. Human immunodeficiency virus-infected macrophages, gp120 and N-methyl D-asparate neurotoxicity. *Annals of Neurology* 33:227-228.

Lipton, S. 1994. Laboratory basis of novel therapeutic strategies to prevent HIV-related neuronal injury. Pp. 183-202 in R. Price and S. Perry, eds. *HIV, AIDS and the Brain*. New York: Raven Press.

Lisansky Gomberg, E. and J. Lisansky. 1984. Antecedents of Alcohol Problems in

Women. Pp. 233-259 in S. Wilsnack and L. Beckman, eds. *Alcohol Problems in Women.* New York: Guilford Press.

Louria, D. 1970. Sexual use of amyl nitrite. *Medical Aspects of Human Sexuality* 4:89.

Lu, B., M. Yokoyama, C. Dreyfus, et al. 1991. NGF gene expression in actively growing brain glia. *Journal of Neuroscience* 11:318-326.

Lurie, P. and A. Reingold, eds. 1993. *The Public Health Impact of Needle Exchange Programs in the United States and Abroad.* San Francisco, CA: University of California.

Lyketsos, C., D. Hoover, M. Guccione, et al. 1993. Depressive symptoms as predictors of medical outcomes in HIV infection. *Journal of the American Medical Association* 270:2563-2567.

Lyness, W., N. Friedle, and K. Moore. 1979. Destruction of dopaminergic nerve terminals in nucleus accumbers: Effect on d-amphetamine self-administration. *Pharmacological Biochemical Behavior* 11:553-556.

MacDonald, P., D. Waldorf, C. Reinarman, et al. 1988. Heavy cocaine use and sexual behavior. *Journal of Drug Issues* 18:437-455.

Magana, J. 1991. Sex, drugs and HIV: An ethnographic approach. *Social Science and Medicine* 33:5-9.

Magura, S., Q. Siddiqi, R. Freeman, et al. 1991. Changes in cocaine use after entry to methadone treatment. *Journal of Addictive Diseases* 10:31-45.

Magura, S., Q. Siddiqi, J. Shapiro, et al. 1991. Outcomes of an AIDS prevention program for methadone patients. *The International Journal of the Addictions* 26:629-655.

Mahler, J., D. Yi, M. Sacks, et al. 1994. Undetected HIV infection among patients admitted to an alcohol rehabilitation unit. *American Journal of Psychiatry* 151:439-440.

Maiman, L. and M. Becker. 1974. The health belief model: Origins and correlates in psychological theory. *Health Education Monographs* 2:336-353.

Malow, R., S. Corrigan, S. Cunningham, et al. 1993. Psychosocial factors associated with condom use among African-American drug abusers in treatment. *AIDS Education and Prevention* 5:244-253.

Mann, J., J. Chin, P. Piot, et al. 1989. The International Epidemiology of AIDS. Pp. 51-61 in J. Piel, ed. *The Science of AIDS.* New York: W. H. Freeman.

Mantell, J. and A. DiVitts. 1990. AIDS Prevention Programs: The Need for Evaluation in the Context of Community Partnership. Pp. 51-61 in L. Leviton, A. Hegedus, and A. Rubrin, eds. *Evaluating AIDS Prevention: Contributions of Multiple Disciplines.* San Francisco, CA: Jossey-Bass.

Marin, B., C. Gomez, and N. Hearst. 1993. Prevalence of multiple heterosexual partners and condom use among Hispanics and non-Hispanic whites. *Family Planning Perspectives* 25:170-174.

Marin, B., C. Gomez, and J. Tschann. 1993. Condom use among hispanic men with multiple female partners: A nine-state study. *Public Health Reports* 108:742-750.

Marmor, M., D. Des Jarlais, H. Cohen, et al. 1987. Risk factors for infection with human immunodeficiency virus among intravenous drug abusers in New York City. *AIDS* 1:39-44.

Martin, J. 1990. Drug use and unprotected anal intercourse among gay men. *Health Psychology* 9:450-465.

Martin, J. 1988. Psychological consequences of AIDS-related bereavement among gay men. *Journal of Consulting and Clinical Psychology* 56:856-862.

Martin, L., J. McDougal, and S. Lsokoski. 1985. Disinfection and inactivation of the Human T Lymphotropic Virus Type III/lymphadenopathy-associated virus. *Journal of Infectious Diseases* 152:400-403.

Martin, W. and J. Sloan. 1977. Neuropharmacology and neurochemistry of subjective effects, analgesia, tolerance, and dependence produced by narcotic analgesics. *Handbook of Experimental Pharmacology* 45:43-158.

Masliah, E., C. Achim, N. Ge, et al. 1994. Cellular neuropathology in HIV encephalitis. Pp. 119-131 in R. Price and S. Perry, eds. *HIV, AIDS and the Brain.* New York: Raven Press.

McCann, K. and E. Wadsworth. 1992. The role of informal caregivers in supporting gay men who have HIV-related illness. *AIDS Care* 4:25-34.

McCoy, H. V. and C. Miles. 1992. A gender comparison of health status among users of crack cocaine. *Journal of Psychoactive Drugs* 24:389-397.

McCoy, H. V. and J. Inciardi. 1993. Women and AIDS: Social determinants of sex-related activities. *Women and Health* 20:69-86.

McCusker, J., A. Stoddard, K. Mayer, et al. 1988. Effects of HIV antibody test knowledge on subsequent sexual behaviors in a cohort of homosexually active men. *American Journal of Public Health* 78:462-467.

McCusker, J., A. Stoddard, J. Zapka, et al. 1992. AIDS education for drug abusers: Evaluation of short-term effectiveness. *American Journal of Public Health* 82:533-540.

McEwan, R., A. McCallum, R. Bhopal, et al. 1992. Sex and the risk of HIV infection: The role of alcohol. *British Journal of Addiction* 87:577-584.

McEwen, B., V. Luine, and C. Fischette. 1988. Pp. 272-281 in S. Easter, K. Barald, and B. Carlson, eds. *Message to Mind.* Sunderland, MA: Sinauer Associates.

McKusick, L., ed. 1986. *What To Do About AIDS? Physicians and Mental Health Professionals Discuss the Issues.* Berkeley, CA: University of California Press.

McKusick, L. and R. Hilliard. 1991. Multiple loss accounts for worsening distress in community hard hit by AIDS. Paper presented: VIIth International AIDS Conference. Florence.

McKusick, L., C. Hoff, R. Stall, et al. 1991. Tailoring AIDS prevention: Differences in behavioral strategies among heterosexual and gay bar patrons in San Francisco. *AIDS Education and Prevention* 3:1-9.

Meisel, R. and D. Pfaff. 1985. Specificity and neural sites of action of anisomycin in the reduction or facilitation of female sexual behavior in rats. *Hormones and Behavior* 19:237-251.

Mellins, C. and A. Ehrhardt. 1993. Families Affected by Pediatric AIDS: Sources of Stress and Coping. Paper presented: IXth International Conference on AIDS. Berlin. Abstract WS-D17-5.

Merchenthaler, I. and J. Maderdrut. 1985. Pp. 273-334 in A. Bjorklund, and T. Hokfelt, eds. *Handbook of Chemical Neuroanatomy.* New York: Elsevier.

Metzger, D., G. Woody, D. De Philipps, et al. 1991. Risk factors for needle sharing among methadone-treated patients. *American Journal of Psychiatry* 148:636-640.

Metzger, D., G. Woody, A. McLellan, et al. 1993. Human immunodeficiency virus seroconversion among intravenous drug users in- and out-of-treatment: An 18-month prospective follow-up. *Journal of Acquired Immune Deficiency Syndromes* 6:1049-1056.

Meyer, I., K. McKinnon, F. Cournos, et al. 1993. HIV seroprevalence among long-stay psychiatric inpatients. *Hospital and Community Psychiatry* 44:282-284.

Mientjes, G., E. van Ameijden, A. van den Hoeck, et al. 1992. Increasing morbidity without rise in non-AIDS mortality among HIV-infected intravenous drug users in Amsterdam. *AIDS* 6:207-212.

Miller, E. 1986. *Street Women*. Philadelphia, PA: Temple University Press.

Mills, S., M. Campbell, and W. Waters. 1986. Public knowledge of AIDS and the DHSS advertisement campaign. *British Medical Journal* 293:1089-1090.

Minerbrook, S. 1989. A night in a crack house: Meet Snookie and the denizens of her world. *U.S. News and World Report* (April 10):29(1).

Moatti, P., W. Dab, H. Loundou, et al. 1992. Impact on the general public of media campaigns against AIDS: A French evaluation. *Health Policy* 21:233-247.

Mondanaro, J. 1990. Community-Based AIDS Prevention Interventions: Special Issues of Women Intravenous Drug Users. Pp. 68-82 in C.G. Leukefeld, R.J. Battjes, and Z. Amsel, eds. *AIDS and Intravenous Drug Use, Community Intervention and Prevention*. New York: Hemisphere Publishing.

Moore, R., J. Hidalgo, and B. Sugland. 1991. Zidovudine and the natural history of the Acquired Immune Deficiency Syndrome. *New England Journal of Medicine* 324:1412-1416.

Moore, R., J. Keruly, D. Richman, et al. 1992. Natural history of advanced HIV disease in patients treated with zidovudine. *AIDS* 6:671-677.

Moreno, S., J. Baraia-Extaburu, E. Bouza, et al. 1993. Risk for developing tuberculosis among anergic patients infected with HIV. *Annals of Internal Medicine* 119:194-198.

Morganthau, T. and P. McKillop, P. 1986. Crack and crime. *Newsweek* (June 16):16(6).

Moses, S., F. Plummer, E. Ngugi, et al. 1991. Controlling HIV in Africa: Effectiveness and cost of an intervention in high-frequency STD transmitter core group. *AIDS* 5:407-411.

Moss, A. 1990. Control of HIV Infection in Injecting Drug Users in San Francisco. Pp. 77-85 in J. Strang and G. Stimson, eds. *AIDS and Drug Misuse: The Challenge for Policy and Practice in the 1990s*. London: Routledge.

Moss, A., K. Vranizan, R. Gorter, et al. 1994. HIV seroconversion in intravenous drug users in San Francisco, 1985-1990. *AIDS* 8:223-231.

Munoz, A., D. Vlahov, L. Solomon, et al. 1992. Prognostic indicators for development of AIDS among intravenous drug users. *Journal of Acquired Immune Deficiency Syndromes* 5:694-700.

Murphy, S. and D. Waldorf. 1991. Kickin' down to the street doc: Shooting galleries in the San Francisco Bay area. *Contemporary Drug Problems* 18:9-29.

Myers, S., R. Heimer, D. Liu, et al. 1993. HIV DNA and antibodies in syringes from injecting drug users: A comparison of detection techniques. *AIDS* 7:925-931.

Namir, S., D. Wolcott, I. Fawzy, et al. 1987. Coping with AIDS: Psychological and health implications. *Journal of Applied Social Psychology* 17:309-328.

National Association of People With AIDS (NAPWA). 1992. *HIV In America: A Profile of the Challenges Facing Americans Living with HIV*. Washington, DC: NAPWA.

National Commission on AIDS. 1990. *Annual Report to the President and the Congress*. Washington, DC: U.S. Government Printing Office.

National Commission on AIDS. 1991a. *America Living With AIDS*. Washington, DC: U.S. Government Printing Office.

National Commission on AIDS. 1991b. *The Twin Epidemics of Substance Use and HIV*. Washington, DC: U.S. Government Printing Office.

National Commission on AIDS. 1993a. *AIDS: An Expanding Tragedy*. Washington, DC: U.S. Government Printing Office.

National Commission on AIDS. 1993b. *Behavioral and Social Sciences and the HIV/AIDS Epidemic*. Washington, DC: U.S. Government Printing Office.

National Institute of Mental Health (NIMH). 1993a. *AIDS Research: An NIMH Blueprint for the Second Decade.* Rockville, MD: NIMH.

National Institute of Mental Health (NIMH). 1993b. *Strategic Plan for AIDS Research: Neuroscience, Neurobehavior, and Behavior Change/Prevention Initiatives, 1993-1988.* Rockville, MD: NIMH.

National Institute of Mental Health (NIMH). 1994. W. Pequegnat and E. Stover, eds. *NIMH Handbook on Developing a Successful Research Application.* Rockville, MD: NIMH.

National Institute on Drug Abuse (NIDA). 1993. *Five Year Strategic Plan for AIDS Research, 1993-1998.* Rockville, MD: NIDA.

National Institute on Drug Abuse (NIDA). Cooperative Agreement Steering Committee. 1992. *The Standard Intervention of the Cooperative Agreement Program for AIDS Community-Based Outreach/Intervention Research.* Rockville, MD: NIDA.

National Research Council (NRC). 1990a. H. Miller, C. Turner, and L. Moses, eds. *AIDS: The Second Decade.* Washington, DC: National Academy Press.

National Research Council (NRC). 1990b. C. Turner, H. Miller, and L. Moses, eds. *AIDS, Sexual Behavior, and Intravenous Drug Use.* Washington, DC: National Academy Press.

National Research Council (NRC). 1991. S. Coyle, R. Boruch, and C. Turner, eds. *Evaluating AIDS Prevention Programs.* Washington, DC: National Academy Press.

National Research Council (NRC). 1993. A. Jonsen and J. Stryker, eds. *The Social Impact of AIDS in the United States.* Washington, DC: National Academy Press.

Navia, B., E-W. Cho, C. Petito, et al. 1986. The AIDS dementia complex II, Neuropathology. *Annals of Neurology* 19:525-535.

Navia, B., B. Jordan, and R. Price. 1986. The AIDS dementia complex. *Annals of Neurology* 19:517-524.

Neaigus, A., S. Friedman, R. Curtis, et al. 1994. The relevance of drug injectors social and risk networks for understanding and preventing HIV infection. *Social Science and Medicine* 38:67-78.

Neugebauer, R., J. Rabkin, J. Williams, et al. 1992. Bereavement reactions among homosexual men experiencing multiple losses in the AIDS epidemic. *American Journal of Psychiatry* 149:1374-1379.

Ngugi, E., J. Simonsen, M. Bosire, et al. 1988. Prevention of transmission of human immunodeficiency virus in Africa: Effectiveness of condom promotion and health education among prostitutes. *Lancet* 15:887-890.

Nicholson, W. and B. Long. 1990. Self-esteem, social support, internalized homophobia, and coping strategies of HIV+ gay men. *Journal of Consulting and Clinical Psychology* 58:873-876.

Nickerson, M. 1975. Vasodilator Drugs. Pp. 727-743 in L. Goodman and A. Gilman, eds. *The Pharmacological Basis of Therapeutics.* New York: Macmillan.

Novick, D., P. Farci, T. Croxsan, et al. 1988. Hepatitis d virus and human immunodeficiency virus antibodies in parenteral drug abusers who are hepatitis b surface antigen positive. *Journal of Infectious Diseases* 158:795-803.

Nyamathi, A., C. Bennett, B. Leake, et al. 1993. AIDS-related knowledge, perceptions, and behaviors among impoverished minority women. *American Journal of Public Health* 83:65-71.

Nyamathi, A., B. Leake, J. Flaskerud, et al. 1993. Outcomes of specialized and traditional AIDS counseling programs for impoverished women of color. *Research in Nursing and Health* 16:11-21.

Oakley, A. 1989. Who's afraid of the randomized controlled trial? Some dilemmas of the scientific method and "good" research practice. *Women and Health* 15: 25-29.

Obbo, C. 1993. HIV transmission through social and geographical networks in Uganda. *Social Science and Medicine* 36:949-955.

O'Brien, M., J. Murray, and W. Wiebel. 1993. Household Seroprevalence Survey in Two High-Risk Chicago Neighborhoods: HIV Pathways Between High-Risk and General Populations. Paper presented: IXth International Conference on AIDS. Berlin.

O'Brien, W. 1994. Genetic and biologic basis of HIV-1 neurotropism. Pp. 47-70 in R. Price and S. Perry, eds. *HIV, AIDS and the Brain*. New York: Raven Press.

O'Connor, P., S. Molde, S. Henry, et al. 1992. Human immunodeficiency, virus infection in intravenous drug users: A model for primary care. *American Journal of Medicine* 93:382-386.

O'Farrell, N. 1989. Transmission of HIV: Genital ulceration, sexual behavior, and circumcision. *Lancet* 2:1157.

Oppenheimer, G. 1992. Causes, cases, and cohorts: The role of epidemiology in the historical construction of AIDS. Pp. 49-83 in E. Fee and D. Fox, eds. *AIDS: The Making of a Chronic Disease*. Berkeley, CA: University of California Press.

O'Reilly, K. and D. Higgins. 1991. AIDS community demonstration projects for HIV prevention among hard-to-reach groups. *Public Health Reports* 106:714-720.

O'Reilly, K., D. Higgins, C. Galavotti, et al. 1990. Relapse from safer sex among homosexual men: Evidence from four cohorts in the AIDS community demonstration projects. Poster presented: VIth International Conference on AIDS. San Francisco. FC717.

Osborne, N. and M. Feit. 1992. The use of race in medical research. *Journal of the American Medical Association* 267:275-279.

Osmond, D. 1990. Heterosexual Transmission of HIV. Pp. 1-9 in P. Cohen, M. Sande, and P. Volberding, eds. *The AIDS Knowledge Base*. Waltham, MA: Massachusetts Medical Society.

Ostrow, D., J. Joseph, R. Kessler, et al. 1989. Disclosure of HIV antibody status: Behavioral and mental health correlates. *AIDS Education and Prevention* 1:1-11.

Ostrow, D., M. Van Raden, R. Fox, et al. 1990. Recreational drug use and sexual behavior change in a cohort of homosexual men. *AIDS* 4:759-765.

Ouellet, L., A. Jimenez, W. Johnson, et al. 1991. Shooting galleries and HIV disease: Variations in places for injecting illicit drugs. *Crime and Delinquency* 37:64-85.

Padian, N. 1988. Prostitute women and AIDS: Epidemiology. *AIDS* 2:413-419.

Padian, N., T. O'Brien, Y. Chang, et al. 1993. Prevention of heterosexual transmission of human immunodeficiency virus through couple counseling. *Journal of Acquired Immune Deficiency Syndromes* 6:1043-1048.

Padian, N., S. Shiboski, and N. Jewell. 1990. The effect of number of exposures on the risk of heterosexual HIV transmission. *Journal of Infectious Diseases* 161:883-887.

Padian, N., J. Wiley, and S. Glass. 1988. Anomalies of Infectivity in the Heterosexual Transmission of HIV. Paper presented: IVth International Conference on AIDS. Stockholm.

Panlilio, L., J. Hill, D. Brenneman, et al. 1990. GP120 and a VIP receptor antagonist impair morris water maze performance in rats. *Society for Neuroscience Abstracts* 16:1330.

Panos Institute. 1988. *AIDS and the Third World.* London: Panos Publications.

Papaevangelou, G., A. Roumeliotou, G. Kallinikos, et al. 1988. Education in preventing HIV infection in Greek registered prostitutes. *Journal of Acquired Immune Deficiency Syndromes* 1:386-389.

Parsons, B., T. Rainbow, D. Pfaff, et al. 1982. Hypothalamic protein synthesis essential for the activation of the lordosis reflex in the female rat. *Endocrinology* 110:620-624.

Paul, J., R. Stall, and F. Davies. 1993. Sexual risk for HIV transmission among gay/bisexual men in substance-abuse treatment. *AIDS Education and Prevention* 5:11-24.

Perry, S. 1994. HIV-related depression. Pp. 223-238 in R. Price and S. Perry, eds. *HIV, AIDS and the Brain.* New York: Raven Press.

Perry, S., B. Fishman, L. Jacobsberg, et al. 1991. Effectiveness of psychoeducational interventions in reducing emotional distress after human immunodeficiency virus antibody testing. *Archives of General Psychiatry* 48:143-147.

Perry, S., L. Jacobsberg, B. Fishman, et al. 1990. Psychological responses to serological testing for HIV. *AIDS* 4:145-152.

Pert, C., R. Mervis, J. Hill, et al. 1989. Morphological and behavioral response to acute and subacute I.C.V. GP120 administration in the rat. *Society for Neuroscience Abstracts* 15:1387.

Peterman, T., R. Stoneburner, and J. Allen. 1988. Risk of human immunodeficiency transmission from heterosexual adults with transfusion associated infections. *Journal of the American Medical Association* 259:55-58.

Peterson, J., J. Catania, M. Dolcini, et al. 1993. Multiple sexual partners among heterosexual African Americans in high risk cities of the United States: The National AIDS Behavioral Surveys. *Family Planning Perspectives* 25:263-267.

Peterson, J., T. Coates, J. Catania, et al. 1990. To Be or Not To Be Tested? Racial, Ethnic and Sexual Orientation Differences in Obtaining HIV Antibody Testing and Receiving Test Results. Paper presented: VIth International Conference on AIDS. San Francisco. Abstract S.C. 101.

Peterson, J., T. Coates, J. Catania, et al. 1992. High-risk sexual behavior and condom use among gay and bisexual African-American men. *American Journal of Public Health* 82:1490-1494.

Pfaff, D. and M. Reiner. 1973. Atlas of estradiol-concentrating cells in the central nervous system of the female rat. *Journal of Comparative Neurology* 151:121-158.

Pfaff, D. and Y. Sakuma. 1979. Deficit in the lordosis reflex of female rats caused by lesions in the ventromedial nucleus of the hypothalamus. *Journal of Physiology (London)* 288:203-210.

Pfaff, D. and S. Schwartz-Giblin. 1988. Pp. 1487-1568 in E. Knobil, and J. Neill, eds. *The Physiology of Reproduction.* New York: Raven Press.

Pickens, R., R. Meisch, and J. Dougherty, Jr. 1968. Chemical interactions in methamphetamine reinforcement. *Psychological Reports* 23:1267-1270.

Pivnick, A., A. Jacobson, K. Eric, et al. 1994. AIDS, HIV infection, and illicit drug use within inner-city families and social networks. *American Journal of Public Health* 84:271-274.

Plummer, F., J. Simonsen, D. Cameron, et al. 1991. Cofactors in male-female sexual transmission of human immunodeficiency virus type 1. *Journal of Infectious Diseases* 163:233-239.

Polk, B., R. Fox, R. Brookmeyer, et al. 1987. Predictors of acquired immunodeficiency syndrome developing in a cohort of seropositive homosexual men. *New England Journal of Medicine* 316:61-66.

Portegies, P., J. de Gans, D. Lange, et al. 1989. Declining incidence of AIDS dementia complex after introduction of zidovudine treatment. *British Medical Journal* 299:819-821.

Potterat, J., R. Rothenberg, D. Woodhouse, et al. 1985. Gonorrhea as a social disease. *Sexually Transmitted Disease* 12:25-32.

Price, R. 1994. Understanding the AIDS Dementia Complex (ADC), The challenge of HIV and its effect on the central nervous system. Pp. 1-45 in R. Price and S. Perry, eds. *HIV, AIDS and the Brain*. New York: Raven Press.

Price, R. and B. Brew. 1988. The AIDS dementia complex. *Journal of Infectious Diseases* 158:1079-1083.

Price, R., B. Brew, J. Sidtis, et al. 1988. The brain in AIDS: Central nervous system HIV-1 infection and AIDS dementia complex. *Science* 239:586-592.

Price, R. and S. Perry, eds. 1994. *HIV, AIDS and the Brain*. New York: Raven Press.

Price, R. and J. Sidtis. 1990. Evaluation of the AIDS dementia complex in clincial trials. *Journal of AIDS* 3:S51-S60.

Price, R. and J. Sidtis. 1992. The AIDS Dementia Complex. Second edition. Pp. 373-382 in G. Wormser, ed. *AIDS and Other Manifestations of HIV Infection*. New York: Raven Press.

Price, R. and J. Worley. 1994. Neurological Complications of HIV-1 Infection and AIDS. Pp. 489-505 in S. Broder, T. Merigan, Jr., and D. Bolognesi, eds. *Textbook of AIDS Medicine*. Baltimore, MD: Williams and Wilkins.

Prochaska, J. In press. Strong and weak principles for progressing from precontemplation to action based on twelve problem behaviors. *Health Psychology*.

Prochaska, J. and C. DiClemente. 1983. Stages and processes of self-change in smoking: Toward an integrative model of change. *Journal of Consulting and Clinical Psychology* 5:390-395.

Prochaska, J., C. DiClemente, and J. Norcross. 1992. In search of how people change. *American Psychologist* 47:1102-1114.

Pruchno, R., M. Kleban, and J. Michaels. 1990. Mental and physical health of caregiving spouses: Development of a causal model. *Journal of Gerontological Science* 45:192-199.

Pulliam, L., B. Herndler, N. Tang, et al. 1991. Human immunodeficiency virus-infected macrophages produce soluble factors that cause histological and neuro-chemical alterations in cultured human brains. *Journal of Clinical Investigation* 87:503-512.

Raab, N.I. and P. Selwyn. 1988. The ruthless young crack gangsters: Links to 200 murders in New York City last year. *New York Times* (March 20):E9.

Rabkin, J., R. Remien, L. Katoff, et al. 1991. AIDS long term survivors: A clinical assessment. Paper presented: American Psychiatric Association annual meeting. May, 1991. New Orleans, LA.

Rabkin, J., J. Williams, R. Neugebauer, et al. 1990. Maintenance of hope in HIV-spectrum homosexual men. *American Journal of Psychiatry* 147:1322-1326.

Raisman, G. and P. Field. 1971. Sexual dimorphism in the preoptic area of the rat. *Science* 173:731-733.

Ratner, M., ed. 1993. *Crack Pipe as Pimp: An Ethnographic Investigation of Sex-for-Crack Exchanges*. New York: Lexington Books.

Raveis, V. and K. Siegel. 1991. The impact of care giving on informal or familial care givers. *AIDS Patient Care* (February):39-43.

Reardon, J., M. Wilson, G. Lemp, et al. 1992. HIV-1 Infection Among Female Injection Drug Users (IDU) in the San Francisco Bay Area, California, 1989-1991: Increased Seroprevalence Rates for IDU Who are Lesbian/Bisexual, Racial/Ethnic Minorities or Cocaine Injectors. Paper presented: VIIIth International Conference on AIDS. Amsterdam. Abstract ThC 1553.

Reichman, L., C. Felton, and J. Edsall. 1979. Drug dependence a possible new risk factor for tuberculosis disease. *Archives of Internal Medicine* 139:337-339.

Resnick, L., S. Veren, S. Salahuddin, et al. 1986. Stability and inactivation of HTLV-III/LAV under clinical and laboratory environments. *Journal of the American Medical Association* 255:1887-1891.

Rettig, R., M. Torres, and G. Garrett. 1977. *Manny: A Criminal Addict's Story.* Boston: Houghton Mifflin.

Rezza, G., A. Lazzarin, G. Angarano, et al. 1989. The natural history of early HIV infection in intravenous drug users: Risk of disease progression in a cohort of seroconvertors. *AIDS* 3:87-90.

Rezza, G., A. Lazzarin, G. Angarano, et al. 1990. Risk of AIDS in HIV seroconverters: A comparison between intravenous drug users and homosexual males. *European Journal of Epidemiology* 6:99-101.

Rhodes, F. and R. Wolitski. 1989. Effect of instructional videotapes on AIDS knowledge and attitudes. *Journal of American College Health* 37:266-271.

Rhodes, F., R. Wolitski, and S. Thornton-Johnson. 1992. An experiential program to reduce AIDS risk among female sex partners of injection-drug users. *Health and Social Work* 17:261-272.

Ritz, M., R. Lamb, S. Goldberg, et al. 1987. Cocaine receptors on dopamine transporters are related to self-administration of cocaine. *Science* 237:1219-1223.

Roberts, D., M. Corcoran, and H. Fibiger. 1977. On the role of ascending catecholaminergic systems in intravenous self-administration of cocaine. *Pharmacology, Biochemistry and Behavior* 6:615-620.

Roberts, D. and G. Koob. 1982. Disruption of cocaine self-administration following 6-hydroxydopamine lesions of the ventral tegmental area in rats. *Pharmacology, Biochemistry and Behavior* 17:901-904.

Roberts, D., G. Koob, P. Klonoff, et al. 1980. Extinction and recovery of cocaine self-administration following 6-hydroxydopamine lesions of the nucleus accumbens. *Pharmacology, Biochemistry and Behavior* 12:781-787.

Rogers, D. and J. Osborn. 1993. AIDS policy—Two divisive issues. *Journal of the American Medical Association* 270:494-495.

Rogers, E. 1983. *Diffusion of Innovations.* New York: Free Press.

Rolf, J. 1993. Working Paper on Methodological Themes. NIAAA Workshop on Alcohol, HIV/AIDS, and Behavioral Risks: Theories and Interventions. May 20-21, 1993. Bethesda, MD.

Rolf, J., J. Baldwin, R. Trotter, et al. 1991. AIDS prevention for youth of rural Native American tribes. Paper presented: VIIth International Conference on AIDS. Florence. Abstract WD 4030.

Rolfs, R., M. Goldberg, and R. Sharrar. 1990. Risk factors for syphilis: Cocaine use and prostitution. *American Journal of Public Health* 80:853-857.

Rosenbaum, M. 1981. *Women on Heroin.* New Brunswick, NJ: Rutgers University Press.

Rosenberg, M. and E. Gollub. 1992. Commentary: Methods women can use that may prevent sexually transmitted disease, including HIV. *American Journal of Public Health* 82:1473-1478.

Rosenberg, P., M. Gail, L. Schrager, et al. 1991. National AIDS incidence trends and the extent of zidovudine therapy in selected demographic and transmission groups. *Journal of the Acquired Immune Deficiency Syndromes* 4:392-411.

Rosenblum, L., J. Buehler, M. Morgan, et al. 1993. Drug dependence: A leading diagnosis in hospitalized HIV-infected women. *Journal of Women's Health* 2:35-40.

Rosenstock, I. 1974. The health belief model and preventive health behavior. *Health Education Monographs* 2:328-335.

Ross, M. and P. Drew. 1991. Effects of nitrite use on lymphocyte mitogenesis in homosexual men. *International Journal of STD and AIDS* 2:133-135.

Rotheram-Borus, M., C. Koopman, C. Haignere, et al. 1991. Reducing HIV sexual risk behaviors among runaway adolescents. *Journal of the American Medical Association* 266:1237-1241.

Rottenberg, D., J. Moeller, S. Strother, et al. 1987. The metabolic pathology of the AIDS dementia complex. *Annals of Neurology* 22:700-706.

Rounsaville, B., S. Anton, K. Carroll, et al. 1991. Psychiatric diagnosis of treatment seeking cocaine abusers. *Archives of General Psychiatry* 48:43-51.

Routtenberg, A. 1972. Intracranial chemical injection and behavior: A critical review. *Behavioral Biology* 7:601-641.

Russell, J., A. Fatatis, P. Nelson, et al. 1990. Vasoactive intestinal polypeptide (VIP) causes intracellular calcium oscillations in astrocytes. *Society for Neuroscience Abstracts* 16:994.

Saad, A. and T. Jerrells. 1991. Flow cytometric and immunohistochemical evaluation of ethanol-induced changes in splenic and thymic lymphoid cell populations. *Alcoholism: Clinical and Experimental Research* 15:796-803.

Saah, A., A. Munoz, V. Kuo, et al. 1992. Predictors of the risk of development of acquired immunodeficiency syndrome within 24 months among gay men seropositive for human immunodeficiency virus type 1: A report from the Multicenter AIDS Cohort Study. *American Journal of Epidemiology* 135:1147-1155.

Sabatier, J., E. Vives, K. Mabrouk, et al. 1991. Evidence for neurotoxic activity of tat from human immunodeficiency virus type 1. *Journal of Virology* 65:961-967.

Sabogal, F., B. Faigeles, and J. Catania. 1993. Data from the National AIDS Behavioral Surveys II: Multiple sexual partners among Hispanics in high-risk cities. *Family Planning Perspectives* 25:257-262.

Sacks, M., H. Dermatis, S. Looser-Ott, et al. 1992. Seroprevalence of HIV and risk factors for AIDS in psychiatric inpatients. *Hospital and Community Psychiatry* 43:736-737.

Sakondhavat, C. 1990. Further testing of female condoms. *British Journal of Family Planning* 15:129.

Samet, H., H. Libman, K. Steger, et al. 1992. Compliance with zidovudine therapy in patients infected with human immunodeficiency virus, type 1: A cross-sectional study in a municipal hospital clinic. *American Journal of Medicine* 92:495-501.

San Francisco Department of Public Health. 1994. *Projections of the AIDS Epidemic in San Francisco: 1994-1997*. Seroepidemiology and Surveillance Branch, AIDS Office. San Francisco, CA: San Francisco Department of Public Health.

Sar, M. and W. Stumpf. 1975. Pp. 120-133 in W. Stumpf and L. Grant, eds. *Anatomical Endocrinology*. Basel, Switzerland: Karger.

Satriano, J. and M. Karp. 1993. AIDS and the Chronic Mentally Ill: Legal and Ethical Issues. Paper presented: Columbia University College of Physicians and Surgeons, Columbia University HIV Mental Health Training Project, and New York State Psychiatric Institute. HIV/AIDS and People With Serious Mental Illness. October 20, 1993. Albany, New York.

Sawyer, R., L. Brown, P. Narong, et al. 1993. Evaluation of a Possible Pharmacologic Interaction between Refabutin and Methadone in HIV-Seropositive Injecting

Drug Users. Paper presented: IXth International Conference on AIDS. Berlin. Abstract P0-B30-2197.

Schensul, J. and S. Schensul. 1990. Ethnographic Evaluation of AIDS Prevention Programs: Better Data for Better Programs. New Directions for Program Evaluation. Pp. 51-62 in L. Leviton, A. Hegedus and A. Kubrin, eds. *Evaluating AIDS Prevention: Contributions of Multiple Disciplines.* San Francisco, CA: Jossey-Bass.

Schiller, N., S. Crystal, and D. Karus. 1990. The role of kin in care giving for persons with AIDS in New Jersey. Paper presented: VIth International Conference on AIDS. San Francisco. Abstract Th.D. 822.

Schilling, R., N. El-Bassel, and L. Gilbert. 1993. Predictors of changes in sexual behavior among women on methadone. *American Journal of Drug and Alcohol Abuse* 19:409-422.

Schilling, R., N. El-Bassel, L. Gilbert, et al. 1991. Correlates of drug use, sexual behavior, and attitudes toward safer sex among African-American and Hispanic women in methadone maintenance. *Journal of Drug Issues* 21:685-698.

Schilling, R., N. El-Bassel, M. Leeper, et al. 1991. Acceptance of the female condom by Latin- and African-American women. *American Journal of Public Health* 81:1345-1346.

Schilling, R., N. El-Bassel, S. Schinke, et al. 1991. Building skills of recovering women drug users to reduce heterosexual AIDS transmission. *Public Health Reports* 106:297-304.

Schinke, S., G. Botvin, M. Orlandi, et al. 1990. African-American and Hispanic-American adolescents, HIV infection, and preventive intervention. *AIDS Education and Prevention* 2:305-312.

Schneider, B. 1991. Women, Children, and AIDS: Research Suggestions. Pp. 134-148 in R. Ulack, and W. Skinner, eds. *AIDS and the Social Sciences: Common Threads.* Lexington, KY: The University Press of Kentucky.

Schneider, B. 1992. AIDS and class, gender, and race relations. Pp. 19-43 in J. Huber and B. Schneider, eds. *The Social Context of AIDS.* Newbury Park, CA: Sage Publications.

Schoenbaum, E., D. Hartel, P. Selwyn, et al. 1989. Risk factors for human immunodeficiency virus infection in intravenous drug users. *New England Journal of Medicine* 321:874-879.

Schreeder, M., S. Thompson, S. Hadler, et al. 1980. Epidemiology of hepatitis b infection in gay men. *Journal of Homosexuality* 5:307-310.

Schuster, C., W. Dockens, and J. Woods. 1966. Behavioral variables affecting the development of amphetamine tolerance. *Psychopharmacologia* 9:170-182.

Schwartz, E., A. Brechbuhl, P. Kahl, et al. 1992. Pharmocokinetics interactions of zidovudine and methadone in intravenous drug-using patient with HIV infection. *AIDS* 5:619-626.

Sechrest, L., H. Freeman, and A. Mulley, eds. 1989. *Health Services Research Methodology: A Focus on AIDS.* Washington, DC: NCHSR.

Seidman, S., W. Mosher, and S. Aral. 1992. Women with multiple sexual partners: United States, 1988. *American Journal of Public Health* 82:1388.

Seligman, J. 1986. Crack: The road back; rehabilitation centers are straining under the load of the new drug epidemic. *Newsweek* (June 30):52(2).

Selik, R., K. Castro, and M. Pappaioanou. 1988. Distribution of AIDS cases, by racial/ethnic group and exposure category, United States, June 1, 1981-July 4, 1988. *Morbidity and Mortality Weekly Report* 37:1-10.

Selwyn, P., P. Alcabes, D. Hartel, et al. 1992. Clinical manifestations and predictors of disease progression in drug users with human immunodeficiency virus infection. *New England Journal of Medicine* 327:1697-1703.

Selwyn, P., N. Budner, W. Wasserman, et al. 1993. Utilization of on-site primary care services by HIV-seropositive and seronegative drug users in a methadone maintenance program. *Public Health Reports* 108:492-500.

Selwyn, P., C. Feiner, C. Cox, et al. 1988. Knowledge About AIDS and High-Risk Behavior Among Intravenous Drug Users in New York City. Pp. 215-227 in R. Galea, B. Lewis, and L. Baker, eds. *AIDS and IV Drug Abusers: Current Perspectives*. Owings Mills, MD: National Health Publishing.

Selwyn, P., A. Feingold, A. Iezza, et al. 1989. Primary care for patients with human immunodeficiency virus (HIV) infection in a methadone maintenance treatment program. *Annals of Internal Medicine* 111:761-763.

Selwyn, P., D. Hartel, V. Lewis, et al. 1989. A prospective study on the risk of tuberculosis among intravenous drug users with HIV infection. *New England Journal of Medicine* 320:545-550.

Selwyn, P., B. Sckell, P. Alcabes, et al. 1992. High risk of active tuberculosis in HIV-infected drug users with cutaneous anergy. *Journal of the American Medical Association* 268:504-509.

Seymour, R. and D. Smith. 1987. *Guide to Psychoactive Drugs*. New York: Harrington Park Press.

Shannon, G., G. Pyle, and R. Bashshur. 1991. *The Geography of AIDS: Origins and Course of the Epidemic*. New York: Guilford Press.

Shaw, G., M. Harper, B. Hahn, et al. 1985. HTLV-III infection in brains of children and adults with AIDS encephalopathy. *Science* 227:177-182.

Shedlin, M. 1990. An Ethnographic Approach to Understanding HIV High-Risk Behaviors: Prostitution and Drug Abuse. Pp. 134-149 in C. Leukefeld, R. Battjes, and Z. Amsel, eds. *AIDS and Intravenous Drug Use, Community Intervention and Prevention*. New York: Hemisphere Publishing.

Shulman, L. and J. Mantell. 1988. The AIDS crisis: A United States health care perspective. *Social Science and Medicine* 26:979-988.

Sidtis, J. 1994. Evaluation of the AIDS dementia complex in adults. Pp. 273-287 in R. Price and S. Perry, eds. *HIV, AIDS and the Brain*. New York: Raven Press.

Sidtis, J., C. Gatsonis, and R. Price. 1992. Zidovudine treatment of the AIDS dementia complex: Results of a placebo controlled trial. *Annals of Neurology* 33:349.

Siegel, J., M. Weinstein, and H. Fineberg. 1991. Bleach programs for preventing AIDS among IV drug users: Modeling the impact of HIV prevalence. *American Journal of Public Health* 81:1273-1279.

Siegel, K., M. Levine, C. Brooks, et al. 1989. The motives of gay men for taking or not taking the HIV antibody test. *Social Problems* 36:368-383.

Siegel, S. 1976. Morphine analgesic tolerance: Its situation specificity supports a Pavlovian conditioning model. *Science* 193:323-325.

Siegel, S. 1978. Morphine tolerance—Is there evidence for a conditioning model? *Science* 200:344-345.

Siegel, S. and K. Sdao-Jarvie. 1986. Attentuation of ethanol tolerance by a novel stimulus. *Psychopharmacology (Berlin)* 88:258-261.

Silverman, D. 1993. Psychosocial impact of HIV-related caregiving on health providers: A review and recommendation for the role of psychiatry. *American Journal of Psychiatry* 150:705-712.

Singer, M. 1991. Confronting the AIDS epidemic among IV drug users: Does ethnic culture matter? *AIDS Education and Prevention* 3:258-283.

Snider, W., D. Simpson, S. Neilsen, et al. 1983. Neurological complications of acquired immune deficiency syndrome: Analysis of 50 patients. *Annals of Neurology* 14:403-418.

Solomon, L., J. Astemborski, D. Warren, et al. 1993. Differences in risk factors for human immunodeficiency virus type 1 seroconversion among male and female intravenous drug users. *American Journal of Epidemiology* 137:892-898.

Solomon, M. and W. DeJong. 1989. Preventing AIDS and other STDs through condom promotion: A patient education intervention. *American Journal of Public Health* 79:453-458.

Solomon, R. 1977. An Opponent Process Theory of Motivation. The Affective Dynamics of Drug Addiction. Pp. 66-103 in J. Maser and M. Seligman, eds. *Psychopathology: Experimental Models*. San Francisco, CA: Freeman.

Sorensen, J., J. London, C. Heitzmann, et al. In press. Psychoeducational group approach: HIV risk reduction in drug users. *AIDS Education and Prevention*.

Sorensen, J., L. Wermuth, R. Gibson, et al. 1991. *Preventing AIDS in Drug Users and Their Sexual Partners*. New York: Guilford Press.

Soskolne, V., S. Aral., L. Magder, et al. 1991. Condom use with regular and casual partners among women attending family planning clinics. *Family Planning Perspectives* 23:223.

Sosnowitz, B. and D. Kovacs. 1992. From Burying to Caring: Family AIDS Support Groups. Pp. 131-144 in J. Huber and B. Schneider, eds. *The Social Context of AIDS*. Newbury Park, CA: Sage Publications.

Spencer, D. and R. Price. 1993. Human immunodeficiency virus and the central nervous system. *Annual Review of Microbiology* 46:655-693.

Stall, R. 1991. An Anthropological Research Agenda for an AIDS Epicenter within the United States. Pp. 100-123 in R. Ulack and W. Skinner, eds. *AIDS and the Social Sciences: Common Threads*. Lexington, KY: The University Press of Kentucky.

Stall, R. and J. Catania. 1994. AIDS risk behaviors among late middle-aged and elderly Americans: The National AIDS Behavioral Surveys. *Archives of Internal Medicine* 154:57-63.

Stall, R., T. Coates, and C. Hoff. 1988. Behavioral risk reduction for HIV infection among gay and bisexual men: A review of results from the United States. *American Psychologist* 43:878-885.

Stall, R., M. Cohen, G. Dowsett, et al. 1992. Pp. 653-667 in J. Mann, D. Tarantola and T. Netter, eds. *AIDS in the World*. Cambridge, MA: Harvard University Press.

Stall, R., M. Ekstrand, L. Pollack, et al. 1990. Relapse from safer sex: The next challenge for AIDS prevention efforts. *Journal of Acquired Immune Deficiency Syndromes* 3:1181-1187.

Stall, R. and B. Leigh. 1994. Understanding the relationship between drug or alcohol use and high risk sexual activity for HIV transmission: Where do we go from here? *Addiction* 89:149-152.

Stein, M., J. Piette, V. Mor, et al. 1991. Differences in access to zidovudine (AZT) among symptomatic HIV-infected persons. *Journal of General Internal Medicine* 6:35-40.

Stein, Z. 1992. Editorial: The double bind in science policy and the protection of women from HIV infection. *American Journal of Public Health* 82:1471-1472.

Stephens, R., T. Feucht, and S. Roman. 1991. Effects of an intervention program on AIDS-related drug and needle behavior among intravenous drug users. *American Journal of Public Health* 81:568-571.

Stephens, R., D. Simpson, S. Coyle, et al. 1993. Comparative Effectiveness of

NADR Interventions. In B. Brown and G. Beschner, eds. *Handbook on Risk of AIDS*. Westport, CT: Greenwood Press.

Stimmel, B., S. Vernace, and F. Schaffner. 1975. Hepatitis b surface antigen and antibody in asymptomatic drug users. *Journal of the American Medical Association* 243:1135-1138.

Stoneburner, R., D. Des Jarlais, D. Benezra, et al. 1988. A larger spectrum of severe HIV-1 related disease in intravenous drug users in New York City. *Science* 242:916-919.

Storosum, J., F. Van Den Boom, and M. Beauzekom. 1990. Stress and coping in people with HIV infection. Paper presented: VIth International Conference on AIDS. San Francisco. Abstract S.B.365.

Stoto, M., D. Blumenthal, J. Durch, et al. 1988. Federal funding for AIDS research: Decision process and results in fiscal year 1986. *Review of Infections Diseases* 10:406-419.

Substance Abuse and Mental Health Services Administrations (SAMHSA). 1993. *Strategic Plan for HIV/AIDS*. Rockville, MD: SAMHSA.

Surrey, J. 1991. The "self-in-relation": A theory of women's development. Pp. 162-180 in J. Gordon, A. Kaplan, J. Miller, et al., eds. *Women's Growth in Connection*. New York, NY: Guilford Press.

San Francisco Department of Public Health. 1992. HIV Incidence and Prevalence in San Francisco in 1992. Summary report: HIV Consensus Meeting. February, 1992. San Francisco, CA.

Susser, E., E. Valencia, and S. Conover. 1993. Prevalence of HIV infection among psychiatric patients in a New York City men's shelter. *American Journal of Public Health* 83:568-570.

Susser, P., S. Miller, M. Bortner, et al. 1992. Affective States and Caregivers of HIV Infected Children. Paper presented: VIIIth International Conference on AIDS. Amsterdam. Abstract POB3852.

Tabakoff, B. and P. Hoffman. 1988. Tolerance and the etiology of alcoholism: Hypothesis and mechanism. *Alcoholism, Clinical and Experimental Research* 12:184-186.

Takigiku, S., T. Brubaker, and C. Hennon. Spring 1993. *AIDS: Education and Prevention* 5:25-42.

Tanfer, K., W. Grady, D. Klepinger, et al. 1993. Condom use among U.S. men. *Family Planning Perspectives* 25:61-66.

Tanner, W. and R. Pollack. 1988. The effect of condom use and erotic instructions on attitudes towards condoms. *The Journal of Sex Research* 25:537-541.

Test, M. and S. Berlin. 1981. Issues of special concern to chronically mentally ill women. *Professional Psychology* 12:136-145.

Thomas, S. and S. Quinn. 1991. The Tuskegee syphilis study, 1932 to 1972: Implications for HIV education and AIDS risk education programs in the black community. *American Journal of Public Health* 81:1498-1505.

Thomas, S. and S. Quinn. 1992. The Attitudes of Black Americans Toward Prevention of HIV Disease through Needle and Syringe Exchange Programs. The Needle Exchange and HIV Prevention Forum. December 10-11, 1992. The Henry J. Kaiser Family Foundation, Menlo Park, CA.

Time. 1988. Slaughter in the streets; crack touches off a homicide epidemic. (December 5):12(3).

Toggas, S., E. Masliah, E. Rockenstein, et al. 1994. Central nervous system damage produced by expression of the HIV-1 coat protein gp120 in transgenic mice. *Nature* 367:188-193.

Tong, T., S. Pond, M. Kreek, et al. 1981. Phenytoin induced methadone withdrawal. *Annals of Internal Medicine* 94:349-351.

Trapido, E., N. Lewis, and M. Comerford. 1990. HIV-1 and AIDS in Belle Glade, Florida: A reexamination of the issues. *American Behavioral Scientist* 33:451-464.

Treaster, J. 1991. New York Times. Inside a crack house: How drug use is changing. *New York Times* (April 6):1,10.

Treisman, G., M. Fishman, C. Lyketsos, et al. 1994. Evaluation and treatment of psychiatric disorders associated with HIV infection. Pp. 239-250 in R. Price and S. Perry, eds. *HIV, AIDS and the Brain*. New York: Raven Press.

Tross, S., D. Hirsch, J. Rabkin, et al. 1987. Determinants of current psychiatric disorder in AIDS spectrum patients. Paper presented: IIIrd International Conference on AIDS. Washington, DC. Abstract T.10.5.

Turner, H. 1988. Stress and coping among AIDS care-givers. Paper presented: The Annual Meeting of the Society for the Study of Social Problems. Atlanta, GA.

Turner, H., J. Catania, and J. Gagnon. 1994. The prevalence of informal caregiving to persons with AIDS in the United States: Caregiver characteristics and their implications. *Social Science and Medicine* 38:1543-1552.

Turner, H. and L. Pearlin. 1989. Informal support of people with AIDS: Issues of age, stress and caregiving. *Generations* 13:56-59.

Tyor, W., J. Glass, J. Griffin, et al. 1991. Cytokine expression the brain during the acquired immunodefiency syndrome. *Annals of Neurology* 31:349-360.

U.S. Congress, Committee on Government Operations. 1992. The Politics of AIDS Prevention: Science Takes A Time Out. House Report 102-1047. Washington, DC: U.S. Government Printing Office.

U.S. Department of Health and Human Services (DHHS). 1992. *The Public Health Service Strategic Plan to Combat HIV and AIDS in the United States*. Washington, DC: U.S. Government Printing Office.

Valdiserri, R., V. Arena, D. Proctor, et al. 1989. The relationship between women's attitudes about condoms and their use: Implications for condom promotion programs. *American Journal of Public Health* 79:499-501.

Valdiserri, R., D. Lyter, L. Leviton, et al. 1989. AIDS prevention in homosexual and bisexual men: results of a randomized trial evaluating two risk reduction interventions. *AIDS* 3:21-26.

van Ameijden, E., A. van den Hoek, H. van Haastrecht, et al. 1994. Trends in sexual behavior and the incidence of sexually transmitted diseases and HIV among drug-using prostitutes, Amsterdam 1986-1992. *AIDS* 8:213-221.

van Ameijden, E., J. van den Hoek, H. van Haastrecht, et al. 1992. The harm reduction approach and risk factors for Human Immunodeficiency Virus (HIV) seroconversion in injecting drug users, Amsterdam. *American Journal of Epidemiology* 1:111-125.

van den Hoek, J., J. van Haastrecht, J. Goudsmit, et al. 1990. Prevalence, incidence, and risk factors of hepatitis C virus infection among drug users in Amsterdam. *Journal of Infectious Diseases* 162:823-826.

van Griensven, G., E. De Vroome, F. De Wolf, et al. 1990. Risk factors for progression of human immunodeficiency virus infection among seroconverted and seropositive homosexual men. *American Journal of Epidemiology* 132:203-210.

Vlahov, D. 1994. HIV seroconversion studies among intravenous drug users. *AIDS* 8:263-265.

Vlahov, D., A. Munoz, S. Cohn, et al. 1990. Seroconversion for HIV-1 in Intravenous Drug Users in Baltimore. Paper presented: VIth International Conference on AIDS. San Francisco. Abstract F.C.557.

Voeller, B. 1991. Gas, dye, and viral transport through polyurethane condoms. *Journal of the American Medical Association* 266:2986-2987.

Vogt, M., D. Craven, D. Crawford, et al. 1986. Isolation of HTLV-III/LAV from cervical secretions of women at risk for AIDS. *Lancet* 1:525-527.

Vogt, M., D. Witt, D. Craven, et al. 1987. Isolation patterns of the human immunodeficiency virus from cervical secretions during the menstrual cycle of women at risk for the acquired immunodeficiency syndrome. *Annals of Internal Medicine* 106:380-383.

Volavka, J., A. Convit, P. Czober, et al. 1991. HIV seroprevalence and risk behaviors in psychiatric inpatients. *Psychiatry Research* 39:109-114.

Wahl, L., M. Corcoran, S. Pyle, et al. 1989. Human immunodeficiency virus glycoprotein (gp 120) induction of monocyte arachidonic acid metabolites and interleukin. *Proceedings of the National Academy of Sciences* 86:621-625.

Waight, P. and E. Miller. 1991. Incidence of HIV infection among homosexual men. *British Medical Journal* 303:311.

Wallace, B. 1991. *Crack Cocaine: A Practical Treatment Approach for the Chemically Dependent*. New York: Brunner/Mazel.

Wallace, R. 1988. A synergism of plagues, planned shrinkage, contagious housing destruction, and AIDS in the Bronx. *Environmental Research* 47:1-33.

Walter, H. and R. Vaughan. 1993. AIDS risk reduction among a multiethnic sample of urban high school students. *Journal of the American Medical Association* 270:725-730.

Walter, H., R. Vaughan, M. Gladis, et al. 1992. Factors associated with AIDS risk behaviors among high school students in an AIDS epicenter. *American Journal of Public Health* 82:528-532.

Wartenberg, A. 1994. "Into whatever houses I enter": HIV and injecting drug use. *Journal of the American Medical Association* 271:151-152.

Washton, A. and M. Gold. 1987. *Cocaine: A Clinician's Handbook*. New York: Guilford Press.

Watters, J., M. Estilo, G. Clark, et al. 1994. Syringe and needle exchange as HIV/AIDS prevention for injection drug users. *Journal of the American Medical Association* 271:115-120.

Weatherburn, P., P. Davies, F. Hickson, et al. 1993. No connection between alcohol use and unsafe sex among gay and bisexual men. *AIDS* 7:115-119.

Weber, R., B. Ledergerber, M. Opravil, et al. 1990. HIV infection in misusers of injected drugs who stop injecting or follow a programme of maintenance treatment with methadone. *British Medical Journal* 301:1362-1365.

Weinstock, H., C. Lindan, G. Bolan, et al. 1993. Factors associated with condom use in a high-risk heterosexual population. *Sexually Transmitted Diseases* 20:14-20.

Weiss, R. and S. Mirin. 1987. *Cocaine*. Washington, DC: American Psychiatric Press.

Weissman, G. and National AIDS Research Consortium. 1991. AIDS prevention for women at risk: Experience from a national demonstration research program. *Journal of Primary Prevention* 12:49-63.

Weitz, R. 1989. Uncertainty and the lives of persons with AIDS. *Journal of Health and Social Behavior* 30:270-281.

Weitz, R. 1993. Powerlessness, Invisibility, and the Lives of Women with HIV Disease. Pp. 101-121 in G. Albrecht and R. Zimmerman, eds. *The Social and Behavioral Aspects of AIDS. Advances in Medical Sociology*, Vol. III. Greenwich, CT: JAI Press.

Welsh, M., S. Boring, R. Oliver, et al. 1992. Peer Education. Paper presented: VIIIth International Conference on AIDS. Amsterdam. Abstract PoD5347.

Wenger, J., T. Tiffany, C. Bombaidier, et al. 1981. Ethanol tolerance in the rat is learned. *Science* 213:575-577.

Wenger, N., L. Linn, M. Epstein, et al. 1991. Reduction of high-risk sexual behavior among heterosexuals undergoing HIV antibody testing: A randomized clinical trial. *American Journal of Public Health* 81:1580-1585.

Wermuth, L., J. Ham, and R. Robbins. 1992. Women Don't Wear Condoms: AIDS Risk Among Sexual Partners of IV Drug Users. Pp. 72-94 in J. Huber and B. Schneider, eds. *The Social Context of AIDS*. Newbury Park, CA: Sage.

Werner, T., S. Ferroni, T. Saermark, et al. 1991. HIV-1 Nef protein exhibits structural and functional similarity to scorpion peptides interacting with K+ channels. *AIDS* 5:1301-1308.

Wesselingh, S., C. Power, J. Glass, et al. 1993. Intracerebral cytokine mRNA expression in AIDS. *Annals of Neurology* 33:576-582.

Westerberg, V. 1992. Alcohol measuring scales may influence conclusions about the role of alcohol in human immunodeficiency virus (HIV) risk and progression to acquired immunodeficiency syndrome (AIDS). *American Journal of Epidemiology* 135:719-725.

Wiebel, W., A. Jimenez, W. Johnson, et al. 1993. Positive Effect on HIV Seroconversion of Street Outreach Intervention with IDUs in Chicago: 1988-1992. Paper presented: IXth International Conference on AIDS. Berlin.

Wiebel, W. and M. O'Brien. 1993. The Indigenous Leader AIDS Outreach Model: Intervention Manual. NIH Pub. 93-3581. Rockville, MD: National Institutes of Health.

Wiley, C., E. Masliah, M. Morey, et al. 1991. Neocortical damage during HIV infection. *Annals of Neurology* 29:651-657.

Wiley, C., R. Schrier, J. Nelson, et al. 1986. Cellular localization of human immunodeficiency virus infection within the brains of acquired immunodeficiency syndrome patients. *Proceedings of the National Academy of Sciences* 83:7089-7093.

Williams, E., N. Lamson, S. Efem, et al. 1992. Implementation of an AIDS prevention program among prostitutes in the Cross River State of Nigeria. *AIDS* 6:229-230.

Williams, J., J. Rabkin, R. Remein, et al. 1991. Multidisciplinary baseline assessment of homosexual men with and without human immunodeficiency virus infection. *Archives of General Psychiatry* 48:124-130.

Williams, T. 1992. *Crackhouse: Notes from the End of the Line*. Reading, MA: Addison-Wesley.

Willocks, L., F. Cowan, P. Glegg, et al. 1990. Natural History of Early HIV Infection. Paper presented: VIth International Conference on AIDS. San Francisco. Abstract S.D.806.

Willocks, L., F. Cowan, R. Brettle, et al. 1992. The spectrum of chest infections in HIV positive patients in Edinburgh. *Journal of Infection* 24:37-42.

Willoughby, B., M. Schecter, K. Craib, et al. 1990. Characteristics of Recent Seroconverters in a Cohort of Homosexual Men: Who are the Prevention Failures? Paper presented: VIth International Conference on AIDS. San Francisco. Abstract FC45.

Wilson, D., B. Nyathi, M. Nhariwa, et al. 1993. A community-level AIDS prevention programme among sexually vulnerable groups and the general population in Bulawayo and Zimbabwe. Unpublished manuscript.

Windle, M. 1993. Some Conceptual and Methodological Considerations for Research on AIDS and Alcohol. Paper presented: NIAAA Workshop on AIDS and Alcohol. May 20-21, 1993. Bethesda, MD.

Windle, M., P. Carlisle-Frank, L. Azizy, et al. 1992. Women and Health-Related Behaviors: Interrelations Among Substance Use, Sexual Behaviors, and Acquired Immunodeficiency Syndrome (AIDS). In R. Watson. ed. *Addictive Behaviors in Women.* Clifton, NJ: Humana Press.

Winkelstein, W., D. Lyman, N. Padian, et al. 1987. Sexual practices and risk of infection by human immunodeficiency virus: The San Francisco men's health study. *Journal of the American Medical Association* 257:321-325.

Winkelstein, W., N. Padian, G. Rutherford, et al. 1989. Homosexual Men. Pp. 117-135 in R. Kaslow and D. Francis, eds. *The Epidemiology of AIDS: Expression, Occurrence, and Control of Human Immunodeficiency Virus Type 1 Infection.* New York: Oxford University Press.

Wober, J. 1988. Informing the British public about AIDS. *Health Education Research* 3:19-24.

Wofsy, C., J. Cohen, L. Hauer, et al. 1986. Isolation of AIDS-associated retrovirus from genital secretions of women with antibodies to the virus. *Lancet* 1:527-529.

Woodman, N. 1985. Parents of Lesbians and Gays: Concerns and Intervention. Pp. 21-26 in N. Hidalgo, T. Peterson, and N. Woodman, eds. *Lesbian and Gay Issues: A Resource Manual for Social Workers.* Silver Spring, MD: National Association of Social Workers.

Woolverton, W. 1986. Effect of D1 and a D2 dopamine antagonist on the self-administration of cocaine and piribedil by rhesus monkeys. *Pharmacology, Biochemistry and Behavior* 24:531-535.

Worth, D. and R. Rodriguez. 1987. Latina women and AIDS. *Radical America* 20:63-67.

Wortman, C., R. Silver, and R. Kessler. In press. The Meaning of Loss and Adjustment to Bereavement. In M. Stroebe, W. Stoebe, and R. Hansson, eds. *Handbook of Bereavement.* New York: Cambridge University Press.

Yancovitz, S., J. Des, N. Peyser, et al. 1991. A randomized trial of an interim methadone maintenance clinic. *American Journal of Public Health* 81:1185-1191.

Yokel, R. and Wise, R. 1975. Increased lever pressing for amphetamine after pimozide in rats: Implications for a dopamine theory of reward. *Science* 187:547-549.

Yokel, R. and Wise, R. 1976. Attenuation of intravenous amphetamine reinforcement by central dopamine blockade in rats. *Psychopharmacology (Berlin)* 48:311-318.

Zamperetti, M., G. Goldurm, E. Abbate, et al. 1990. Attempted suicide and HIV infection: Epidemiological aspects in a psychiatric ward. Paper presented: VIth International Conference on AIDS. San Francisco.

Zenilman, J., B. Erickson, R. Fox, et al. 1992. Effect of HIV post-test counseling on STD incidence. *Journal of the American Medical Association* 267:843-845.

Zwi, A. and A. Cabral. 1991. Identifying "high risk situations" for preventing AIDS. *British Journal of Medicine* 303:1527-1529.

APPENDIXES

A
Grants Analysis Methodology

Τhis appendix provides more detail about the methodology employed by the committee in conducting the analysis of the AIDS grants presented in Chapter 6. Specifically, it reviews sources of information, development of the database, and general limitations of the data.

SOURCES OF INFORMATION

The primary source of grant information for the three institutes came from the CRISP (Computer Retrieval of Information on Scientific Projects) system. CRISP is an on-line computer-based system that contains information on funded extramural and intramural research in the Public Health Service.

Initial requests for grant information were made to the AIDS coordinators at NIAAA, NIDA, and NIMH. Specifically, IOM staff requested information for all extramural AIDS research grants (all mechanisms), cooperative agreements, contracts, and intramural research projects since the institutes' first funded AIDS research (FY 1983). The institutes responded by compiling and submitting CRISP files for all extramural AIDS-related research grants (including cooperative agreements) and contracts. NIMH was the only institute to submit CRISP files for all intramural AIDS-related research projects.

NIDA and NIMH also submitted comprehensive lists of AIDS grants (titles, investigators, ID numbers, and total funding) for FY

1989 through FY 1992. IOM staff cross-checked these lists against all CRISP abstracts received and both of these sets of information against the institutes' historical budget tables for each fiscal year. Although minor discrepancies were found, IOM staff worked with the AIDS offices and the budget offices of each institute to address them and to ensure that the committee ultimately had access to a complete set of AIDS-related grant abstracts with accurate information. Remaining discrepancies are described in the database section, below.

The CRISP files for each AIDS research grant funded by NIAAA, NIDA, and NIMH contained detailed information identifying the principal investigator, institution, project title, project summary abstract, IRG code, program class code, years of funding, and amounts paid in each year. The identification number for each grant (which also appears on the CRISP file) includes: an activity type code to identify the type of application received and processed (e.g., new and competing); an activity code (e.g., funding mechanism) to identify the category of research (e.g., R01); the institute, center, or division (ICD) code to identify the institute (AA = NIAAA; DA = NIDA; MH = NIMH); a five-digit serial number; and suffixes to identify other relevant information such as the grant year. CRISP files for contracts provide the total funding commitment without a breakdown of spending for each fiscal year, whereas CRISP files for intramural research do not provide funding information.

To guide the analysis of the grants data, the IOM staff and committee also reviewed and referred to a number of documents, including formal and informal budget documents, "Moyer Reports" (FY 1989 through FY 1993), AIDS Expenditure Reports from HHS, the NIMH Strategic Plan for AIDS Research (1993-1998), the NIMH AIDS Research Blueprint for the Second Decade, the NIMH HIV Prevention Highlights, the NIMH Handbook on Developing a Successful Research Application, the NIDA Five-Year Strategic Plan, a variety of documents describing program initiatives at all three institutes, and all program announcements (PAs), requests for applications (RFAs), and requests for proposals (RFPs) issued by NIAAA, NIDA, and NIMH since FY 1983.

DATABASE

To facilitate the grants analysis, IOM staff created a database using the Paradox database management system. A form was developed to record pertinent information for each AIDS grant and contract (Box A.1). In addition to information tracked by the

CRISP system (investigator, title, summary abstract, identification number, etc.), the IOM database includes fields to identify domains of science using the committee's matrix codes. Other fields identify whether a project included or targeted homosexuals, women, racial/ethnic minorities, and people of different economic classes in the study sample, whether it included an analysis of gender, race/ethnicity, and class factors, and whether it included qualitative, evaluation, and health services research. Although the committee intended to analyze the grants on these characteristics, the information available from the CRISP abstracts and other data sources was insufficient for this task. Many abstracts did not specify the composition of the study sample, and, even if they did, most did not mention whether an analysis of gender, race/ethnicity, or class factors was part of the project design. Similarly, many did not make clear if an evaluation component was included.

Three IOM staff members were involved in reading the CRISP abstracts and entering key information into the IOM database. Two staff members coded each grant for all new variables—including science categories. One of these staff members checked each entry to ensure consistency.

Efforts were made to ensure a high level of coding reliability. Two IOM staff members reviewed the science categories for each record in the database. In addition, several committee members and additional IOM staff with relevant science expertise reviewed samples of grants from the database to verify appropriate coding.

LIMITATIONS

As mentioned above, the basic grant information that was entered into the IOM database was originally compiled by the AIDS coordinators at each institute. Every effort was made to ensure consistency and comparability between the grant information in the IOM database and institute budget information. Although institute staff from the AIDS offices and budget offices were extremely helpful in providing information when requested, IOM staff could not obtain explanations for all discrepancies that were found.

Specifically, IOM staff was informed that complete and/or accurate information about grants and grant funding was unavailable for the first several years of AIDS funding at the institutes. For example, summary abstracts were not available for grants funded in FY 1983 and FY 1984. Likewise, the institutes could not ex-

Box A.1
Sample Form

Principal Investigator:	J. P.
Institution:	Falling Rock University
Agency Code:	DA
Serial #:	01234
Title:	Reducing high-risk sexual behaviors among injection drug users (IDUs)
Research Subject(s):	Human

Summary: To compare differential effects of two interventions for reducing high-risk sexual behaviors among IDUs in treatment programs. Participants will be randomly assigned to either a standard AIDS education treatment (two informational sessions) or to an enhanced AIDS education treatment (two informational sessions, plus training in negotiation skills and individual counseling). A follow-up survey and interviews will be conducted six months after the interventions.

Race:	N	Biomedical:	N
Gender:	N	Epidemiology:	N
SES:	N	Psychosocial:	Y
Health Services Research:	N	Social:	N
Qualitative:	Y	Code:	Applied

FY	TYPE	Mechanism	Suffix	Award Amount
87	1	R01	01	$256,789
88	5	R01	02	$245,678
89	5	R01	03	$234,567
			Total:	**$737,034**

plicitly state which grants were categorized as AIDS research during the first several years of AIDS funding before systematic record-keeping for AIDS research began. Despite these limitations, the database total dollar amounts were comparable to the amounts reported in the institutes' historical budget tables for FY 1987 through FY 1992. Therefore, the committee's analysis primarily focuses on these years.

Another major limitation of the data was the absence of detailed information on study procedures or outcomes. Although this information was not critical to the basic analysis of balance within the institutes' AIDS programs, it is critical to other aspects of the report, in particular the committee's discussions of research findings from institute-supported AIDS intervention projects. Where possible, the committee turned to the published literature for information.

B

Abbreviations and Acronyms

ACTU	AIDS Clinical Trials Unit
ADAMHA	Alcohol, Drug Abuse, and Mental Health Administration
ADC	AIDS dementia complex
AHCPR	Agency for Health Care Policy and Research
AIDS	acquired immune deficiency syndrome
AMEN	AIDS in Multiethnic Neighborhoods
ARRM	AIDS Risk Reduction Model
AZT	zidovudine
B&F	buildings and facilities
CAIR	Center for AIDS Intervention Research
CAPS	Center for AIDS Prevention Studies
CARE	Community-Based Outreach/Intervention Research
CCTP	Comprehensive Community Treatment Program
CDC	Centers for Disease Control and Prevention
CMHS	Center for Mental Health Services
CMV	cytomegalovirus
CNS	central nervous system
CRISP	Computer Retrieval of Information on Scientific Projects
CSAP	Center for Substance Abuse Prevention
CSAT	Center for Substance Abuse Treatment
CSF	cerebrospinal fluid
DNA	deoxyribonucleic acid
DRG	Division of Research Grants
FDA	Food and Drug Administration

FTE	full-time equivalent
gpl20	HIV-1 envelope glycoprotein
HBV	Hepatitis B virus
HHS	Department of Health and Human Services
HIV	human immunodeficiency virus
HRSA	Health Resources and Services Administration
HTLV-1	human T-cell leukemia/lymphoma/lymphotropic virus
ICD	institutes, centers, and divisions
IDU	injection drug user
IMPAC	Information for Management, Planning, Analysis, and Coordination
IOM	Institute of Medicine
IR	intramural research
IRG	initial review group
IV	intravenous
IVDU	intravenous drug user
JAMA	Journal of the American Medical Association
LAAM	levo-alpha-acetyl methadol
LAV	lymphadenopathy-associated virus
MACS	Multicenter AIDS Cohort Study
MMWR	Morbidity and Mortality Weekly Report
MRI	magnetic resonance imaging
NABS	National AIDS Behavioral Surveys
NADR	National AIDS Demonstration Research Program
NAPO	National AIDS Program Office
NAPPASA	Native American Prevention Project on AIDS and Substance Abuse
NAS	National Academy of Sciences
NASADAD	National Association of State Alcohol and Drug Abuse Directors
NCI	National Cancer Institute
NCRR	National Center for Research Resources
NHLBI	National Heart, Lung, and Blood Institute
NIAAA	National Institute on Alcohol Abuse and Alcoholism
NIAID	National Institute of Allergy and Infectious Diseases
NIDA	National Institute on Drug Abuse
NICHD	National Institute of Child Health and Human Development
NIH	National Institutes of Health
NIMH	National Institute of Mental Health
NINDS	National Institute of Neurological Disorders and Stroke

NMDA	N-methyl-D-aspartate
NRFC	not recommended for further consideration
OA	Office of the Administrator
OAR	Office of AIDS Research
OASH	Office of the Assistant Secretary for Health
OD	Office of the Director
OMB	Office of Management and Budget
ONAP	Office of National AIDS Policy
ONDCP	Office on National Drug Control Policy
OSAP	Office of Substance Abuse Prevention
OTI	Office of Treatment Improvement
P01	research program project
P50	specialized research center
PA	program announcement
PCP	*Pneumocystis carinii* pneumonia
PCR	polymerase chain reaction
PET	positron emission tomography
PHS	Public Health Service
PML	progressive multifocal leukoencephalopathy
PNS	peripheral nervous system
QUIN	quinolinic acid
R01	investigator-initiated grant
R10	cooperative clinical research
R18	research demonstration project
R&D	research and development
RFA	request for application
RFP	request for proposal
RMS	research management and support
RPG	research project grant
SAMHSA	Substance Abuse and Mental Health Services Administration
SBIR	small business innovative research grant
SIV	simian immunodeficiency virus
SRG	special review group
STD	sexually transmitted disease
STT	syringe tracking and testing
tat	*trans*-activator of transcription
TB	tuberculosis
TNF-α	tumor necrosis factor
TRU	treatment research unit
U10	cooperative clinical research
VIP	vasoactive intestinal peptide
WITS	Women and Infants Transmission Study

C

Acknowledgments

The committee would like to thank the people listed below who, through interviews, presentations, conversations, and the submission of written materials, provided information important for our work. Affiliations are those at the time of contact.

John Abbott, National Institute on Drug Abuse

Moises Agosto, National Minority AIDS Council

Zili Amsel, National Institute on Drug Abuse

Bernard Arons, Center for Mental Health Services

J. Hampton Atkinson, HIV Neurobehavioral Research Center, University of California, San Diego

Andy Avins, Center for AIDS Prevention Studies, University of California, San Francisco

William Bailey, American Psychological Association

Robert Battjes, National Institute on Drug Abuse

Ronald Bayer, HIV Center for Clinical and Behavioral Studies, Columbia University

Myron Belfer, Substance Abuse and Mental Health Services Administration

Alison Bennett, National Institute of Mental Health

Diane Binson, Center for AIDS Prevention Studies, University of California, San Francisco

Jack Blaine, National Institute on Drug Abuse

Floyd Bloom, The Scripps Research Institute

Steven Bowen, Health Resources and Services Administration

Kendall Bryant, National Institute on Alcohol Abuse and Alcoholism

Michael Buchmeier, The Scripps Research Institute

William Bukoski, National Institute on Drug Abuse

Iain Campbell, The Scripps Research Institute

Alex Carballo-Dieguez, HIV Center for Clinical and Behavioral Studies, Columbia University

Joseph Catania, Center for AIDS Prevention Studies, University of California, San Francisco

Margaret Chesney, Center for AIDS Prevention Studies, University of California, San Francisco

Kyung-Hee Choi, Center for AIDS Prevention Studies, University of California, San Francisco

Thomas J. Coates, Center for AIDS Prevention Studies, University of California, San Francisco

Jay Coburn, AIDS Action Council

Dave Conrad, National Institute on Drug Abuse

Elaine Corrigan, Center for Mental Health Services

Francine Cournos, Columbia University and New York State Psychiatric Institute

James Curran, Centers for Disease Control and Prevention

Denis Darko, The Scripps Research Institute

William Darrow, Centers for Disease Control and Prevention

Don Des Jarlais, Beth Israel Medical Center

Ralph DiClemente, Center for AIDS Prevention Studies, University of California, San Francisco

Diane di Mauro, Social Science Research Council

Renee Dupont, HIV Neurobehavioral Research Center, University of California, San Diego

Anke Ehrhardt, HIV Center for Clinical and Behavioral Studies, Columbia University

Lee Eiden, National Institute of Mental Health

Maria Ekstrand, Center for AIDS Prevention Studies, University of California, San Francisco

Sandra Estepa, Latino Commission on AIDS

Anthony Fauci, Office of AIDS Research, National Institutes of Health

Isa Fernandez, National Institute of Mental Health

Martin Fishbein, Centers for Disease Control and Prevention

Charles Fitzgerald, National Association of State Alcohol and Drug Abuse Directors

Ripley Forbes, Subcommittee on Health and the Environment, United States Congress

Marshall Forstein, American Psychiatric Association

Howard Fox, The Scripps Research Institute

Eleanor Friedenberg, National Institute on Drug Abuse

Samuel Friedman, National Development and Research Institutes

Paul Gaist, Office of AIDS Research, National Institutes of Health

Kristine Gebbie, Office of National AIDS Policy

Sander Genser, National Institute on Drug Abuse

Peter Ghazal, The Scripps Research Institute

Meyer Glantz, National Institute on Drug Abuse

Lisa Gold, The Scripps Research Institute

Ellen Goldstein, Center for AIDS Prevention Studies, University of California, San Francisco

Cynthia Gomez, Center for AIDS Prevention Studies, University of California, San Francisco

Frederick Goodwin, National Institute of Mental Health

Enoch Gordis, National Institute on Alcohol Abuse and Alcoholism

Jack Gorman, Columbia University

Igor Grant, HIV Neurobehavioral Research Center, University of California, San Diego

Mark Green, National Institute on Alcohol Abuse and Alcoholism

Judith Greenberg, Centers for Disease Control and Prevention

Mel Haas, Center for Mental Health Services

Thomas Hall, Center for AIDS Prevention Studies, University of California, San Francisco

Mark Harrington, Treatment Action Group

Christine Hartel, National Institute on Drug Abuse

Harry Haverkos, National Institute on Drug Abuse

Cheryl Healton, Columbia University, School of Public Health

Steve Henriksen, The Scripps Research Institute

Warren Hewitt, Center for Substance Abuse Treatment

Dan Hicks, American Psychiatric Association

Derek Hodel, AIDS Action Foundation

David Holtgrave, Centers for Disease Control and Prevention

Nancy Hondros, National Institute on Alcohol Abuse and Alcoholism

Stephen Hulley, Center for AIDS Prevention Studies, University of California, San Francisco

Joyce Hunter, HIV Center for Clinical and Behavioral Studies, Columbia University

Leslie Isaki, National Institute on Alcohol Abuse and Alcoholism

Terry Jernigan, HIV Neurobiological Research Center, University of California, San Diego

Stephen Jones, Centers for Disease Control and Prevention

Daryl Kade, Substance Abuse and Mental Health Services Administration

Susan Kegeles, Center for AIDS Prevention Studies, University of California, San Francisco

Jeffrey Kelly, Medical College of Wisconsin

May Kennedy, Emory University

George Koob, The Scripps Research Institute

Stephen Koslow, National Institute of Mental Health

Carl Latkin, Johns Hopkins University

Art Lawrence, Office of National AIDS Policy

Jeff Levi, AIDS Action Foundation

Felice Levine, American Sociological Association

Richard Levinson, Emory University

Trenece Lewis, National Institute of Mental Health

Markku Linnoila, National Institute on Alcohol Abuse and Alcoholism

Ed Long, Labor, Health and Human Services, and Education Appropriations Subcommittee, United States Senate

Peter Lurie, Center for AIDS Prevention Studies, University of California, San Francisco

Eliezer Masliah, HIV Neurobehavioral Research Center, University of California, San Diego

Jack Maser, National Institute of Mental Health

Claude Ann Mellins, HIV Center for Clinical and Behavioral Studies, Columbia University

Miriam Messinger, Boston University

Heino Meyer-Bahlberg, HIV Center for Clinical and Behavioral Studies, Columbia University

Heather Miller, National Institute of Allergy and Infectious Diseases

Randy Miller, National Task Force on AIDS Prevention

Sutherland Miller, HIV Center for Clinical and Behavioral Studies, Columbia University

Richard Millstein, National Institute on Drug Abuse

Merrill Mitler, The Scripps Research Institute

Leonard Mitnick, National Institute of Mental Health

Robert Moore, National Institutes of Health

Donna Moreau, Columbia University

Steve Morin, Office of Representative Nancy Pelosi, United States Congress

Lennart Mucke, The Scripps Research Institute

William Narrow, National Institute of Mental Health

Richard Needle, National Institute on Drug Abuse

Sondra Nelson, National Association of State Alcohol and Drug Abuse Directors

Mary Ellen Oliveri, National Institute of Mental Health

Peggy Overbey, American Anthropological Association

Maria Oziemkowska, Johns Hopkins University

Willo Pequegnat, National Institute of Mental Health

Lucille Perez, Center for Substance Abuse Prevention

Susan Persons, Consortium of Social Science Associations

John Peterson, Center for AIDS Prevention Studies, University of California, San Francisco

Tom Phillips, The Scripps Research Institute

Richard Pine, National Institute of Mental Health

Dianne Rausch, National Institute of Mental Health

Robert Remien, HIV Center for Clinical and Behavioral Studies, Columbia University

Carmen Richardson, National Institute on Alcohol Abuse and Alcoholism

Sherry Roberts, National Institute of Mental Health

Margaret Rosario, HIV Center for Clinical and Behavioral Studies, Columbia University

Mary Jane Rotheram-Borus, University of California, Los Angeles

Katherine Haynes Sanstad, Center for AIDS Prevention Studies, University of California, San Francisco

James Satriano, New York State Psychiatric Institute and Columbia University

Karen Shangraw, National Institute of Mental Health

Charles Sharp, National Institute on Drug Abuse

Amy Shultz, Labor, Health and Human Services, and Education Appropriations Subcommittee, United States Senate

George Siggins, The Scripps Research Institute

George Sonsel, Health Resources and Services Administration

James Sorensen, Center for AIDS Prevention Studies, University of California, San Francisco

Ron Stall, Center for AIDS Prevention Studies, University of California, San Francisco

Hugh Stamper, National Institute of Mental Health

Beth Steel, National Institute on Drug Abuse

Zena Stein, HIV Center for Clinical and Behavioral Studies, Columbia University

Mike Stephens, Committee on Appropriations, United States Congress

Yaakov Stern, HIV Center for Clinical and Behavioral Studies, Columbia University

Ellen Stover, National Institute of Mental Health

Jeff Stryker, Center for AIDS Prevention Studies, University of California, San Francisco

Ezra Susser, HIV Center for Clinical and Behavioral Studies, Columbia University

Sandy Thananant, National Institutes of Health

Frank Tims, National Institute on Drug Abuse

Susan Tross, HIV Center for Clinical and Behavioral Studies, Columbia University

Charles Turner, Research Triangle Institute

Ljubisa Vitkovic, National Institute of Mental Health

Marina Volkov, Federation of Behavioral, Psychological and Cognitive Sciences

Patricia Warne, HIV Center for Clinical and Behavioral Studies, Columbia University

Ken Warren, National Institute on Alcohol Abuse and Alcoholism

John Watters, Center for AIDS Prevention Studies, University of California, San Francisco

Karen Weidenheim, Albert Einstein School of Medicine

Wendy Wertheimer, Office of AIDS Research, National Institutes of Health

Tim Westmoreland, Office of Representative Henry Waxman, United States Congress

Jack Whitescarver, Office of AIDS Research, National Institutes of Health

Roy Widdus, National Commission on AIDS

Wayne Wiebel, University of Illinois, Chicago

Brian Wilcox, American Psychological Association

Charles Willoughby, National Institute of Mental Health

Mike Wilson, The Scripps Research Institute

Flossie Wong-Staal, HIV Neurobiological Research Center, University of California, San Diego

D
Contributors

HORTENSIA DE LOS ANGELES AMARO, Ph.D. is professor of social and behavioral sciences at the Boston University School of Public Health. She received the Ph.D. degree in psychology from the University of California, Los Angeles in 1982. She has authored over 40 publications in scientific journals and books in the areas of substance use, reproductive health, and mental health. Dr. Amaro is currently the principal investigator of several research projects including a community-based prevention program to reduce drug use and risk of infection among pregnant women, a study of drug use among adult mothers, a study on intergenerational gaps between parents and children and substance use among Hispanic youth, and a qualitative study of the meaning of health and well-being in five ethnic groups. She has held leadership positions within the American Psychological Association, and served on the editorial board of the *American Journal of Public Health* and as associate editor of the *Psychology of Women Quarterly*. She has served on the Massachusetts Governor's Task Force on AIDS, managed the Board of Regents of Higher Education, and was a member of the IOM Committee on Women in Clinical Research. Dr. Amaro has received awards for her work from the American Psychological Association and the Massachusetts Public Health Association and an honorary degree from Summors College.

IRA B. BLACK, M.D. is professor and chairman, Department of

Neuroscience and Cell Biology, University of Medicine and Dentistry of New Jersey (UMDNJ)-Robert Wood Johnson Medical School, director of the Joint Graduate Program in Physiology and Neurobiology of UMDNJ-Robert Wood Johnson Medical School and Rutgers University, and past president of the Society for Neuroscience of North America. He is a clinical neurologist and neuroscientist who is studying regulation by the environment of brain genes encoding growth factors, survival factors, and neurotransmitters. This work is being applied to the treatment of late-life degenerative neurologic diseases, including Alzheimer's disease and Parkinson's disease. Dr. Black has served on numerous international and national panels and advisory committees and is presently a member of the Scientific Advisory Board of the Center for Advanced Biotechnology and Medicine of New Jersey, a member of the Mental Health Special Projects Review Committee of NIMH, and director of the Princeton-Robert Wood Johnson-Rutgers University Consortium in Neuroscience. He is the recent recipient of a McKnight Foundation Award in Neuroscience, a Jacob Javits Award in Neuroscience from NINDS, the Viktor Hamburger Award, and the New Jersey Pride Award in Science. He is the author of approximately two hundred articles in neuroscience and of two books, *Cellular and Molecular Biology of Neuronal Development* and *Information in the Brain: A Molecular Perspective*.

H. KEITH H. BRODIE, M.D. is president emeritus of Duke University, James B. Duke Professor of Psychiatry, and professor of law and experimental psychology. He received the M.D. degree from the Columbia University College of Physicians and Surgeons in 1965 and completed his residency in psychiatry at Columbia Presbyterian Medical Center. Dr. Brodie's career in medical research has been focused on the biochemistry of mental illness, a subject in which he has published over 60 articles and book chapters. In addition, he is joint author or co-editor of 11 books, including 3 volumes of the *American Handbook of Psychiatry*. Dr. Brodie has also served on the editorial board of the *American Journal of Psychiatry*. He has contributed to his profession and to the community at large as a practicing physician, as a member and officer of numerous professional associations, and as a consultant to national organizations concerned with health care. Dr. Brodie is the youngest president ever to have served the American Psychiatric Association and was the only psychiatrist to head an Association of American Universities institution.

COLLEEN CONWAY-WELCH, Ph.D., C.N.M., F.A.A.N. is professor and dean at the Vanderbilt University School of Nursing in Nashville, Tennessee. She came to Vanderbilt in November, 1984 from the School of Nursing at the University of Colorado Health Sciences Center, where she was professor of nursing and director of the Nurse-Midwifery Graduate Program. Prior to her appointment at Colorado in 1980, Dr. Conway-Welch served on the faculties of the California State University Department of Nursing in Long Beach, California, George Mason University Department of Nursing in Fairfax, Virginia, Georgetown University School of Nursing in Washington, D.C., and the State University of New York Downstate Medical Center College of Nursing in Brooklyn. She has also held a number of nursing service staff positions in labor and delivery in emergency rooms, operating rooms, and intensive care units. Dr. Conway-Welch received her B.S.N. from Georgetown University, her M.S.N. from Catholic University, and her Ph.D. in nursing from New York University. She completed her nurse-midwifery education at the Catholic Maternity Institute in Santa Fe, New Mexico. Dr. Conway-Welch was the recipient of the Jack Dempsey Award for Humanitarianism at the Seventh Annual Helen Hayes Community Award Dinner benefiting St. Clare's Hospital Spellman Center for AIDS, and received the March of Dimes Service Award. She participates in a number of community and professional activities as well as serving on several corporate boards.

CURTIS L. DECKER, J.D. is executive director of the National Association of Protection and Advocacy Systems (NAPAS). NAPAS represents 190 agencies throughout the country that provide legal advocacy services for persons with disabilities, including persons with HIV infection. After graduating from Hamilton College and Cornell Law School, Mr. Decker served as a VISTA volunteer, senior attorney at the Baltimore Legal Aid Bureau, executive director of a child abuse and neglect resource project in Maryland, and executive director of the Maryland Disability Law Center. He has served on the AIDS councils of both Maryland Governors Hughes and Schaeffer and as co-chair of the Rights Task Force of the National Organizations Responding to AIDS (NORA) from 1984 to 1992. He has written several articles on legal issues relating to HIV infection funded by the Robert Wood Johnson Foundation and the Institute on Rehabilitative Issues Report on HIV and Vocational Rehabilitation (1989). Mr. Decker also served as chair of the community advisory committee of the Baltimore component of the multicenter AIDS cohort study.

BARUCH FISCHHOFF, Ph.D. is professor of social and decision sciences and of engineering and public policy at Carnegie Mellon University. He received the Ph.D. degree in psychology from the Hebrew University of Jerusalem. Dr. Fischhoff is a nationally recognized expert on risk assessment and communication and on decision making under uncertainty and has over 170 scientific publications to his credit, including *Acceptable Risk* (Cambridge University Press). He is a member of the Institute of Medicine. At the National Research Council, Dr. Fischhoff has participated in eight committees and panels, including the Ad Hoc Panel on Behavioral Science Contributions to AIDS (1987), the Committee on Human Factors (1980-1987), and the Committee on Risk Perception and Communication (1987-1989). As a consultant, Dr. Fischhoff has served the U.S. Nuclear Regulatory Commission, the Environmental Protection Agency, the Departments of Energy and Justice, the Centers for Disease Control and Prevention (AIDS communication program), the World Wildlife Fund/Conservation Foundation, and many more. Dr. Fischhoff is consulting editor for *Organizational Behavior and Human Decision Processes* and *Accident Analysis and Prevention* and is associate editor of *The Journal of Risk and Uncertainty* and *Cognitive Psychology.* He has been honored by the American Psychological Association, the Society for Risk Analysis, and the Society for Judgement and Decision Making.

SUSAN FOLKMAN, Ph.D. is professor of medicine at the University of California, San Francisco, and a senior scientist and co-director of the Center for AIDS Prevention Studies (CAPS). She received the Ph.D. degree from the University of California, Berkeley, in 1979. Dr. Folkman is internationally recognized for her theoretical and empirical work on psychological stress and the coping process. This work appears in numerous peer-reviewed journal articles and books, including the well-known volume *Stress, Appraisal, and Coping,* co-authored with Richard Lazarus. She is currently principal investigator on four grants from the National Institute of Mental Health that focus on stress and coping in the context of HIV disease. Dr. Folkman has major interests in caregivers of persons with AIDS, who are becoming an increasingly important link in the health care delivery system, and in interventions designed to help people cope effectively with HIV disease. She is also director of the science core at CAPS, which involves her in review, mentoring, and assistance to junior scientists at CAPS engaging in research on primary prevention and early intervention in HIV disease. She has served on the NIMH Mental Health in AIDS Study Section and chaired the NIMH AIDS Psychosocial Assessment Work Group.

MINDY FULLILOVE, M.D. is associate professor of clinical psychiatry and public health at Columbia University and New York State Psychiatric Institute. She received the M.D. degree from the Columbia University College of Physicians and Surgeons and completed her psychiatric residency at New York Hospital-Westchester division and Montefiore Hospital. Dr. Fullilove's current research focuses on the epidemiology of HIV infection in minority communities and trauma as a co-factor in drug abuse. From 1986 to 1990 she served as director of Multicultural Inquiry and Research on AIDS (MIRA), a component of the University of California, San Francisco (UCSF) Center for AIDS Prevention Studies, located at the Bayview-Hunter's Point Foundation. Dr. Fullilove has a particular interest in preparing minority students to participate in academic medicine, and to that end founded and directed the UCSF Medical Scholars Program and the Columbia University College of Physicians and Surgeons Student Success Network. She was a member of the National Academy of Sciences panel on AIDS Intervention and Research in 1990, has served on ADAMHA's AIDS Advisory Committee, and is a member of the National AIDS Drug Development Task Force.

MARGARET A. HAMBURG, M.D. is the commissioner of health for New York City. She received the M.D. degree from Harvard Medical School and completed her residency in internal medicine at the New York Hospital-Cornell Medical Center. Dr. Hamburg began her service in the New York City Department of Health in June 1990 as deputy commissioner for family health services. In that position she was responsible for child health, school and adolescent health, day care, dental health services, lead poisoning control, families with special needs, maternity services and family planning, and substance abuse services. Between 1986 and 1988, Dr. Hamburg worked for the federal assistant secretary for health in the areas of disease prevention and health promotion. From 1988 to 1990, Dr. Hamburg was a senior member of the National Institute of Allergy and Infectious Diseases, first as special assistant to the director and then as the assistant director of the institute. While at the National Institutes of Health she was instrumental in shaping AIDS research strategies and policies. Dr. Hamburg has extensive research experience in the areas of biology of addictions, behavioral sciences, and child development. She serves on many health-related committees and organizations and is the author of numerous scientific articles.

JAMES G. HAUGHTON, M.D., M.P.H. is senior health services policy advisor to the Los Angeles County Department of Health Services. In this capacity he has responsibility for assisting the department in preparing for the delivery of managed care. Prior to assuming these responsibilities in May, 1993, he served for six and a half years as medical director and chief of staff of the King/ Drew Medical Center of the Los Angeles County Department of Health Services and associate dean for postgraduate medical education at the Charles R. Drew University of Medicine and Sciences. After ten years as a private practitioner of obstetrics and gynecology in Brooklyn, New York, he began his medical administrative and public health career in the New York City Health Department, where he served for eight years. He then moved to Chicago where he served for ten years as executive director of the Health and Hospitals Governing Commission of Cook County. Dr. Haughton is a diplomate of the American Board of Preventive Medicine and a fellow of the American College of Preventive Medicine. He has been awarded a Rosenhaus Lectureship by the American Public Health Association and an honorary doctor of science degree by the Chicago Medical School, University of Health Sciences. He is a member of the Institute of Medicine and in that capacity has served as a member of several study committees. Dr. Haughton currently serves as a member of the Editorial Advisory Board of the Journal of Community Health and as a member of the Medical Advisory Committee to the AIDS Program Office of the Los Angeles County Department of Health Services.

JAMES A. INCIARDI, Ph.D. is director of the Center for Drug and Alcohol Studies at the University of Delaware; professor in the Department of Sociology and Criminal Justice at Delaware; adjunct professor in the Department of Epidemiology and Public Health at the University of Miami School of Medicine; and distinguished professor at the State University of Rio de Janeiro. Dr. Inciardi received a Ph.D. in sociology from New York University and has extensive research, clinical, field, and teaching experience in the areas of AIDS, substance abuse, and criminal justice. He currently chairs the National Institute on Drug Abuse AIDS Research Review Committee. Dr. Inciardi has been director of the National Center for the Study of Acute Drug Reactions at the

University of Miami School of Medicine; vice-president of the Washington, D.C.-based Resource Planning Corporation; associate director of Research for the New York State Narcotic Addiction Control Commission; and director of the Division of Criminal Justice at the University of Delaware. He has done extensive consulting work nationally and internationally and has published some 35 books and more than 170 articles and chapters in the areas of substance abuse, criminology, criminal justice, history, folklore, social policy, AIDS, medicine, and law.

EDWARD H. KAPLAN, Ph.D. is professor of management sciences at the Yale School of Management, professor of medicine at the Yale School of Medicine, and Lady Davis Visiting Professor at the Hebrew University of Jerusalem, Hadassah Medical Center. He received the Ph.D. degree in urban studies and planning from the Massachusetts Institute of Technology in 1984. Prior to his arrival at Yale in 1987, Dr. Kaplan was assistant professor of management sciences at the University of Massachusetts, Boston (1985-1987) and adjunct lecturer/research associate at the Harvard John F. Kennedy School of Government (1984-1985). Dr. Kaplan has long been dedicated to the application of operations research methods to the analysis of public policy problems. Since 1987 his research has been devoted almost exclusively to modeling HIV transmission dynamics and to using these models in the design and evaluation of AIDS intervention programs. He has published over 35 papers in peer-reviewed journals since beginning his AIDS research in 1987, and his book *Modeling the AIDS Epidemic: Planning, Policy and Prediction*, co-edited with Margaret Brandeau, has just been published. Dr. Kaplan continues to serve *pro bono* as the principal investigator evaluating New Haven's legal needle exchange program, for which he designed a unique syringe tracking and testing system. For this work he received the 1992 Franz Edelman Award from the Institute of Management Sciences and a 1991 Connecticut Health Commissioner's AIDS Leadership Award. An active member of several professional societies, Dr. Kaplan currently serves as departmental editor for *Management Science*, associate editor for *Operations Research*, and associate editor for the *Journal of Acquired Immune Deficiency Syndromes*.

RICHARD W. PRICE, M.D. is professor and head of the Department of Neurology, University of Minnesota. He received the M.D. degree from Albany Medical College in 1967 and completed his neurology residency at Cornell University Medical College in

1972. Dr. Price has a history of research and publication in the areas of HIV infection, AIDS, and neurology. He has served on the editorial boards of *AIDS* (from 1986 to 1990) and *Neurology*, and is editor of the *Journal of Neuro-AIDS*. Dr. Price was chair of the Neurology Committee of the National Institute of Allergy and Infectious Diseases AIDS Clinical Trials Group from 1986 to 1990 and was a member of the NIAID AIDS Research Review Committee from 1987 to 1989. He also served on the Psychobiological, Biological, and Neuroscience Subcommittee of the Mental Health AIDS Research Review Committee from 1991 to 1992.

ALFRED SAAH, M.D., M.P.H. is associate professor of the Infectious Diseases Program at the Johns Hopkins University School of Hygiene and Public Health. He received the M.D. degree from the University of Maryland School of Medicine, Baltimore, in 1973 and the M.P.H. from the Johns Hopkins University School of Hygiene and Public Health in 1981. While at the National Institutes of Health, Dr. Saah served as medical epidemiologist, Epidemiology and Biometry Section, and as attending physician, Infectious Diseases Service, National Institute of Allergy and Infectious Diseases (1981-1987). He was Epidemiologist and project director for Rickettsial Diseases, Egyptian/Israeli Regional Project on Control of Arthropod-Borne Diseases from 1983 to 1989. Since 1983, Dr. Saah has been a collaborator in the Multicenter AIDS Cohort Study. Since 1987, he has been associate professor of medicine at the School of Medicine, Johns Hopkins University, and associate professor of epidemiology at the School of Hygiene and Public Health, Johns Hopkins University. From 1989 to 1992, he was director, Infectious Diseases Program, Department of Epidemiology, at the School of Hygiene and Public Health at Johns Hopkins University. Dr. Saah is a fellow of the American College of Physicians, the Infectious Diseases Society of America, and the American Public Health Association, as well as other professional societies. Since 1989 he has been associate editor of *AIDS Targeted Information*. Dr. Saah is author of numerous articles in professional journals and book chapters.

PETER SELWYN, M.D., M.P.H. is currently the associate director of the Yale AIDS Program, director of the HIV/AIDS Clinic, and associate professor of medicine, epidemiology, and public health at Yale University School of Medicine and Yale-New Haven Hospital. He received the M.D. degree from Harvard Medical School in 1981 and the M.P.H. degree in epidemiology from Columbia

University in 1989. He completed his residency in the Residency Program in Social Medicine at Montefiore Medical Center, Bronx, New York in 1984. From 1984 until 1992, Dr. Selwyn was the medical director of the Drug Abuse Treatment Program at Montefiore Medical Center in Bronx, New York, where he helped to develop clinical care programs and a variety of research projects concerning HIV infection among drug users. These projects included studies of the natural history of HIV infection among drug users, studies of pregnancy and reproductive decision making in drug-using women, and the development of integrated primary care and substance abuse treatment services for HIV-infected drug users. Dr. Selwyn has served as an ad hoc and permanent member of numerous scientific, advisory, and review committees in the areas of HIV infection and drug abuse, and has been a consultant on AIDS and substance abuse to the New York State Health Department and the Global Program on AIDS of the World Health Organization. He is the author of over 50 scientific articles, book chapters, review articles, and monographs concerning medical, epidemiologic, and social aspects of HIV infection and drug use.

JUDITH D. AUERBACH, Ph.D. is currently a senior program officer at the Institute of Medicine, where she is study director for the Committee on Substance Abuse and Mental Health Issues in AIDS Research. Previously, she was associate director for government affairs of the Consortium of Social Science Associations (COSSA). During her tenure at COSSA, Dr. Auerbach was involved in educational and advocacy activities directed at the inclusion of social science perspectives in the health research enterprise of the federal government (especially NIH and the former ADAMHA). She was instrumental in coordinating efforts to end prohibitions on sexual behavior studies, to focus on social and behavioral research on AIDS, and to enhance attention to women's health issues. Dr. Auerbach began her policy work in Washington in 1988 as a Congressional Science Fellow, sponsored by the Society for Research in Child Development, when she worked on child, family and health policy issues in the office of Representative Pat Schroeder. From 1989 to 1990, she was director of the Institute for the Study of Women and Men at the University of Southern California. Dr. Auerbach received her Ph.D. in sociology from the University of California, Berkeley, in 1986, and taught sociology at Widener University and the University of California, Los Angeles. She has published and presented in the fields of child care, family leave, gender issues, health research, and science policy, including the book, *In the Business of Child Care: Employer Initiatives and Working Women* (Praeger).

KAREN AUTREY is the project assistant and senior secretary at the Institute of Medicine for the Committee on Substance Abuse and Mental Health Issues in AIDS Research. Ms. Autrey has been with the National Academy of Sciences for three years. She previously worked as project assistant with the Film Office of the Office of Government and External Affairs. The Film Office, as liaison between prominent scientists and production companies, participates in the development and production of films for public television and ensures that the information used in the films is scientifically sound. Ms. Autrey worked in the Film Office during the production of *The Infinite Voyage* and *Space Age*. Before coming to NAS, Ms. Autrey worked at The Wilderness Society and the Electronic Industries Association. As a volunteer, Ms. Autrey tutors underprivileged five-, six-, and seven-year-olds through the Black Diamonds Organization and helps mentally retarded adults at the Northern Virginia Training Center. In 1987, Ms. Autrey received her B.S. in psychology at James Madison University in Harrisonburg, Virginia.

ROBERT MULLAN COOK-DEEGAN, M.D. is the director of the Division of Biobehavioral Sciences and Mental Disorders at the Institute of Medicine, National Academy of Sciences. He was previously an expert (consultant advisor) to the National Center for Human Genome Research at the National Institutes of Health. Dr. Cook-Deegan served as the acting executive director of the Biomedical Ethics Advisory Committee of the U.S. Congress throughout its active life, from December 1988 to October 1989. Before that, he was a senior associate at the Office of Technology Assessment, U.S. Congress, for six years. He is the author of *The Gene Wars: Science, Politics and the Human Genome* (Norton).

HOLLY DAWKINS is a research assistant at the Institute of Medicine for the Committee on Substance Abuse and Mental Health Issues in AIDS Research. In her five years at IOM, Ms. Dawkins has worked in six IOM units on over a dozen projects. The projects range from assessing modern methods of clinical investigation, to investigating decision-making processes for the adoption and coverage of medical technologies, to evaluating the development and use of clinical practice guidelines. In 1991 she received an Institute of Medicine staff award for her work on the IOM study to evaluate the artificial heart program of the National Heart, Lung, and Blood Institute. Ms. Dawkins has three publications in IOM reports. In 1986 she received the A.B. degree in English Literature, with honors, from Brown University.

LESLIE M. HARDY, M.H.S. is currently director of the Institute of Medicine's Roundtable for the Development of Drugs and Vaccines Against AIDS, a group composed of leaders from government, the pharmaceutical industry, academia, and patient advocacy. The roundtable convenes workshops and conferences to identify and help resolve impediments to the rapid availability of safe, effective drugs and vaccines for HIV infection and AIDS. Previously, Ms. Hardy directed the IOM study of prenatal and newborn screening for HIV infection, which resulted in the 1991 report *HIV Screening of Pregnant Women and Newborns*. She also formerly served as staff officer for the IOM/NAS AIDS Activities Oversight Committee, which produced the study report *Confronting AIDS: Update 1988*. During her work with the AIDS Oversight Committee, she focused on issues pertaining to the delivery and financing of health care for people with HIV infection and AIDS, stress among AIDS care providers, and the care of neuropsychologically impaired people with AIDS. Ms. Hardy received her bachelor of arts degree in zoology and botany from Duke University and her master of health science degree in maternal and child health from the Johns Hopkins University School of Hygiene and Public Health.

CONSTANCE M. PECHURA, Ph.D. has been at the Institute of Medicine since 1988 and is presently associate director of the Division of Biobehavioral Sciences and Mental Disorders. She has directed a number of projects on topics including assessing health effects of chemical weapons exposure on World War II human subjects, integrating computer technologies to map the human brain, microbial pathogenesis, developmental neurobiology, sleep research, psychoneuroimmunology, science base of medically assisted conception, mental and addictive disorders in women, fetal research, and health and human rights. After earning a B.S. degree in psychology from the Virginia Commonwealth University, Dr. Pechura received a Ph.D. in anatomy, with a specialization in neuroscience, from the F. Edward Hebert School of Medicine of the Uniformed Services University of the Health Sciences (USUHS). A recipient of a National Science Foundation Graduate Fellowship, Dr. Pechura has taught medical school courses in gross anatomy, microscopic anatomy, and neuroanatomy at USUHS, where she was awarded an outstanding teaching award in 1985. Her postdoctoral training was at the National Institute of Neurological Disorders and Stroke. Currently, she is a health policy tutor at Stanford in Washington. Her published laboratory research has included studies of blood-brain barrier function, glucose utilization in experimental head injury, and the neuroanatomy of pain sensation.

MICHAEL A. STOTO, Ph.D. is the director of the Division of Health Promotion and Disease Prevention of the Institute of Medicine. He received an A.B. in statistics from Princeton University and a Ph.D. in statistics and demography from Harvard University, and was formerly an associate professor of public policy at the Harvard University John F. Kennedy School of Government. A member of the professional staff since 1987, Dr. Stoto directed the IOM's effort in support of the Public Health Service's *Healthy People 2000* project and has worked on IOM projects addressing a number of issues in public health, health statistics, health promotion and disease prevention, vaccine safety and policy, and AIDS. Dr. Stoto is co-author of *Data for Decisions: Information Strategies for Policy Makers* and numerous articles in statistics, demography, health policy, and other fields. He is a member of the American Public Health Association, the American Statistical Association, the International Union for the Scientific Study of Population, the Population Association of America, and other organizations.

CHRISTINA WYPIJEWSKA, M.P.H. is a program officer at the Institute of Medicine for the Committee on Substance Abuse and Mental Health Issues in AIDS Research. Prior to joining the IOM, she worked in the Public Health Service for the Office of the Assistant Secretary for Health in the areas of disease prevention and health promotion. As prevention policy advisor, Ms. Wypijewska coordinated PHS implementation strategies for *Healthy People 2000* and contributed to worksite health promotion initiatives, including the *1992 National Survey of Worksite Health Promotion Activities*. When she first joined the PHS, Ms. Wypijewska worked as the special assistant for the deputy assistant secretary for health, providing research, writing, and editorial assistance for a variety of articles and publications. Ms. Wypijewska received her M.P.H. degree from Yale University and her undergraduate degree in biology from Vassar College. In the D.C. community, she has volunteered as a counselor with the D.C. Rape Crisis Center and the Prenatal Program of the Washington Free Clinic, where she currently serves on the Board of Directors.

Index

A

Abusive relationships, 96-97

ACT-UP, 93

ADAMHA. *See* Alcohol, Drug Abuse, and Mental Health Administration

ADAMHA Reorganization Act of 1992 (PL 102-321), 19, 157, 158, 162, 165, 166

and grant review process, 22, 176-177

implications for services and research, 35-36, 245

Addiction. *See* Alcohol use; Injection drug use; Substance abuse; Withdrawal syndrome

Advisory councils, 22, 170, 176, 177-178, 179, 181

Africa, 51, 52, 60, 100-101, 112, 115

African Americans, 39-40, 67, 90, 94, 97

in research, 34, 95, 102-103, 106-107, 204, 239, 248

AIDS Advisory Council, 170

AIDS clinical trials units (ACTUs), 226

AIDS dementia complex (ADC), 12-13, 31, 42, 125-134, 141

research recommendations, 17-18, 151

treatment, 13, 134

AIDS in Multiethnic Neighborhoods (AMEN) study, 73-74, 230

AIDS Risk Reduction Model (ARRM), 85

Alcohol, Drug Abuse, and Mental Health Administration (ADAMHA), *v*, 35, 37

budget process, 21, 171, 172-175

grant review process, 22, 177

history of, 159-162

reorganization, *vi-vii*, 3, 19, 20, 21, 35, 36, 37, 42, 43, 158-168, 171, 174-175, 185, 240, 245

See also National Institute of Mental Health; National Institute on Alcohol Abuse and Alcoholism; National Institute on Drug Abuse; Office of Substance Abuse Prevention; Office of Treatment Improvement; Substance Abuse and Mental Health Services Administration

Alcohol Research Centers, 201, 203

Alcohol use, 61, 69, 70, 73

immune system effects, 13-14, 26, 134-135, 198, 201, 202

intervention and outreach, 106-107, 247-248

Center for Substance Abuse Prevention
(CSAP), *vi*, 35, 240, 244
Center for Substance Abuse Treatment
(CSAT), *vi*, 20, 35, 163, 240, 241,
243, 248, 249, 251
Centers for Disease Control and
Prevention (CDC), 38, 62, 85, 95,
252, 253, 254
Central nervous system (CNS), 12-13,
15, 17-18, 30, 34, 124, 125-134,
151, 209, 225-226, 238-239
opportunistic infections of, 12, 125,
126
and sexual behavior, 10, 122
See also AIDS dementia complex;
Brain; Neurobiology
Cerebral toxoplasmosis, 12, 125
Cerebrospinal fluid (CSF), 13, 127, 128
Cervical secretions, 50
Class. *See* Socioeconomic status
Clinical trials, 226
Cocaine, 10, 53, 54, 55, 61, 81, 82,
118, 122. *See also* Crack
cocaine
Cofactors of transmission, 48
in sexual practices, 48-51, 53, 59-66
Cognitive coping strategies, 16, 143,
144. *See also* Avoidant coping;
Coping behavior
Cognitive impairment, 6, 77. *See also*
AIDS dementia complex; Mental
health and illness; Seriously
mentally ill
Collaborative research, 30-31, 34,
229-232, 238-239
and grant review process, 23, 185
and service programs, 34, 36-37, 43,
240, 245-254
Commercial sex workers, 52, 69, 96,
110-111, 113, 115. *See also*
Sex-for-crack exchanges
Community factors, 5, 8-9, 10-11, 24,
76, 88-89, 93-94, 118, 123
activism, 93-94
high-risk settings, 4-5, 56-57, 71-75,
76
See also Cultural factors; Social
networks; Social norms; Social
science research; Social-
structural research
Community intervention and outreach,

10-11, 88, 102-103, 104-105,
108-109, 114-116, 123, 228
for alcohol users, 247-248
for commercial sex workers, 115
for drug users, 5, 28, 116, 212-213,
214, 216, 241, 243, 249-250
for gay men, 91, 93-94, 114
and mental health services, 241,
243-244, 252-253
models of, 86-87
for Native Americans, 247-248
stress among workers, 17, 150-151
for youth, 244, 248, 251
See also Demonstration projects;
National AIDS Demonstration
Research Program
Comprehensive Community Treatment
Program (CCTP), 35, 241, 243
Concurrent epidemics and health
events, 5, 6, 50, 71, 75, 76, 77
Condoms, 51, 83, 84, 92, 97, 111, 114,
115
and drug use, 60, 75, 116
female, 111, 112-113
Contracts and contract proposals, 181,
192, 193
Cookers, 54-55
Cooperative agreements (U01s), 181,
192, 193
Cooperative clinical research (R10/
U10) awards, 192
Coping behavior, 15, 16, 19, 30, 141,
142-145, 153
of caregivers, 19, 141, 147, 148, 153
NIMH research, 19, 153
Cortical dementias, 128
Cost-effectiveness of interventions, 9,
11, 33, 121, 122, 123, 238
Cost-to-benefit ratio, 121, 122
Cottons, 54, 55
Counseling services, 99, 110, 244
Couples, 8, 11, 55-56, 89, 91, 92, 110,
123. *See also* Drug-running
partners; Sexual partners
Crack cocaine, 34, 59-63, 210, 211, 238
and sexual behavior, 28, 59, 60-63,
75, 211
Crack houses, 4-5, 59, 76
CRISP (Computer Retrieval of Information
on Scientific Projects) system, 177,
299-300, 301

intervention and outreach, 241, 243-245, 252-253
research recommendations, 6, 18, 77
seroprevalence among patients, 40, 69, 70, 71, 73
See also AIDS dementia complex; Depression; Emotional distress; Psychoneuroimmunology; Seriously mentally ill; Stress
Methadone, 14, 18, 82, 111, 138, 152, 251
Methods to extend research in time (MERIT) awards, 192
Microglia, 13, 131
Military recruits and personnel, 69
Motherhood, 97
Multicenter AIDS Cohort Study (MACS), 118, 142, 226
Multi-disciplinary research. *See* Cross-disciplinary research
Multi-Site HIV Prevention Trial, 227

N

National AIDS Behavioral Surveys (NABS), 230
National AIDS Demonstration Research Program (NADR), 116, 191, 212-213, 214, 217, 220, 249
National AIDS Program Office (NAPO), 38, 172, 254
National Cancer Institute, 232, 233
National Center for Research Resources, 233, 234
National Heart, Lung, and Blood Institute, 233, 234
National Institute of Allergies and Infectious Diseases, 232, 233, 234
National Institute of Mental Health (NIMH), *vi, vii, viii,* 2, 3, 4, 5, 6, 10, 11, 16, 40, 41, 42, 43, 47, 76, 77, 78, 122, 123, 151, 152, 153, 157, 158, 159, 160, 161, 162, 163, 236-237, 238, 239, 255, 256
AIDS coordinator position, 20, 29, 31, 33, 165, 168, 223, 237
budget process, 21, 174, 175-176
collaborative activities, 17-18, 19, 30-31, 34, 37, 38, 151, 152, 229-232, 254, 255

grant review process, 22-23, 179, 181-183, 185
research portfolio and funding allocations, 23-24, 25, 29-30, 31, 42, 189-191 192, 193, 221-229, 232, 233, 234, 235
service linkages, 240, 243, 247, 251-253
National Institute on Alcohol Abuse and Alcoholism (NIAAA), *vi, vii, viii,* 2, 3, 4, 5, 6, 10, 11, 18, 19, 40, 41, 42, 43, 76, 77, 78, 122, 123, 151, 152, 153, 157, 158, 160, 161, 162, 163, 236-237, 238, 239, 255, 256
AIDS coordinator position, 20, 25-26, 31, 33, 165, 168, 237
budget process, 21, 174, 175-176
collaborative activities, 17, 18, 19, 30-31, 34, 37, 38, 151, 229-232, 254, 255
grant review process, 22-23, 179, 180, 181, 182-183, 185
research portfolio and funding allocations, 23-24, 25-26, 31, 42, 189-191, 193, 198-204, 232, 233, 234, 235
service linkages, 240, 247-248
National Institute on Child Health and Human Development, 225, 233, 234
National Institute on Drug Abuse (NIDA), *vi, vii, viii,* 2, 3, 4, 5, 6, 10, 11, 18, 19, 40, 41, 42, 43, 47, 62, 76, 77, 78, 122, 123, 151, 152, 153, 157, 158, 160, 161, 162, 163, 236-237, 238, 239, 255, 256
AIDS coordinator position, 20, 26-27, 31, 33, 165, 168, 199, 200, 208-209, 237
budget process, 21, 174, 175-176
collaborative research activities, 18, 19, 20, 30-31, 34, 37, 38, 229-232, 254, 255
grant review process, 22-23, 179, 180, 181, 182-183, 185
research portfolio and funding allocations, 23-24, 25, 26-28, 31, 42, 189-191, 192, 193, 205-221, 232, 233, 234, 235
service linkages, 240, 241, 247, 248-251